"In *Neurobiology Essentials*, Montgomery displays her gift for making extremely complex concepts clear and accessible. Her extensive use of case material makes for a compelling read and explicates otherwise inscrutable neurobiological processes; she guides her reader through "moment to moment" interactions with clients, elucidating the neurobiological underpinnings of theories and interventions along the way. The result is a contemporary, innovative, research-based framework for clinical practice that will be the "go-to" neurobiological text for practitioners and students alike. This is an impressively scholarly work that makes a neurobiological perspective human."

—Susan Bliss, Ph.D., L.C.S.W., Assistant Professor, Molloy College

Neurobiology Essentials
for Clinicians

The Norton Series on Interpersonal Neurobiology

Allan N. Shore, PhD, Series Editor
Daniel J. Siegel, MD, Founding Editor

The field of mental health is in a tremendously exciting period of growth and conceptual reorganization. Independent findings from a variety of scientific endeavors are converging in an interdisciplinary view of the mind and mental well-being. An interpersonal neurobiology of human development enables us to understand that the structure and function of the mind and brain are shaped by experiences, especially those involving emotional relationships.

The Norton Series on Interpersonal Neurobiology provides cutting-edge, multidisciplinary views that further our understanding of the complex neurobiology of the human mind. By drawing on a wide range of traditionally independent fields of research—such as neurobiology, genetics, memory, attachment, complex systems, anthropology, and evolutionary psychology—these texts offer mental health professionals a review and synthesis of scientific findings often inaccessible to clinicians. The books advance our understanding of human experience by finding the unity of knowledge, or consilience, that emerges with the translation of findings from numerous domains of study into a common language and conceptual framework. The series integrates the best of modern science with the healing art of psychotherapy.

A Norton Professional Book

Neurobiology Essentials for Clinicians

What Every Therapist Needs to Know

Arlene Montgomery

Foreword by Allan N. Schore

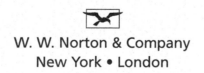

W. W. Norton & Company
New York • London

All material in Appendix B is reprinted with permission from the *Diagnostic and Statistical Manual of Mental Disorders*, Fourth Edition, Text Revision, (Copyright © 2000). American Psychiatric Association.

Copyright © 2013 by Arlene Montgomery

All rights reserved
Printed in the United States of America
First Edition

For information about permission to reproduce selections from this book, write to Permissions, W. W. Norton & Company, Inc., 500 Fifth Avenue, New York, NY 10110

For information about special discounts for bulk purchases, please contact W. W. Norton Special Sales at specialsales@wwnorton.com or 800-233-4830

Manufacturing by LSC Communications, North Chelmsford
Book design by Paradigm Graphics
Production manager: Leeann Graham

Library of Congress Cataloging-in-Publication Data

Montgomery, Arlene, author.
 Neurobiology essentials for clinicians : what every therapist needs to know / Arlene Montgomery ; foreword by Allan N. Schore. — First edition.
     p. ; cm. — (Norton series on interpersonal neurobiology)
"Norton professional book."
 Includes bibliographical references and index.
 ISBN 978-0-393-70602-4 (pbk.)
 I. Title. II. Series: Norton series on interpersonal neurobiology.
 [DNLM: 1. Nervous System Physiological Phenomena. 2. Brain—physiology.
3. Interpersonal Relations. 4. Neurobiology—methods. 5. Neurons—physiology.
6. Psychotherapeutic Processes. WL 102]

 616.8—dc23

                    2012047711

W. W. Norton & Company, Inc. 500 Fifth Avenue, New York, N.Y. 10110
www.wwnorton.com

W. W. Norton & Company Ltd. 15 Carlisle Street, London W1D 3BS

   5 6 7 8 9 0

To my husband, Seth H. Montgomery.
Thank you. Really.

CONTENTS

Foreword
Allan N. Schore

For a number of years I have been scouring the planet for potential authors for the Norton Series on Interpersonal Neurobiology. Many of these authors have well-established international reputations as scholars and renowned clinicians, but an equal number of others are new voices in the field. These extremely curious, dedicated individuals have, through their own intensive study, mastered both a large body of interdisciplinary scientific knowledge and a broad and deep range of clinical experience.

Arlene Montgomery is a prime example of a new, exciting voice. For well over a decade, this gifted clinician-academic has been teaching interpersonal neurobiology to students at the University of Texas at Austin's School of Social Work, and continually attracting overflow classes. Over the years the course has been grounded in my first book, *Affect Regulation and the Origin of the Self*, no easy read for first- and second-year graduate students who are just entering the profession. These students are challenged by her course to absorb large amounts of clinical knowledge and to gain an understanding of the relevance of neuroscience to their emerging psychotherapeutic skills.

Montgomery's extraordinary talent as a master teacher and skilled psychodynamic psychotherapist is expressed in her creative use in the classroom of personally relevant, day-to-day and, indeed, moment-to-moment subjective bodily-based emotional experiences that lie at the core of her students' conscious and unconscious worlds. Her teaching style thus encourages more than the accumulation of a large body of explicit knowledge about the connections between psychology and biology—it also calls for an inwardly focused reflective function, one that attends to the student's implicit processes. To demonstrate the ubiquity of these "hidden" nonconscious and nonverbal brain/mind/body processes, she also utilizes an interpersonal neurobiological perspective to analyze the images the culture is generating, (for example, by having the class attend to rapid facial, prosodic, and gestural right-brain communications in highly affective scenes from popular films).

In the following pages Montgomery organizes, synthesizes, and integrates her extensive academic knowledge and clinical skills in order to offer a coherent, well-researched, theoretically based, and clinically relevant volume on neurobiology essentials for clinicians. Although the volume provides a valuable text for the training of mental heath professionals across a wide spectrum of disciplines (social work, psychology, counseling, psychiatry, and psychoanalysis), each chapter breaks new ground in providing fresh and creative interpersonal neurobiological models of a number of complex clinical problems, which advanced clinicians will find provocative and stimulating.

The reader will note that, although Montgomery cites a large number of neuroscientific and clinical authors, she utilizes the perspective of regulation theory to organize both her neurobiological and clinical data. At the very beginning of my most recent volume, in this same IN Series, I stated that regulation theory is offered as a systematic exposition of the general principle of a science. Specifically, it is a formulation of an explanatory conception of the process of development, as it moves along the life span. Thus regulation theory, including its developmental variant, modern attachment theory, serves as a source of testable hypotheses for scientific research, but also as a potential source of more complex and efficient models of clinical intervention.

The opening chapters in the first half of the book (Foundational Neuroscience Concepts) build upon and expand regulation theory's modeling of a number of well-known yet enigmatic clinical phenomena. Utilizing an interpersonal neurobiological lens, Montgomery's curious and synthetic mind focuses upon a number of essential developmental brain/mind/body processes that appear in the therapeutic alliance: the re-expression of right-lateralized autonomic components of the attachment system in heightened affective moments, the role of the right amygdala in unconscious subcortical threat processing, the arousal-regulating functions of a variety of defense mechanisms, and the communication of conscious and unconscious affects via projective identification. In the latter section of the book, regulation theory is used to generate novel interpersonal neurobiological understandings of personality disorders, the adolescent brain, group work, and supervision. Let me provide a glimpse of the upcoming chapters, and speak more to the point of where this book breaks new ground.

Among clinicians of all schools there is currently an intense interest in not only brain but also body. The key to understanding bodily processes is the neural control of bodily processes by the autonomic nervous system (ANS). The nonconscious regulation of bodily-based autonomic arousal is a central aspect of the early developing emotion-communicating attachment mechanism. Indeed this is a central theme of Chapter 1, which overviews the functions of both the right brain and its deep connections to the ANS, and then describes the clinical expressions of this mechanism in a transcript of a psychotherapy session. The author boldly asserts, "Tracking psychophysiological arousal can be a very valuable assessment exercise leading to diagnosis and intervention considerations. . . . This repetitive experience of synchronizing appropriate arousal management strategies with the brain of another has the potential to actually change brain functioning for the better." It is often forgotten that affects have two dimensions, valence (positive–negative, pleasant–unpleasant, approach–avoidance of discrete emotions) and arousal (intensity, energy, calm–excited). My sense is that clinicians have focused too much on the former, which has impacted clinical models. But arousal—especially somatic, peripheral, autonomic arousal—is what is essentially transmitted and regulated in a relational context, and in this book it gets the attention it deserves.

In light of the clinical fact that the patient's defense mechanisms impact what can be taken in relationally, and that defenses themselves can become more complex with clinical work, Montgomery devotes the bulk of the opening chapter to the role of the autonomic nervous system in defense mechanisms. This work builds upon my own earlier model of defense mechanisms as nonconscious strategies of emotional regulation for avoiding, minimizing, or converting affects that are too difficult to tolerate, with an emphasis on dissociation and projective identification that prevents entrance into "dreaded states" charged with intense affects that can potentially traumatically disorganize the self system. Keep in mind that defenses are utilized on both sides of the therapeutic alliance, jointly acting upon the therapeutic change process, and that the earliest core defenses are shaped for better or worse by the patient's and clinician's own attachment experiences. Tying this into early interpersonal neurobiological attachment mechanisms, in my first book I proposed that the insecure-avoidant infant excessively utilizes a parasympathetic-dominant state in passive avoidance, gaze aversion, and conservation-withdrawal, thereby biasing the maturing limbic–autonomic system to low arousal energy-conserving states. On the other hand, at times of relational stress the insecure-resistant infant's maturing ANS is sympathetically based.

Moving the model significantly forward, Montgomery asserts that at the most basic neuropsychobiological level, all defense mechanisms are modulators of emotional arousal. She then presents a model of dividing the defense mechanism into four types of nonconscious arousal strategies used by the various attachment typologies: homeostatically balanced defenses that under stress resiliently shift between sympathetic (SNS) and parasympathetic (PNS) components of the ANS (secure), parasympathetically driven defenses that attempt to decrease arousal but cannot manage higher levels of relational stimulation (insecure-avoidant), sympathetically driven defenses that attempt to increase arousal but cannot easily manage lower levels of relational stimulation (insecure anxious-ambivalent), and disorganized defenses in which the SNS and PNS are frequently uncoupled, arousal levels are extreme, and defenses seem to appear without a predictable strategy (disorganized-disoriented). Regarding these defensive biases Montgomery notes, "What this means in practical terms is the underutilized branch may be avoided in a predictable fashion." Indeed, in an extended table in Chapter 2 the author uses this model to characterize every known defense in terms of these arousal dimensions, including internalization, sublimation, suppression, dissociation, intellectualization, repression, acting out, splitting, and undoing.

To add to the power of the model the author then presents numerous cases that demonstrate the unique forms of expression of arousal modulating defenses with different types of patients in various therapeutic contexts. In this conceptualization, pathology is defined as the rigid use of the same restricted set of defenses, regardless of the context, and resilience is defined as the capacity to manage increasingly difficult intensities of affective arousal without resorting to pathological defense mechanisms and behaviors. To demonstrate the psychoneurobiological model of defenses, she presents the verbatim transcript of various patient-therapist interactions, and then an analysis of the right-brain-to-right-brain limbic-autonomic arousal communications at another preverbal level beneath the words. Montgomery states, "A focus on typical ways that each client manages emotions will generally uncover defense mechanisms that have been used to protect the client emotionally." I would add that the focus is also upon the therapist's defenses against affective arousal. This format of utilizing case descriptions, dozens of them, to demonstrate precisely how regulation theory translates into clinical practice is used throughout the book.

In later chapters Montgomery continues to expand her clinical model, describing, in some detail, the unique role of the right amygdala, a major subcortical center for threat appraisal and management. Noting that threat can originate either from the external environment or from internal thoughts and feelings, she observes, "The personality can eventually become patterned by the level of arousal that is mobilized to meet most situations and can remain dominated by amygdalar functions that respond to the most minimal hint of threat, leading to chronic over/under/ erratic reacting." Keeping in mind that the right amygdala interacts directly with both the sympathetic and parasympathetic components of the ANS, she then discusses the relationship between autonomic arousal and the sympathetic-dominated personality disorders, parasympathetic-dominated personality disorders, and uncoupled ANS oscillating personality disorders. This work represents a significant elaboration of ideas put forth in my first book, that borderline personality disorder reflects an uncoupled nonreciprocal mode of autonomic control, while a parasympathetic-dominant autonomic mode prevails in narcissistic personality disorder. Indeed, in Chapter 5 Montgomery forges an even tighter linkage between the autonomic arousal defenses used in the four attachment typologies and the primary autonomic defenses of thirteen different personality disorders. Along the way she offers rich case examples of ANS arousal in both childhood attachment and equivalent adult attachment categories. To strengthen the argument of continuity of defensive orientations, she frequently offers clinical sessions with the same patient, some over different decades.

The second half of the book (Special Populations and Topics) contains chapters on the application of regulation theory to three other areas of clinical import. A chapter on the continual evolution of the early forming attachment limbic-autonomic circuits in the adolescent brain includes an extended table summarizing selected functions of the adolescent and adult brain. Most models of the development of the adolescent brain focus on cognitions and behavior, but here Montgomery highlights the changes in the "emotional brain," both cortically and, even more important, subcortically. She notes that particular circuits that psychobiologically support defensive strategies are epigenetically sculpted in infancy, but in adolescence they are further pruned by the social environment. In this manner the autonomic bias resulting from the early critical period over- or under-pruning of SNS and PNS circuits influences the nature of the later adolescent pruning. This limbic-autonomic circuit pruning is a central mechanism that impacts the emergence of Axis I psychiatric and Axis II personality disorders in adolescence.

The later chapters discuss the use of regulation theory in understanding group dynamics and the change mechanism embedded in group psychotherapy, an area that has been overlooked by most writers, and in exploring "the professional use of the self" in the supervisory process. Here the author discusses the role of autonomic arousal in adaptive and defensive projective identification in the parallel process between the supervisee and supervisor and the client-clinician relationship. Again, she uses an analysis of clinical material with an adult–most fascinatingly, the same patient who was seen as a child in an earlier chapter. A bonus is that throughout the book the patients represent a broad spectrum of different cultural backgrounds and varying socioeconomic levels.

In addition to the considerable advances in theory and practice to the discipline of interpersonal neurobiology, another significant contribution of this work is reflected in Montgomery's creative, innovative, and synthetic structural organization of the book. Numerous extensive tables summarize a large body of interdisciplinary research that directly relates to various clinical processes, including functions and characteristics of the amygdala, selected functions of the upper right cortex, comparison of selected functions of the adolescent and adult brain, attachment categories of childhood as managed by the autonomic nervous system, relationship between arousal branches of the autonomic nervous system and various personality disorders, the arousal modulating biases of a spectrum of different defense mechanisms, and steps involved in projective identification during a therapeutic encounter. Montgomery states that these can be used for teaching purposes with therapists at all levels of clinical experience. The presentation of data in this holistic form is an efficient strategy for portraying the integrative functions of the right lateralized neurobiological mechanisms that operate in the rapid, nonlinear, nonconscious subjective realm. An appendix includes a worksheet on identifying defense mechanisms in any clinical encounter.

A second creative contribution of the book is the novel method by which the author describes the rapid nonverbal right-brain dynamics that underlie and precede later left-brain verbalizations and behavioral actions. The author asserts, "Almost line by line, each case examines the clinician and client interactions in terms of related neuroscience knowledge in an attempt to explain the kind of interaction, the intensity of the affect, or what the client is unconsciously trying to elicit from the clinician." Indeed, throughout the book, Montgomery's focus is on the structures and functions of the right lateralized system that operates beneath awareness, at a level deeper than the conscious minds and spoken words of both members of the therapeutic dyad. Toward that end, each vignette is accompanied by a dual tracking of both the conscious verbal and nonconscious nonverbal emotional communications between client and therapist. Thus, beneath each segment of a verbal transcript, Montgomery offers a simultaneous analysis of the affective arousal alterations associated with the right-brain-to-right-brain communications of one relational unconscious to another relational unconscious. This format highlights the energetic transmissions embedded with transfers of emotion within a co-created intersubjective field, and it demonstrates how nonconscious defenses alter the expression and reception of these affective communications.

The ambitious goal of the book is to more deeply understand the nonlinear bodily-based dynamics of the "social," "emotional" right brain, the biological substrate of the human unconscious. Arlene Montgomery has herein made a number of important contributions toward that goal.

Allan N. Schore

PREFACE

Working as a clinical social worker has been one of the most gratifying and frustrating experiences in my life. It has been gratifying to be part of experiences that were clearly helpful, if not healing, for clients; the frustration has come from efforts to explain why that help or healing was the case without relying on "practice wisdom," an oft-criticized source of data. In the mental health field there were many ways to acquire the wisdom of our clinical foremothers and forefathers, but until the past two decades, there was scant scientific support for what experienced practitioners knew significantly helped those struggling with biopsychosocial issues. There was also much criticism for interventions that did not have scientific support, particularly those therapies of longer duration. The hard sciences have not traditionally been particularly accessible to those who studied the social sciences. Though a wealth of information that could have explained, from a neurobiological perspective, the personal psychology of clients who sought help with their emotional and behavioral issues, until recently, that interface was not readily available.

I imagine that for many of us in the field, there were turning points that led to our pursuing training as mental health practitioners. Looking back on my own experience, I remember the day—actually, the moment—that I changed my major from nursing (I was in my last semester in the program) to social work. I was going through my mental checklist preparatory to moving to another city to finish the last rotation in nursing. I remember walking to my car from a weekend of work with emotionally disturbed adolescents at a residential psychiatric hospital. At 21 years old, I was still an adolescent myself, but working my way through college at the hospital made me feel years older that my teenage charges. I looked around the campus at the kids eating their supper in the dining hall, and it hit me that I was much more interested in their psychological world than I was in their blood pressure and heart rate. I realized that I had been working for several years in the environment in which I was best suited to work as a professional.

Although the social workers, psychologists, psychiatrists, and nurses had less contact with the residents than I did as a child-care staff member, nonetheless I could see that they were helping them and that their patients were bonded to them. I was already (fairly unconsciously) trying to reconcile the therapists' influence with what I was seeing in the relationships with those of us who actually lived in their lives on the dorm, the soccer field, the classroom, and various off-campus activities that we chaperoned. It is still surprising to me now how little we can "know" and still have a positive impact on another person's compromised psychological organization.

Later, after I was a social worker working in yet another residential psychiatric hospital, I read Trieschmann's *The Other 23 Hours*. I knew that my musings and intuition about the possibility of the healing potential of relationships (not simply techniques) was beautifully captured in Trieschmann's insistence that no child could recover from his or her traumatic experiences with just 1 hour of therapy per week. It would take the entire milieu. Today, I translate the writings of Trieschmann and others (e.g., Redl and Winemann) into the current findings on the neurobiology of attachment. The "practice wisdom" of those with years of success in treating people with all manner of developmental insults is supported by the explosion of current research on the brain revealing the physiology through which humans attune and connect. How to integrate scientific findings about the nervous system with the multiplicity of treatment theories is the current challenge in the mental health field.

As have many other clinicians, I have eagerly tried to keep up with the rich research and literature on the ways neurophysiology affects clinical work—a sometimes discouraging yet also satisfying endeavor. The reason for the excitement is obvious. The discouragement comes from there being so many discoveries every day and in fields in which most social scientists have little or no scientific background to understand. This book represents an effort to choose a few vital functions of the brain and nervous system that critically impact psychological clinical interventions. It is not an exhaustive catalogue or discussion, but a selective one, with multiple references provided for those who wish to read more extensively on various related topics.

In an intellectually friendly way, I want to share my experience in trying to teach students and supervise interns and new licensees about basic and important neurobiological facts as related to such areas as child development, attachment, personality development, and resilience in the face of various kinds of trauma. The more I have tried to integrate relevant scientific findings with clinical work, teaching, and supervision, the more convinced I have become that the information cuts across most, if not all, theoretical treatment strategies and interventions. The usefulness of learning basic brain functions and applying that knowledge to most current theories is exciting and inclusive. My hope is that graduate students, their faculty, agency supervisors, and those in practice whose education or training did not include the current neuroscience research will find this book an easy reference. I have tried to provide something for a variety of interests.

For example, the beginning of each chapter addresses certain related brain structures and their functions. I recommend that those who are not comfortable starting with the science proceed to the second part of each chapter and read the case. Almost line by line, each case examines the clinician and client interactions in terms of related neuroscience knowledge in an attempt to explain the kind of interaction, the intensity of affect, or what the client is unconsciously trying to elicit from the clinician. After reading the case, the beginning of the chapters may seem more user-friendly, as many examples of the neuroscience were detailed in the case notes. There are also tables that can be used on clinical material of all kinds. I like to use, for example, a list of right-brain functions (Table 6.1) to study various Hollywood movies because the facial expressions and body language are easy to see. I rewind many times for teaching purposes. I have come to prefer this format to that of printed cases because the students or workshop participants can also focus on their own reactions to the evocative characters and situations, as we examine the brain-to-brain interactions in the movie.

Part I covers the topics of affect regulation, defense mechanisms, threat management, and therapeutic engagement issues in terms of their neurological underpinnings. Chapter 1 illustrates the functioning of the autonomic nervous system through the history of Cori, a 15-year-old girl whose family lost everything in Hurricanes Katrina and Rita. The affect regulation strategies of Cori and other family members were altered by a series of losses that included her stepfather, the family dog, the city of New Orleans, the state of Louisiana, their home, and all their belongings. Despite also having experienced the loss of her father as a child, from the history, the family's resilience via family and community support seemed clear. However, as the family tried to establish roots in Texas, their emotional management strategies underwent changes such that Cori began faltering in school.

Chapter 2 continues to try to understand Cori by examining the defense mechanisms (managed by the limbic system) she exhibits in a therapy session.

The brain-to-brain neurobiological experiences of the therapist in relation to Cori is the focus.

Chapter 3 examines a session between a medical doctor and his patient, Mr. Ryan, who is a fireman whose uncharacteristically poor judgment contributed to severe burns. The exercise speculates on Mr. Ryan's emotional self states and somatic (bodily) states as managed by the amygdala and also speculates on his doctor's various ways of processing affect-related meaning as expressed by Mr. Ryan's behavior.

Two case illustrations in Chapter 4 attempt to explain issues of social engagement as enhanced or hindered by "neuroception" (Porges, 2011), which is a subtle, out-of-consciousness assessment of safety or danger indicating approach or avoidance, respectively. One case considers Baby Ruth, a career criminal who may be a psychopath or at least an antisocial personality organization. This is in contrast to Bebe, who has some similar, but not as severe, automatic and unconscious ways of managing unbearable affect via the vagal system.

Personality organization as an affect management strategy is the topic explored in Chapter 5. Using 14 cases, we consider the physiological arousal system when it has become organized into certain expectable, rigid behaviors. The secure and insecure attachment strategies of childhood and adulthood are each explored via a case example. The attachment strategy is compared to certain diagnosable disordered personality organizations. The arousal strategies to manage affect are seen to be quite similar in the attachment strategies and the personality organization. For example, the childhood avoidant attachment style relies on defense mechanisms that attempt to keep affect quite low; therefore, the low arousal branch of the autonomic nervous system, the parasympathetic branch, is the more reliable branch for affect management. In adulthood, the avoidant behaviors may become organized in a schizoid personality organization, among other possible personality disorders. It seems to be the case that all attachment categories (which are essentially affect management strategies) are affected by the high or low arousal systems.

Part II examines special populations, including adolescents, group work, and clinical supervision. In Chapter 6, the session notes of Cori from Chapter 2 are examined a second time to contrast adolescent and adult brain functioning. Table 6.2 compares adolescent and adult neurobiology. It is intended to be used for teaching or other purposes.

Chapter 7 selects a recent textbook on group psychotherapy (Rutan, Stone, & Shay, 2007) to review how selected neurobiological principles of regulation theory (Schore, 2003b, pp. 279–281) undergird stages of group development (i.e., formative, reactive, mature, termination); group dynamics (i.e., group culture, norms, roles); therapeutic factors (i.e., supportive factors, learning factors); mechanisms of change (i.e., internalization, transference); and therapeutic processes of change (i.e., confrontation, clarification, interpretation, working through).

Integrating selected neurobiological concepts into the clinical supervisory process is the focus of Chapter 8. Explored are such concepts as projective identification and dissociation and ways they are related to the transference and countertransference experiences of two dyads: the intern–client and the supervisor–intern relationships. Ways that neurobiological processes support the clinical work and the clinical supervision are examined via case material between the student intern and also through a recording of supervision between the supervisor and intern.

My personal goal is to bring certain information to bear on "practice wisdom," which I now consider to be both an oral and written tradition of socializing new clinicians into techniques and strategies that seemed to have stood the test of time in helping people, but which did not have a body of scientific measurement or testing behind them until recently. A large research literature exists for evidence-based short-term cognitive and behavioral techniques and strategies. To date, little of this research has included an extensive look at the neurobiology, particularly those right-hemispheric functions underpinning the interventions. The material in this book aims to detail experiences common to any type of face-to-face therapy and has an interpersonal component, regardless of theoretical orientation. I hope that many of the tables will be used to study and teach the neurobiology of clinical material. For me, the learning has come about from the repetition of applying to clinical examples the information about how structures in the brain function to promote or create obstacles to constructive and satisfying interpersonal contact and personal functioning.

Neurobiology Essentials
for Clinicians

PART I
Foundational Neuroscience Concepts

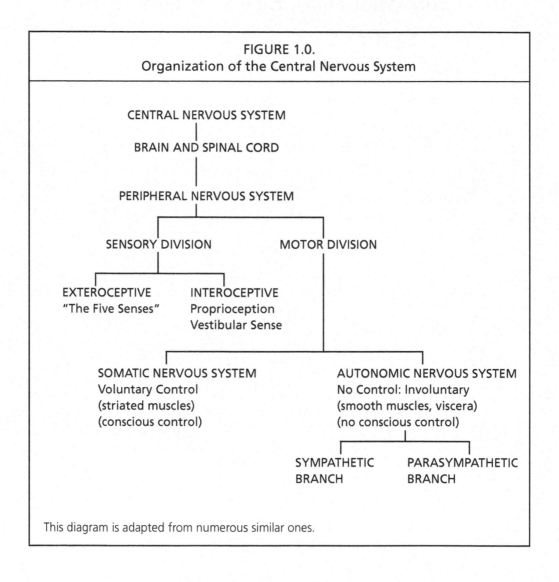

FIGURE 1.0.
Organization of the Central Nervous System

CENTRAL NERVOUS SYSTEM

BRAIN AND SPINAL CORD

PERIPHERAL NERVOUS SYSTEM

SENSORY DIVISION   MOTOR DIVISION

EXTEROCEPTIVE   INTEROCEPTIVE
"The Five Senses"   Proprioception
                      Vestibular Sense

SOMATIC NERVOUS SYSTEM   AUTONOMIC NERVOUS SYSTEM
Voluntary Control   No Control: Involuntary
(striated muscles)   (smooth muscles, viscera)
(conscious control)   (no conscious control)

                      SYMPATHETIC   PARASYMPATHETIC
                      BRANCH   BRANCH

This diagram is adapted from numerous similar ones.

CHAPTER 1

Affect Regulation and the Autonomic Nervous System

Illustrations from a Case History

This chapter focuses primarily on the clinical usefulness of learning about the functions of the autonomic nervous system and its branches, the sympathetic nervous system and parasympathetic nervous system. Certain other areas and functions of the brain are briefly addressed as well, including left–right hemisphere specialization and the major divisions of the brain, including the cerebral cortex. The neurobiological substrates of selected phenomena are illustrated in case material. These clinical phenomena include interactive, self- and autoregulation; attunement, bonding, and attachment; cultural issues; resiliency; shame; and protective behaviors, particularly defense mechanisms.

Throughout this chapter a clinical case history is used to speculate on how certain experiences of the client and her family may exemplify neurobiological processes, particularly the management of emotional arousal. Most clinicians know that the application to clinical work of information about brain structure and function can be a tedious and daunting undertaking, particularly in the moment-to-moment tracking of client and clinician interactions. And to what end, anyway? Tracking psychophysiological arousal can be a valuable assessment exercise leading to diagnosis and intervention considerations. Some clients' brains will need to repetitively "borrow" the arousal system management of the clinician in order to manage arousal in nonproblematic ways. This repetitive experience of synchronizing appropriate arousal management strategies with the brain of another has the potential to actually change brain functioning for the better. Some clients will not need to make such basic changes, but rather will need to reestablish a previous level of arousal management that was temporarily disrupted. And, of course, many clients will fall somewhere in the middle.

Below is a brief history of Cori, who was referred to the school counselor because her grades had "dropped off" after making all A's the first 6 weeks she was in school. The commentary on Cori's family history and recent traumatic experiences is similar to any clinician's thinking process. As an outside observer, the initial effort involves trying to speculate on explanations for certain behaviors of clinical interest. At this point in most clinical encounters, the attempt to understand the significance of a client's history can be a rather distant, intellectual effort—in contrast to deconstructing the actual experience between the client and the clinician, especially regarding emotional arousal management issues as related to behavior, defense mechanisms, or symptoms. As the evaluation continues, more information is collected about how events, stressors, and other relevant factors have influenced the management of emotions. At issue is discerning the degree and kind of corrections, changes, or improvements needed in the client's emotional management system. Will the initial intervention consist of problem-solving and psychoeducation components, which tend to be more intellectual and cognitive in nature? Or will there be a need to use the treatment relationship to change and improve the client's brain capacity to manage arousal in nontroublesome ways? Or something in between?

When first making tentative hypotheses about linking neurobiological concepts to clinical dynamics, I recommend working with others, whether you are a teacher, supervisor, and/or clinician or student, intern, or supervisee. For handy reference, helpful tables, figures, and summaries of brain structure and function are provided throughout the chapters. Throughout this chapter, selected neurobiological concepts are often illustrated with case history about an adolescent whose family had survived Hurricanes Katrina and Rita.

Case of Cori

At the time of treatment, Cori was a 15-year-old girl whose family had settled in Austin, Texas, after fleeing Hurricanes Katrina and Rita in August of 2005. She lived with her 12-year-old sister, her mother, and her paternal grandmother. Cori was in the eighth grade of a local middle school, though she should have been in the ninth grade. Her family was bussed to Houston, where they lived in FEMA (Federal Emergency Management Administration) housing for several months after leaving the New Orleans area. Obviously, this relocation was disruptive to Cori's schooling, so she was a grade behind, as was her sister.

Cori's mother and grandmother found work quickly in Austin. Her mother worked at a nursing home as an LVN (licensed vocational nurse) and her grandmother found work as a seamstress and worked for several cleaners and dance studios, sewing recital costumes and making evening gowns for formal events in the African American community. Cori and her sister babysat for several families in the neighborhood. They had not affiliated with a local Catholic Church comfortably because there were so few African American parishioners, unlike in New Orleans. Her grandmother had attended a nearby Baptist church, which she and her granddaughters liked, but Cori's mother was not happy with that idea for some reason.

Clinicians may wonder how Cori's cognitive functions have been impacted by her doubtlessly traumatic experiences and what may have contributed to, or compromised, her coping skills. What is required of a counselor to address the presenting problem of the falling grades? A brief review of the functions of each hemisphere, the four lobes of the brain, and a major arousal system (the autonomic nervous system) is necessary in order to address the underlying neurobiological functions that may guide understanding and intervention regarding emotional arousal management. To provide relief from dense descriptions of psychobiological processes, examples are interspersed throughout the text. Only a passing familiarity with these concepts is necessary to deconstruct the clinical interactions that are described.

Left–Right Hemisphere Specialization

The brain is asymmetrical, meaning that the left and right sides have different functions (Gainotti, 2012; Hellige, 1993; MacNeilage, 1990; MacNeilage, Rogers, & Vallortigara, 2009; McGilchrist, 2009; Semrud-Clikeman, Fine, & Zhu, 2011). Ultimately, however, the two sides of the brain work together as the corpus callosum (a fibrous band of tissue connecting the two sides of the brain) becomes increasingly "practiced" in coordinating communication between the two sides, or hemispheres, of the brain. Each side of the brain controls the other side of the body. An exception is the eyes, which are the source of most nonverbal information in the face; however, "recognizing emotions from visually presented facial expressions requires right somatosensory cortices" (Adolphs, Damasio, Tranel, Cooper, & Damasio, as cited in Schore, 2003b, p. 44; see also Schore, 2003b, pp. 223–228). Some have begun to describe the existence of two separate brains rather than two sides of the brain (Schore, 2003b, p. xv), whereas others have historically focused more on the ways in which the two hemispheres interact to produce unity of thought and action (Hellige, 1993, p. 4). At any rate, the focus of this book is mainly on the functions of the right brain.

Briefly, the left side of the brain controls the conscious, routine, detailed, aware (explicit), cognitive, rational, and verbal mental states whereas the right side detects and responds to unexpected stimuli that are perceived below consciousness (implicit) and mediates perception of spatial relations, global patterns, emotional (affective) experiences, facial recognition, and psychobiological states (MacNeilage, Rogers, & Vallortigara, 2009; Schore, 2003b, pp. xiv–xvii). The evolutionary importance of left–right specialization, which began 500 million years ago in early vertebrates, is to enhance survival (MacNeilage et al., 2009). One side of the body (generally the right side of the body, which is controlled by the left brain) is adept at controlling well-established behaviors—for example, feeding, foraging, and fighting. The other side (the left brain) is specialized to respond to predators quickly. MacNeilage et al. (2009) made the additional point that for both sides of the brain to control the routine as well as the reaction to novelty and possible danger would be inefficient and would negatively affect survival. For details, see MacNeilage (1990).

The mental health field seems to have followed this "left–right specialization." For example, Schore pointed out (2003b, p. xv) that certain treatment strategies primarily focus on the left (verbal) hemisphere, such as the use of verbal reappraisal or mental self-talk to regulate anxiety states, whereas other strategies focus on the right (nonverbal) hemisphere by addressing tone of voice, facial expression, and bodily states reflecting affective states. The referral for services for Cori may reflect problematic hemispheric functioning: Her left-brain cognitive and intellectual capacities had been functioning very well (e.g., Cori made all A's in the initial 6-week grading period), with the subsequent drop in academic functioning suggesting that the right hemisphere's capacity to manage affective states may have become increasingly compromised as the semester wore on. In short, if Cori was beginning to have difficulties regulating her emotions (primarily a right-hemisphere function), those difficulties may have been the cause of her declining school performance.

Major Divisions of the Brain

The human brain is divided into three major parts. From the spinal cord on up are the hindbrain (automatic activity), the midbrain (emotional feelings and reactions), and the forebrain (higher mental processes, such as thinking and language) (Bourne & Russo, 1998, p. 74). See Figure 1.1 to view these three major divisions of the brain. The outer layer (forebrain) of the brain's cerebrum is the cerebral cortex, which is one-fourth-inch thick and composed

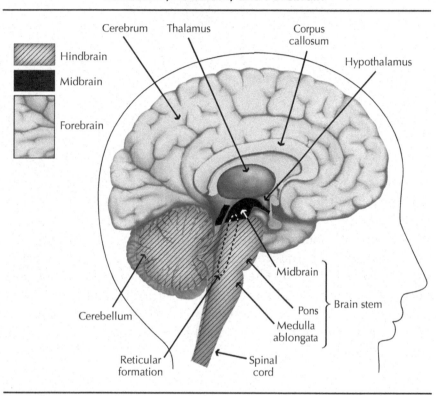

FIGURE 1.1
Hindbrain, Midbrain, and Forebrain

mainly of gray matter, whereas white matter of the cerebrum connects the lower brain areas to the cerebral cortex (Johnson, 2003, pp. 247–249). The cerebral cortex is responsible for integrating and interpreting sensory information, memory storage, abstract thought, conscious awareness, and conscious control of skeletal muscles (Johnson, 2003, p. 248). The four lobes of the cortex in Figure 1.2 are the frontal (conscious thought, speech, and initiates motor activity), temporal (language, interprets auditory information, and perceptual judgment), parietal (sensory information from skin), and occipital (vision) lobes (Johnson, 2003, p. 248). For mental health interventions, it is important to note that all four lobes are involved in memory storage of the specific information for which they are designed. For example, should there be damage to certain areas of the brain, the location-specific nature of infor-

FIGURE 1.2
The Four Lobes of the Cortex

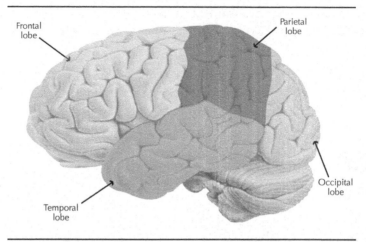

mation processing would be critical to understand so that interventions could take the impairment into account (Johnson, 2003, p. 248).

The human nervous system "consists of two major divisions: the brain and spinal cord . . . and the peripheral nervous system consists of all the nervous tissue outside the central nervous system" (Buelow, Hebert, & Buelow, 2000, pp. 151, 153). The peripheral nervous system is further divided into sensory and motor divisions, and the motor division is divided into the somatic nervous system and the autonomic nervous system. As noted above, the autonomic nervous system is divided into the sympathetic and the para-sympathetic branches (Johnson, 2003; Buelow, 2000). See Figure 1.0.

The Autonomic Nervous System

The right hemisphere is dominant over the left hemisphere in identifying and managing emotional experiences (McGilchrist, 2009; Schore, 2003a, 2003b). This section examines the role of attunement, bonding, and attachment in emotion regulation with an emphasis on the adaptive or maladaptive functioning of the autonomic nervous system as affected by experience during development. The affect management aspects of defense and resilience are discussed as well.

Identification and Management of Emotional Experiences

The case of Cori focuses on the identification of, and management issues around, the intensity (magnitude of emotional feeling or arousal) and/or valence (degree of attractiveness; positive–negative; approach–avoidance) of an emotional experience and its manifestations (see Hariri, Bookheimer, & Mazziotta, 2000, for details on modulation of emotional responses and the limbic system). For example, the ways in which various family members express grief are examined. Any affect could be expressed on a continuum from *not at all*, to *modulated expression*, to a *bidirectional expression* (meaning, oscillating from very high to very low in intensity), and/or to *not modulated* (extremely high arousal or extremely inhibited arousal). *Note*: Some clinicians make a distinction between emotions, feelings, and affects (LeDoux, 1996), whereas others do not (Fosha, 2000, 2010). For the purpose of examining the history of Cori in this chapter, it is easier to track the neurobiology of interactions if there is not a fine distinction made among these terms and to simply think of emotion/feeling/affects as a reaction in the brain that causes a change in the internal state and signals actions, whether the action is completed or not (Applegate & Shapiro, 2005; Cozolino, 2002; Fonagy, Gergely, Jurist, & Target, 2004; Siegel, 2007; Tronick, 2007).

In the initial adjustment to the forced move to Austin, it seems that family members were quite functional, perhaps expressing their grief in modulated ways. They seemed to handle adequately their home, work, and school responsibilities, as far as the counselor knew. This initially stable functioning may have resulted from the family's long history of good to high socioemotional capacity. (See study by Oosterman & Schuengel, 2007, on the role of the autonomic nervous system as a regulatory process in the parent–child relationship.) The dyadic/interactive regulation of emotion is described as the constructive regulation of affect/emotions in a right-brain to right-brain manner with another person (Schore, 2003b, pp. 279–281).

Right-Hemisphere Emotional Management: The Role of Attunement, Bonding, and Attachment

For the purpose of clinical precision, it seems important to differentiate among the right-hemisphere phenomena of attunement, bonding, and attachment, though those terms are often used interchangeably even in the dictionary and thesaurus. In the clinical context, *attunement* is the subtle adjusting that may occur between two brains (especially in relation to arousal and energy shifts; Schore, 2003a, pp. 96–97) and resonating with the internal states of another person (Cozolino, 2002); *bonding* is a connection (a felt experience) between two brains and personalities; and *attachment* is essentially the affect management strategy that develops over time, whose formation depends upon the interaction between an individual and his or her caretaking other(s). These brain–brain interactions promote the development of cerebral circuits (Trevarthen, 1993b).

In my experience, attunement is necessary for bonding, which is itself necessary to an eventual attachment (for details, see Cozolino, 2006, p. 62). Clinical work can be done in any of these states. However, the more the affect management style that characterizes a client's typical way of dealing with emotions needs to be changed and "rewired" neurobiologically, the more at least an experience of *emotional attunement* or *bonding* should occur with the clinician. "Rewiring" likely requires an attachment (neurobiologically regulating affect), which will take time to develop and may be fraught with difficulties. These difficulties often include the client's unconscious translocation of the troublesome past relationship experiences (or aspects of it) into the present relationship in what is termed an *enactment*. This enactment could be an opportunity to engage in a repair of sorts (similar to Tronick's "interactive repair," 1989) or a corrective experience within the "containing" therapeutic relationship (Bion, 1962). The clinician may be drawn into the client's barely conscious hope/need/fear of the possibility for a corrective emotional experience. The client's unconscious reservations to respond to relationship opportunities likely have their origins in past experiences that involved exposing him- or herself to being vulnerable to another person and being disappointed, or worse. Clients with a balanced affect management strategy may require little attunement and bonding for the clinician to grasp the issues, empathize, and properly address the presenting problem.

It now seems clear that the outcomes of techniques that seem to address primarily left-hemisphere cognitions may be enhanced when right-hemisphere emotional management functioning is improved (Siegel, 2007, p. 226; Panksepp, as cited in Fosha, Siegel, & Solomon, 2009). There may be a corollary to that concept in the speculation that, as noted previously, the fact that Cori's grades had "dropped off" may have resulted from compromised left-hemisphere work due to compromised right-hemisphere affect management issues.

As the history and session notes are reviewed in Chapter 2, we will see that Cori may be trying to use the fragile attunement to her therapist to help her regulate her affect somewhat. On the way to attunement, clients can draft the clinician into participating in a psychologically defensive operation (e.g., acting out, projective identification, or dissociation; the topic of defenses is treated in detail in later chapters, especially Chapter 2). This maneuver creates the possibility for the dyadic/interactive regulation of affect to occur between two brains (or the opposite, a therapeutic impasse; see Chapter 8). In the brief history of Cori and her family, it could be assumed that attunement, bonding, and attachment had been normative before the hurricanes and consequent disruptions to their lives.

The right hemisphere is the focus of most therapeutic interventions, regardless of technique (Schore, 2003b, pp. 279–281). The right hemisphere is faster than the left hemisphere in registering the positive or negative intensity of experience—that is, "valence tagging"—and does so without conscious awareness (Pizzagalli, Regard, & Lehmann, 1999). The more sensitive a clinician is about the level of somatopsychological arousal in the client and in him- or herself, the more finely attuned the possible interventions. As discussed in following chapters, though no particular theoretical approach is necessarily recommended, some approaches are more naturally responsive to certain neurobiologically compromised mental conditions. In the case of Cori studied in this chapter, the focus is on using family history to track both the arousal (or lack of arousal) and the psychological defensive maneuvers employed to manage the level of arousal in the client and her family members.

Factors Influencing the Functioning of Autonomic Nervous System

As mentioned briefly above, there are two important systems in the brain and body that manage higher and lower levels of arousal and are connected to every major organ of the body and many glands. These two systems are segments of the autonomic nervous system: The *sympathetic* segment excites, and the *parasympathetic* segment inhibits. These functions may variously be referred to as high/low or up/down-regulated. Branches working smoothly in tandem create what is termed *homeostatically balanced arousal states*.

Ideally, the autonomic nervous system responds to and regulates the internal state of the body to maintain homeostasis; according to Porges (2011), this homeostasis can be disrupted when external needs become more important than the regulation of the internal state (which is regulated by the central nervous system). Proper functioning generally finds "the parasympathetic branch promot[ing] functions associated with growth and restoration . . . and the sympathetic branch promot[ing] increased output of energy to deal with challenges from outside the body" (Porges, 2011, p. 80). In this section of the chapter we examine what happens when homeostatic balance is temporarily disrupted and, most especially, what happens when there is pressure from the environment to activate primarily one or the other of the autonomic nervous system branches as an automatic response to most situations. Additionally, when either too much excitement or too much inhibition occurs, particularly too frequently and/or over too long a time period, the normative use of the branches may become compromised. For example, the same parasympathetic branch that permits a calm approach (inhibition to promote social interaction) may severely inhibit behavior (via freeze) in cases of stress, which temporarily serves as a protective factor and is a learned response resulting from past experiences. Or vice versa, when the extreme activation of the sympathetic branch may have to be utilized to cope (via fight, flight) with unusual stress, instead of the normal actions of daily life.

The sympathetic branch is dominant for the expression of terror, rage, excitement, and elation, and the parasympathetic branch is dominant for the expression of shame, disgust, hopeless despair, and profound detachment (Schore, 2003b, pp. 111, 249; Schore, 2003a, p. 267–268). Additionally, the parasympathetic branch, in coordination with the vagal system (see Chapter 4 for details), makes possible calm approaches in social interactions (Porges, 2011, p. 59).

The caregiving experiences, family, religion, community, subculture, and larger culture can train or "determine the individual's characteristic approach to affect regulation" (Schore, 2003a, p. 83) and emotional nonverbal communication (Tucker, as cited in Schore, 2003a, p. 84; also see Foster, Moskowitz, & Javier, 1996, regarding culture, class, and nonverbal communication). For instance, some cultures are more likely to expect grief experiences that are down-regulated and inhibited as normative. In contrast, some cultures will socialize as appropriate emotionally up-regulated states. On an interesting historical side note, even Freud may have been referring to arousal states long ago in his several considerations of pleasure–unpleasure—for example, when he described states of psychic tension as increasing or decreasing (Brenner, 1974, pp. 66–70). Either state could be sought or avoided because the idiosyncratically experienced arousal states could be either pleasureable or unpleasurable. Freud was surely referring to states of arousal, which we now know are managed in large measure by the branches of the autonomic nervous system.

Cori's family seemed to adjust to the new community, engaging in work and school responsibilities, rather quickly considering their recent displacement and losses. Perhaps their capacity to socially engage was previously functional (homeostatically balanced?), so that they had ample social and emotional skills upon which to draw. However, Cori's grades have declined, and this undesirable shift has precipitated a referral to the counselor to look into the problem (environmental stressors disrupting homeostasis, with one branch of the autonomic nervous system becoming over-used?). To reiterate, an obvious concern is that Cori's emotional instability (right hemisphere) may have affected her intellectual work (left hemisphere, primarily). There are, of course, other possible explanations.

Because affect regulation is so heavily influenced by the autonomic nervous system's two branches, the environmental influences (e.g., sociocultural learning experiences, caregiving experiences, other interpersonal influences, trauma) may create a preference for the automatic, reflexive use of either the sympathetic or parasympathetic segments of the autonomic nervous system (Schore, 2003a, pp. 22, 25). The overuse of either up or down regulation in response to difficult-to-tolerate emotions can make the overly utilized branch the dominant, more-likely-to-be-used branch. Conversely, the other branch will become the nondominant branch. To review, this pattern is in contrast to the autonomic nervous system's employing the excitatory or the inhibitory branch as *appropriate* to the situation, instead of using one branch most of the time.

What is the significance of relying on one branch? This uncoupling means that the two branches do not work together very well to create homeostatic balance in managing levels of affect and their expression (Rothschild, 2000; Schore, 2003a, pp. 82–86; Cozolino, 2002, p. 59). The uncoupled branches of the autonomic nervous system may be a powerful force in influencing a dominant defensive style. This fact may have a profound effect on the creations of attachment styles in childhood (secure; insecure-avoidant; insecure-resistant [also termed *insecure-ambivalent*]; and disorganized [also termed *disoriented* or Type "D"]) (Cozolino, 2002, pp. 208–209); attachment styles of adulthood; as well as on certain psychiatric disorders, including the personality disorders, posttraumatic stress disorder (PTSD), and perhaps certain depressive and anxiety disorders (Schore, 2003a, pp. 32–35, 83–84, 234–307). For example, the depressive disorders are more down-regulated (parasympathetic branch), and the anxiety disorders are more up-regulated (sympathetic branch). Additionally, Schore (2003a) described the autonomic nervous system's regulation effects as biased in the childhood attachment categories as follows: Secure attachment involves a homeostatic balance between the two branches (pp. 277; pp. 180–181); insecure-avoidant attachment is biased toward the parasympathetic branch (pp. 26–28); the insecure resistant/ambivalent category is biased toward the sympathetic branch (pp. 28–29); and the disorganized/disoriented/Type D may involve rapid shifting between the two branches or the branches may be hyperactivated simultaneously (pp. 189–198).

Certain clinical constructs also have embedded within them regulation of affect, including such concepts as the internal working model (Bowlby, 1988), representations of interactions that have been generalized (RIGS, Stern, 1985), selfobject (Kohut, 1977), and internalized object relations (Kernberg, 1976), to name a familiar few (see a later section in this chapter). These constructs may be considered to refer to forms of affect management strategies that may evolve to preferentially manage high or low arousal and avoid the less tolerable or the less comfortable opposite level of arousal.

Conversely, these constructs may also refer to homeostatically balanced arousal management, with the exception of the selfobject, which is, by definition, a balanced, positive internal experience (Kohut, 1977).

Defense and Resilience

Resilience is the capacity of the nervous system to tolerate increasingly difficult levels of affect without resorting to toxic defense mechanisms; it begins with the child and caregiver's interaction capacity to transition between positive affect and negative affect and back to positive affect (Demos, as cited in Schore, 2003b, p. 11). Various maneuvers can be employed to prevent the less-used segment of the autonomic nervous system from being taxed, because the neural circuitry is simply not as hardy and sturdy. To repeat, some of these maneuvers include defenses (adaptive or maladaptive protective actions, beliefs, thoughts, or emotions that serve to protect from psychological distress; Conte & Plutchik, 1995; Vaillant, 1977) or characterological patterns of behavior that may become a certain type of attachment pattern in some cases. The attachment pattern may eventually evolve into predictable but disordered personality organization. For example, the defenses associated with antisocial personality, such as acting out and regression, are up-regulated and driven by the sympathetic branch. A person with antisocial personality traits struggles with the depressive, down-regulated affects, finding them much more difficult to tolerate than exciting affects (see case of Baby Ruth in Chapter 4). The defensive maneuvers are employed to avoid straining the less well-developed parasympathetic branch. In the case of avoidant attachment category of childhood, the parasympathetic branch is more heavily utilized to manage life experiences. Defenses such as denial, suppression, dissociation, and/or blocking of affect are often employed to avoid experiencing the more highly arousing emotions.

Another example of the failure of defensive structures is often found in a person with severe narcissistic personality traits. Common defenses include projection (blaming), denial, intellectualization, devaluation, and isolation of affect (defenses striving for dampening and lowering affect, managed by the parasympathetic branch of the autonomic nervous system). All these defenses attempt to minimize or avoid arousing experiences (managed by the sympathetic branch). Should the person with these traits be humiliated or shamed (an experience that many defensive maneuvers of those with narcissistic traits are designed to avoid), narcissistic rage and aggression may occur. Shame can become an unregulated humiliated state involving anger/rage wherein the brain cannot access a working model of a soothing other (Schore, 2003b, pp. 172–177). The shamed person with narcissistic traits may lose control of his or her emotional expression. This failure of the inhibiting defenses may then permit the activation of the compromised excitatory branch. Should that occur, the person may be unable to contain the high expressions of affect in an acceptable manner (worst case, giving into narcissistic rage), which is a departure from the "cooler" and more detached manner usually in evidence.

The examples of disordered personality functioning such as those with antisocial or narcissistic behaviors are the opposite of the concept of resilience. Being able to tolerate increasingly painful levels of affect without resorting to maladaptive defensive mechanisms is a nonconscious experience-dependent affect regulation capacity (Hofer, 1994; Field, 1985; Greenspan, 1981). Demos (as cited in Schore, 2003b, p. 11) described infant resilience as the capacity of the child and the parent to transition from positive to negative and back to positive affect. Those people who have severe traits of narcissism (e.g., grandiosity) and who experience humiliation may attempt to remain detached and "above it all" and will be relying on the inhibitory (parasympathetic) branch to manage affect. If they become overwhelmed by the dreaded affective state of shame, they may go from positive (i.e., the nonshamed state) to negative (i.e., the shamed state), and not be able to regulate their affect, either by themselves or by using others interactively. Therefore, they often will experience an intolerable up-regulated state beyond their ability to bear, regulate, or terminate easily.

Thinking in terms of levels of arousal, it could be speculated that Cori's initial ability to function in school may have indicated a homeostatically balanced autonomic nervous system, with, perhaps, neither the parasympathetic nor sympathetic being favored; grades that "dropped off" may indicate an imbalance of some sort—perhaps she is beginning to use psychological defenses that impair her academic functioning. Did she withdraw (become down-regulated via the parasympathetic, which inhibits), or did she become more active than usual (via the sympathetic, which excites)? Extreme employment of either branch can compromise functioning, particularly the cognitive functioning necessary for academic work.

Some possible parasympathetically managed defense mechanisms include blocking, denial, inhibition, intellectualization, isolation of affect, passive–aggressive behavior, or repression. Some possible sympathetically managed defenses include acting out, regression, mania, or externalization. Toward the second 6 weeks Cori was in school, these defensive maneuvers may be replacing the more homeostatically balanced and adaptive defenses such as affiliation, altruism, humor, self-assertion, sublimation, or suppression. It is helpful to consider some obvious defenses being employed at the beginning of deconstructing a clinical encounter and the branch of the autonomic nervous system, which may have become the more automatic way of managing affect. As the session unfolds, a clinician may begin to develop a more refined understanding of how the client manages affect (see Chapter 2 for a detailed discussion of arousal management and defense mechanisms).

The level of functionality in this family is obvious: The adults find work right away; they turn to a source of support, the church; and initially at least, Cori functions well in school, despite the traumas. In neurobiolological terms, the family might be described as resilient, a characteristic that Schore translates into the ability to tolerate increasingly higher levels of affect without resorting to maladaptive defense mechanisms and to adaptively shift between interactive regulation in interconnected contexts and autoregulation in autonomous contexts (2003a, pp. 84–85; 2003b, p. 281). The more adaptive defenses (e.g., self-assertion, anticipation, altruism) may indicate that an adaptive level of functioning existed prior to the recent and severe traumas. Additionally, it could be speculated that when first settling in Austin, this hard-working family employed the manic defense. This up-regulated defense allows a person to be quite productive. However the hyperactivated state may not be sustainable for long periods of time.

Speculations on the Intersection of Culture, the Expression of Affect, and Mirror Neurons

Exciting discoveries in the past few years about what have come to be called *mirror neurons* may shed light on the transmittal of social and cultural learning, though that conclusion remains controversial (Hickok, 2008). Mirror neurons are distributed throughout the brain and are closely associated with motor neurons (Stern, 2004, p. 79). Populations of mirror neurons become active within the motor system of the brain when people experience emotion as well as when they see emotion expressed by others. Gallese termed this experience "embodied simulation" in 2010 (p. 79), having used the term *mimesis* in 2009 (p. 4), meaning, basically, "mimicry." Gallese argued that humans' brains are "wired to identify with each other and that such processes of identification can be neurally grounded since the discovery of mirror neurons and other mirroring neural mechanisms" (2009, p. 4). It takes less than 1 second for the faces of two people to register and mimic perceived expressions on the face of the other, all occurring at levels beneath awareness (Stenberg, Wiking, & Dahl, 1998) and thereby facilitating nonverbal communication and unconscious learning.

Mirroring may also provide direct internal experience and therefore understanding of another person's acts and intentions. How? Siegel (2007) defined "mirror properties in the nervous system . . . as the ways in which our social brain has processes in which it perceives the intentional, goal-directed actions of others and links this perception to the priming of the motor systems to engage in that same action" (Siegel, 2007, p. 347). The literal definition of mirroring does not really capture the intentional aspect ascribed to mirror neurons. As the brain can attribute intention from scant information, there is more than an exact replica of an action registering in the brain (Siegel, 2007) that affects social interactions. If mirror neurons help predict what comes next in a familiar series of movements or behaviors, then that function is an economical aspect of socialization. Once something is learned, an indication, clue, or hint will suffice to let it be known what comes next in our dyad, family, or culture.

These nonverbal and beneath-consciousness, but broad, aspects of communication may transmit cultural learning, according to Tucker (as cited in Schore, 2003a, p. 84), in that the brain learns to regulate itself as proscribed by the culture, among many aspects of cultural learning. Ideally, the flexible regulation of emotional states (originally accomplished by successful interactive regulation in interdependent, interconnected, synchronous and attuned contexts) may eventually become a self-regulating, autonomous, and independent governor of the emotions. "Good enough" (Winnicott, 1958) social interactions can promote the kind of brain differentiation that creates a balance between the sympathetic and parasympathetic branches of the autonomic nervous system—a balance that promotes flexibility between the branches rather than ascendance of one branch or the other (Schore, 2003a, p. 85).

The earliest cultural learning experiences involve the affective transactions that influence the balance between the interactive and autoregulation strategies, as described by Schore (2003a, pp. 84–85). Not only is the regulation of emotion/affect heavily influenced by cultural proscriptions, but also by the gradual accretion of preferences for how aroused one should become. In the case illustration in this chapter, tracking the ways that mourning can be expressed may become a matter of speculation because the data are historical and based upon interactions, but worth the time and effort nonetheless. In addition to social interactions, there are many influences on any learned emotional expression, often quite subtle and not conscious. These include the behavioral and affective styles of family members with whom the client identifies (embodied simulation, mimesis), religion, subculture, language, and region, to name a few.

A brief example of how culture socializes the direction and intensity of affective expression is provided by a colleague from Korean culture. This person told me that excited displays of emotion generally are not acceptable, including during mourning. In contrast, another colleague related that her Italian emigrant grandmother was herself, and expected others to be, emotional and expressive, especially around matters involving loss and death. When as an adult, my friend visited her relatives in Italy, she was constantly cried over effusively by relatives whom she had never met, because, they said, she had been "lost" to them (as was her emigrant grandmother) and was now "found." The case example in this chapter examines competing emotional/affective socializing influences on Cori.

Case of Cori, Continued

Cori was 6 years old when her father, Cecil, was lost in the Gulf of Mexico when it is believed that a sudden storm capsized the shrimp boat on which he worked. No one ever actually knew for sure. For several years after his death, the family moved from New Orleans to a more rural area on one of the bays where the paternal grandmother lived. Cori remembered her mother and grandmother talking endlessly about her lost father over coffee at the kitchen table, having Masses said for her father, attending church several times a week to pray for him, and being known in the close-knit community as "Cecil's girl." Cori thought of those years after her father's death as "pretty great" and quickly amends the statement to add, "But, of course we missed my daddy a lot."

Cori described her grandmother's house as small, always smelling like coffee, and filled with remnants from the material that her grand-mother had cut up for her sewing jobs. Cori and her sister Jakki spent most of their time with their grandmother, who worked at home and was known "all over town" for the perfect garments that she sewed. Cori and Jakki spent lazy days making "doll clothes and dog clothes" and eventually "people clothes," which their grandmother taught them to stitch for "fancy people" to help earn money. Though they missed their mother, Cori and Jakki understood that her job in the city as a nurse paid more than she could earn where her grandmother lived. Her grandmother, Mimi, sang Baptist hymns while she sewed. Though she taught them to sing with her, Mimi cautioned them not to sing some of them around the church, because the "Catholics don't approve of those old hymns." Cori and Jakki sat at card tables with their own scissors, pins, needles, and thread as they listened to the radio or sang, all the while under the watchful gaze of big framed pictures of Martin Luther King, Jr., John F. Kennedy, and Jesus on the cross with Mother Mary looking on. Mimi's old dog, Mary, would pace between the sewing room and living room all day.

There seems to have been a support network in the extended family and community that promoted adaptation with resilience in Cori and her family. The family seemed able to easily access and constructively utilize available support for their grief and mourning. There were rituals (religious and family interactions) through which to actively mourn the father's death, perhaps leading to homeostatic balance in the autonomic nervous systems of all family members. Intrapsychically as well as via dyad and group interactions, the grief, sadness, and other emotions of family members for the loss of Cecil seem to have been addressed in the context of emotional warmth, containment of affect, and respect.

We could imagine that both hemispheres were engaged: the right hemisphere in processing the nonverbal, ambient atmosphere among people and the left hemisphere, in the thinking, planning, and implementation of the sewing, chatting around the table, etc. There seems to have been attunement among the family members, leading to a synchronized contact that may had its own rhythm, perhaps comforting, soothing, and enabling all to perform their daily, age-appropriate tasks.

Further, the experience among the family members might be described as the dyadic/interactive regulation of affect, which, for the children, could have led to the appropriate management of their own emotions in an age/stage-appropriate manner—that is, to the autoregulation of affects—without their resorting to maladaptive defense mechanisms. Cori's easy ability to describe in such evocative detail the ambience of the home with its emotional warmth, comfort, and containment of emotions (Bion, 1962) is itself an indication of the effect on her personality organization of the experience-dependent regulation of affect. The dyadic regulation of Cori's emotional states can lead to the formation (over time) of neurocircuitry that endures to become traits (Beebe, 2005; Hebb, 1949; Perry, Pollard, Blakely, Baker, & Vigilante, as cited in Schore, 2003a, p. 252).

Additionally, these affect regulation strategies—which include the appropriate use of reliable others with whom to interact in shared genuine interest and emotional connection through meaningful and routine activities (sewing together and drinking coffee at the kitchen table)—are examples of the following constructs which can be helpful or useful: the function provided by positive helpful selfobjects (Kohut, 1971); the function provided by healthy internal working models (Bowlby, 1988); the internalized positive representation of self and other with the linking affect (Kernberg, 1980); positive RIGs (Stern, 1985); and the secure attachment (Schore, 2003b). It might also be the case that the parasympathetic and sympathetic branches of the autonomic nervous system are working harmoniously to manage the internal experience of emotions as well as the various physiological states (Porges, 2011). When the affect is constructively managed in the right brain, in particular, the employment of compromising compensatory defenses or behaviors is less likely and, ideally, unnecessary. The more homeostatically balanced defenses may instead be in evidence, defense mechanisms such as affiliation, anticipation, humor, self-assertion, self-observation, sublimation, and/or suppression.

Right Hemisphere: Where Affect Regulation Strategies Are Processed

Affect management strategies (i.e., regulatory systems) "are not innate, but a product of the experience-dependent maturation of the right brain" (Schore, 2003a, p. 83). Regulation strategies (processed primarily in the right hemisphere) are the product of implicit learning (procedural learning), which involves the unconscious processing of emotional stimuli (Morris, Ohman, & Dolan, 1998; Wexler, Warrenburg, Schwartz, & Janer, 1992, as cited in Schore, 2003b, p. 35). Dysregulated affect may extend the client beyond the "window of tolerance" (Siegel, 2007), the discomfort or pain of which the brain will attempt to manage. The right hemisphere is also dominant for the production of the neurohormones that mediate coping responses (Wittling & Pfluger, 1990), which are, in part, an affect regulation strategy. These neurohormones— which include cortisol (which stops the activation of the sympathetic branch) and corticotropin releasing factor (facilitates the release of energy; Yehuda, 1999)—are the mediators of the human stress response (Wittling, 1997).

This brings the discussion to the interactions between clients and clinicians. Representative descriptions/conceptualizations of affect management strategies (processed primarily in the right hemisphere; these strategies have the potential to regulate or dysregulate each party) occurring between client and clinician are summarized below:

1. The affect-laden transference–countertransference experience is an attempt to unconsciously restage problematic past relationship experiences with the hope for a different outcome (Weiss & Sampson, 1986). Ideally, these "affectively loaded traumatic interpersonal experiences that can fuel transference reenactments" will become available for learning and change so that the past is updated and not rigidly repeated in current relationships (Levin, 1997, pp. 1140–1141).
2. Kohut (1977) conceptualized selfobject as the experience/function that occurs with a mature brain capable of soothing (down-regulating)

and preventing its opposite, which is fragmentation (stimulating to the point of emotional fracture) (see Charnus & Livingston, as cited in Edward & Sanville, 1996 [pp. 386-403], and Rowe & MacIsaac, 1988, for details).

3. Bion (1962) was one of the first to describe the containment function of an other who returns difficult emotions in a more manageable form to the less sturdy other (in current terms, Bion may have been describing interactive re-regulation to achieve homeostatic balance).

4. Kernberg (1980) described an internalized object relationship as the self representation, the object (other) representation, and the linking affect. Each element (as well as the interaction among the elements of the configuration) of the internalized object relation can be examined in the clinical encounter in order to address the affect regulation or dysregulation potential.

5. Benjamin (1988) stated that the intersubjective position of each person in a dyad must recognize the other as an equivalent center of expression (as cited in Mitchell & Aron, 1999, p. 184), an experience similarly described as "mutual mapping" by Tronick and Weinberg (1997, p. 75, as cited in Schore, 2003b, p. 76). Mutual mapping may "cocreate dyadic amplification of state," which may make possible the "transfer of affect" between two brains (particularly between limbic systems), potentially an adaptive or maladaptive phenomena (Schore, 2003b, p. 76).

6. The Stone Center proposed a relational approach (Jordan, 2000) with an emphasis on connection, disconnection, and reconnection (of affective states). The hope is that the reconnection affectively stabilizes the client and perhaps invites a better experience emotionally to counteract earlier problematic ones.

7. Schore (1994, 2003a, 2003b) emphasizes the neurobiological aspects of attachment that manifest in different types of arousal management styles (i.e., attachment styles). The right hemisphere has control over the bodily components of all emotional states via the sympathetic and parasympathetic branches of the autonomic nervous system (Spencer, 1996, as cited in Schore, 2003a, p. 82), and the right hemisphere "stores an internal working model of the attachment relationship that determines the individual's characteristic approach to affect regulation" (Schore, 2003a, p. 83). Bowlby famously coined the term *internal working model* to describe the unconscious representation of the early family experience (Bowlby, 1988), an idea that has had a profound effect on child development research in attachment (Schore, 2003b, p. 45).

8. Stern (1985) proposed the concept of RIGs, or representations of interactions that have been generalized, likely a right-hemisphere experience. Like the constructs of internalized object relations, internal working model, and attachment strategies, RIGs also describe interpersonal interactions that preserve experiences and may have adaptive or maladaptive consequences regarding affect management. According to Levin (1997, p. 1141), RIGs are "an example of the schema approach" to transference. Schemas are seen "as a way of understanding various mental states and transference experiences of the patient" (Horowitz, p. 43, as cited in Levin, 1997, p. 1140).

9. Freud (1912/1958a, 1915/1959a) described the client's "attachment" to the clinician as a necessary condition for a therapeutic encounter (though Freud used the term attachment, it is unlikely that the current neurobiological meaning of that term was what he meant; it is more likely that he meant some form of attunement or bonding). It is thought that Freud's concept of attachment invites repetition of past stressful experiences, which might be restaged with the possibility of rendering the experiences understandable and verbalizable. In so doing, the unconscious repeating of difficult past relationship elements may be replaced with remembering them on a conscious level. This conscious remembering may master an affectively loaded memory of a traumatic interpersonal experience (Levin, 1997, pp. 1140–1141).

Defense mechanisms are described as "nonconscious strategies of emotional regulation for avoiding, minimizing, or converting affects that are too difficult to tolerate, with an emphasis on dissociation and projective identification; these right-brain defenses prevent the entrance into 'dreaded states' charged with intense affects that can potentially traumatically disorganize the self system" (Schore, 2003b, p. 280). Projective identification is an example of the arousal management function of a defense mechanism. It could be described as the experience between two right hemispheres as one brain needs to "download" intolerable affects into another brain so that an unbearable affective experience is avoided (L. Horowitz, 1983; Kernberg, 1980). Dissociation (another defense mechanism) may occur at the moment of the "download" so that the projected affects or other psychological material can be disavowed and actually assigned to the recipient of the projection(s) (Schore, 2003b). An early template for this dynamic may be the concept of the caregiver serving as an "auxillary cortex" for the child (Diamond, Krech, & Rosensweig, as cited in Schore, 2003b, p. 13) or Bion's (1962) concept of the "container" function as one person holds emotions for another.

10. Cognitive behavior therapies also address the effect of affect regulation. For a discussion of several studies supporting its efficacy in this area, see Farmer (2009, pp. 109–112).

Clinical Implications of Learned Management Preferences Via the Autonomic Nervous System

What are the clinical implications of the brain being trained to prefer one way of managing certain affects or even all affects? Affect tolerance issues—depression, anxiety, alexithymia (not being able to put into words one's inner experiences), or impulse control problems—can be one reason for seeking psychotherapy. To the degree that the client has environmentally induced preferences for emotional intensity that travel down one of the segments (i.e., either the excitatory sympathetic or the inhibitory parasympathetic segment of the autonomic nervous system), the other segment is likely compromised.

The clinical implication of this brain-based understanding is to utilize a therapeutic intervention that is intended to increase the tolerance of affects that are generally warded off. For example, in grief, if a person is so down-regulated that he or she is unable to engage in mourning, interventions that help this person experience and express grief may be indicated. The person may need to grieve in the presence of another who is able to allow feelings of arousal and empathically "be with" the client, right hemisphere to right hemisphere. Of course, cultural considerations and family ways of grieving may play a critical role in choosing an intervention that is also sensitive to existing neurobiology regarding affective expression of grief.

It is a critical clinical skill of the clinician to make him- or herself available to experience the same feelings (synchrony) as the client (right hemisphere to right hemisphere), at least temporarily. This synchrony is the experience of fine-tuning and resonating with the internal state of another person (Schore, 2003a, p. 38). Staying in emotional contact (synchrony) may avoid a potentially dysregulating state of asynchrony, which is a break or rupture in attunement (Schore, 2003b, pp. 38–41; see also Beebe, 2005). Fosha (2000) uses the phrase "goes beyond mirroring," which I take to mean that once there is synchrony, the clinician may be participating in new experiences with the client. Just the fact of another person resonating with the client's state may be quite new and, to take the experience to a new level, the client may have the sense that the clinician is helping with arousal management. Ultimately, the client may have the experience that formerly unbearable affects can be self-regulated. This self-regulation would occur as new neural structures were created by the client's brain, resulting from the synchrony and resonance. The clinical goal is to improve or augment the client's previous ways of regulating affect via psychological defensive maneuvers, which eventually may have become problematic.

At this point in the therapeutic encounter a new possibility is introduced: that is, of interactively regulating what the client has previously experienced as unbearable affects, however briefly, by providing contact with the brain and personality of an other (Bebee & Lachmann, 2002). The overarching goal of self-regulation (regulation of internal states) can be achieved via two modes: interactive regulation (of arousal, stress affect) with others in a connected context, and autoregulation, without others in autonomous contexts (Schore, March 21, 2011, personal communication). The end result is that the underutilized branch (whether sympathetic or parasympathetic) is strengthened and little used neurocircuitry is made more adequate. This connection of neural circuits via synapse formation may happen quickly, within 10–15 minutes of having an experience (Greenough, 2011). The strengthening via increased opportunities for positive development is possible via neural plasticity (Aoki & Stekevitz, 1988; Cicchetti, 2004; Greenough, 1986).

The interpersonal brain-to-brain contact may create dendrites and other related structures to connect and/or strengthen neural circuitry (Schore, 2003b, p. 220) so that, in this case, difficult affects can be increasingly tolerated. According to Schore (2003b, pp. 279–281), the long-term goal of psychotherapy is to reorganize insecure working models of affect management such that an "earned secure model" of affect management replaces the previous model (see Chapter 5 for descriptions of different neurobiology of attachment categories). In order for an improved model of attachment to be created, new neural circuitry can be created by the growth of new connections (via dendritic growth and synaptogenesis, in part).

The Case of Cori, Continued

The summer before Cori entered the sixth grade, her mother married a man who moved them all back to their former neighborhood in New Orleans. Cori and Jakki were surprised by this new union because they did not know that their mother was even interested in anyone; they thought she was still mourning their father. Their grandmother at first did not say anything, but in the sewing room, the girls could hear her crying, turning up the radio, and crying some more.

For the next few years the family was fairly comfortable. The mother did not talk about their father, Cecil, any more. The stepfather had adult children who lived nearby and were friendly, the family attended the Catholic Church from their childhood, and Cori and Jakki were award-winning students. Cori was a pom-pom girl as well as the class president; her grandmother made all the uniforms for the cheer squad, not to mention costumes for some of the school plays and a formal dress for a banquet where Cori and other students were honored. The girls spent the summers with Mimi on one of the bays on the Gulf of Mexico.

The family had to cope with a dramatic and traumatic change, with its potential for destabilizing the individual members and the family unit itself. The grandmother's reaction was an uncharacteristic withdrawal into her own sadness, and perhaps grief, over the girls moving away. The grandmother's response was unlike the coping strategy Cori remembered when her father's boat had disappeared; at that time feelings were shared openly within the family, church, and neighborhood. In this circumstance, however, the grandmother had sequestered herself, although Cori was aware of her grandmother's crying.

At this point in the history, helpful data have been gathered about at least two models of handling sadness and grief over loss: one within relationships and one alone. The grandmother's solitary crying and attempts to hide her feelings is not, in itself, necessarily problematic. Perhaps this behavior was part of autoregulation (autonomous) for Mimi. Although Mimi's avoidance of others may have been a departure from previous examples of her emotional coping responses, perhaps she feared hurting the children by her reactions. She may have been attempting, and failing, to utilize the defenses of sublimation, repression, and/or denial. Perhaps recognizing that her own efforts to down-regulate (parasympathetic branch) had failed her, she chose to remove herself from the girls' presence. She may have been utilizing the defense mechanism of altruism (a more homeostatically balanced defense, depending on the context).

We could speculate that Cori may have deeply identified with her grandmother, particularly around the loss of Cecil (attunement and bonding leading to attachment). Therefore, Cori's right hemisphere (seat of affect management strategies) would have been molded by the constant example of her grandmother's affect management strategies (experience-dependent). We might speculate that the subculture in which Cori was reared proscribed interactive regulation of emotion as a function of the situation. Perhaps communally addressing Cecil's loss was appropriate, but it may have been deemed selfish for the grandmother to impose her personal emotions on others in response to the girls' leaving. Only questioning closely over time can address these suppositions.

The resilience of the family seems clear from the level of functionality implicit in their lives. There is the example of the mother not mentioning Cecil in their new life back in New Orleans; it remains to be seen if this was adaptive or not. The grandmother remained an integral part of the family, as she still sewed festive garments for Cori and others, though located in another town. Cori and Jakki's returning to their grandmother's home for the summers seems like a stabilizing experience, reminiscent of earlier times that may have been critical to the girls' implicit learning of affect management strategies. In the summers, at least, there was the likelihood of soothing, comforting, containing, connected, and regulated affective experiences. The chances were good that the girls would have had many ways to "download" any intolerable affects into another more mature brain, given the way in which the grandmother's home and community functioned. It is likely that during the summers, the girls experienced emotional regulation within the multiple relational connections among family and friends.

When the hurricane (Katrina) was predicted to hit New Orleans Parish, Cori's mother and stepfather decided to pack up some food and a few clothes, pick up their grandmother, and go to Port Arthur, Texas, to stay with her stepfather's relatives. When they got to their grandmother's house there was flooding, and they could not decide whether to stay or get out. There was no way to know about the flooded roads on the way to Texas. Finally, they decided to leave. Those few hours of indecision were costly. The delay would put the family in the path of the second hurricane, Rita. Their grandmother had an argument with their stepfather over taking a little portable sewing machine, but he finally relented. Mary, the dog, was in the car, but as they slowly made their way toward Texas, Mary got away from the stepfather at a rest stop and disappeared. They had to leave the dog in the storm. When they got to the Texas Gulf Coast, Hurricane Rita hit and their stepfather was killed by a collapsing shed as he tried to help his relatives pen up some livestock. The family then went to Houston to federally funded disaster management apartments and after a few months, settled in Austin, Texas.

The examination of Cori's situation continues in Chapter 2, as a session with the school counselor is described.

Concluding Comments

The history of the stressors on Cori's family system has been the focus of this chapter, which is more intellectualized and academic an exercise (the left hemisphere) than in the subsequent chapters. The effort is to examine emotions in real time with a focus not so much on words as on the nonverbal emotional communication beneath the words (right hemisphere). Nonetheless, even from a systemic and global perspective, many worthwhile clinical speculations can be made that may contribute to understanding Cori's behavior and interactions with the clinician.

Again, I recommend that you refer to the schematic of the nervous system and the autonomic nervous system as well as the definitions of salient terms/concepts and use them as a reference and reminder of the possible neurobiological forces that may be influencing the interpersonal interactions in a therapeutic encounter. In addition, lists of the defense mechanisms (Tables 2.2, 2.3, and 2.4 in Chapter 2) are intended to link the concept of level of arousal with the function of the particular defense (e.g., decrease in arousal linked to avoidance or numbness; increase in arousal linked to excessive activation). Only time will tell if the speculations and their implications are correct.

CHAPTER 2

Defense Mechanisms and the Limbic System

FIGURE 2.0
The Limbic System

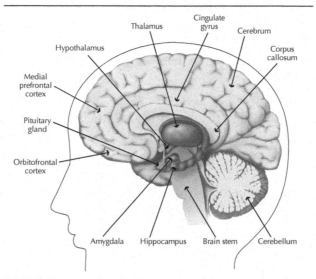

This chapter addresses the functions of the limbic system as they are related to the regulation of emotions, feelings, and affects. There are many regulatory systems in the body that manage the physiological functions such as heart rate, blood pressure, or respiration. However, this chapter has a narrower focus on the clinical significance of selected defense mechanisms that regulate emotional arousal via the autonomic nervous system.

Location in the Brain of the Limbic System and Selected Structures Involved in Processing Emotion and Memory

The *limbic system* is a theoretical concept about several structures in the brain that feature prominently in the processing of emotion and memory (Solms & Turnbull, 2002, p. 17). Because it is a theoretical concept rather than one discrete structure, various scientists consider different structures as composing the limbic system. Figure 2.1 provides an overview of the structures and their functions that are usually included in descriptions of the limbic system. For those readers whose interest is not keenly focused upon the technical details of the structures but rather the functions of the limbic system in relation to psychological defenses, a reading of the case in the second part of the chapter may be a more useful place to begin. After reading the case and the neurobiological explanations of interactions between clinician and therapist that are interspersed within the dialogue, the technical information at the beginning of this chapter may be more usable.

FIGURE 2.1
Anatomy of the Hippocampal Formation

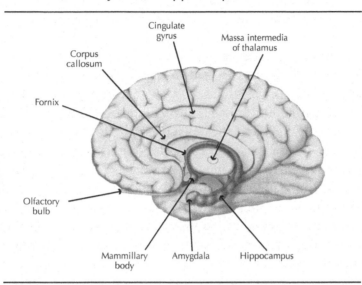

The limbic system, a group of interconnected structures located underneath the cerebral cortex, includes the amygdala (which processes fear, safety–danger, attachment, early memory, emotional experience, implicit memory) and the hippocampus (explicit memory working with cerebral cortex) (see Greatrex [2002] for the relationship between amygdalar functioning and traumatic memories, dissociation, and projective identification). The amygdala connects to the hypothalamus, which controls the autonomic nervous system and the endocrine system, both of which control internal and surface organs (e.g., the skin) and act in synergy (Furness, 2006, p. 24). In turn, the hypothalamus connects to septal areas (which play a key role in inhibiting aggression; Sapolsky, 2005, p. 145) and to the fornix (fiberous pathway under the corpus callosum linking to diencephalon, which includes the thalamus and hypothalamus; Carter, 2009, p. 53), then joins the hippocampus to the mamillary bodies (associated with episodic memory; Carter, 2009, p. 154; Solms & Turnbull, 2002, pp. 17–18). Ratey (2001) includes the medial thalamus as part of the limbic system. The thalamus is the major relay station for nerve signals coming from the senses (except for smell); the medial thalamus is situated approximately in the middle of the thalamus (Carter, 2009, p. 60). According to Green and Ostrander (2009, p. 46), the "thalamus has substantial interactions with all brain regions widely regarded as components of the limbic system." Schore also includes the orbitofrontal (ventromedial) cortex as well (personal communication, March 12, 2011). It should also be noted that the endocrine system (or neuroendocrine system) manufactures and secretes hormones into the bloodstream that help maintain an optimal internal environment; the levels of hormone within the bloodstream are regulated by feedback mechanisms that are located, in most cases, in the hypothalamus–pituitary unit. (For nonmedical mental health practitioners who want extensive but easy-to-read information on locations in the body and functions of various hormones, see Carter, 2009, p. 112; Farmer, 2009; Green & Ostrander, 2009; Johnson, 2003; Stauffer, 2010, p. 234.)

Though located in both the left and right hemispheres of the brain, the limbic system is neuroanatomically elaborated in the right hemisphere, which is dominant for the processing of affect (Schore, 2003b, p. xv) and other information in a holistic fashion (Nebes, as cited in Cozolino, 2002, p. 110). The right hemisphere processes physiological sensory information that can become experienced as emotions/feelings/affects (Schore, 2003b, p. 225). In contrast, the left hemisphere, which is dominant for language as well as analytical and linear thinking (Schore, 2003b, p. xv), is not as "densely connected" to the body as the right hemisphere (Cozolino, 2002, p. 110).

It is now well known clinically that stress may degrade normative coping abilities (Sapolsky, 1994), in part, by diminishing the brain's capacity to maintain homeostatic balance in the autonomic nervous system. Furthermore, memory systems just beneath consciousness, which resonate with current fearful experiences, may also account for diminished coping to stressors. LeDoux (1996, pp. 200–201) differentiates between *emotional memory* (processed in the amygdala) and the *memory of emotion* (processed in the hippocampus and related structures). Memories of emotions are more matter-of-fact and calmly recalled; emotional memories, in contrast, are experienced as "raw" and intense, perhaps as when the original affects were first experienced. Emotional memories are more likely to be relived (reenacted in flashback form, as if the past experience were occurring in the present), whereas memories of emotions are more likely to be verbalizable in summary form.

The explicit (hippocampus) and implicit (amygdala) memory systems, although similar to Freud's concept of the conscious (explicit) and unconscious (implicit), do not, according to Cozolino (2002, p. 87), overlap entirely. Implicit knowledge is associated with the right hemisphere. The early developing, implicit self represents the biological substrate of the human unconscious mind and is intimately involved in the processing of bodily based affective information associated with various motivational states. Dissociated affects are located in the right hemisphere outside of awareness (Schore, 1994, 2003a, 2003b); subcortical amygdalar-centered memories include attachment schema and transference. Implicit memory is context-free with no source attribution (Cozolino, 2006, p. 129). Explicit knowledge, in contrast, has a cortical and left-hemisphere bias; it is contextualized with a known memory source; memories include identity and social information, narratives, autobiographical descriptions, social rules, norms, and expectations (Cozolino, 2006, p. 129).

A related dual-system concept (i.e., the implicit–explicit memory systems) for the processing of experience is LeDoux's model of fast and slow fear circuitry (1996), paralleling Jacobs and Nadal's (1985) taxon (amygdala) and locale (hippocampus) systems. Processing experiences with more primitive systems (e.g., the amygdala) can indicate overwhelming stress and/or an impaired sophisticated regulatory process (Cozolino, 2002, p. 247).

What Are Emotions/Feelings/Affects? How Is the Appraisal of Emotion Related to Affect Management?

The research and literature on emotions/feelings/affects have a rich history both in the fields of biology and psychology. For simplicity's sake in this book, these terms are considered more or less interchangeable. (For a comprehensive discussion on the differences, see LeDoux, 1996; Rothschild, 2000, pp. 56–64; Sheafor & Horejsi, 2008, pp. 160–163, 393–394). Darwin (1872) speculated that there are basic emotions that have recognizable expressions irrespective of culture (joy, surprise, fear, sadness, anger, contempt, shame); and later Tomkins (1962, 1963, 1970) added another innate emotion, interest. Panksepp (2009, pp. 1–6) has identified (from animal models) circuitry within the brain of seven emotional dispositions of critical importance for generating primary-process affective states: seeking, fear, rage, lust, care, panic (separation distress), and play. Current literature in affective neuroscience typically refers to the expression of emotions/feelings/affects as *affect management*. Some affects are internally managed without an external manifestation whereas other affective experiences are quite obviously externally managed via certain behaviors (e.g., via many of the defense mechanisms discussed in this chapter).

How have emotions been described? Emotions are currently viewed as biological functions of the nervous system rather than merely psychological states that are independent of the underlying brain mechanisms (LeDoux, 1996, p. 12). More specifically, emotions are described as a way of communicating important internal states and needs (Ratey, 2001, p. 227) whose function is one of "action readiness" (Panksepp, 2000, p. 37). Solms and Turnbull (2002) described emotions as comprised by an "internally directed sensory modality that provides information about the current state of the bodily self" (p. 105) which makes people want to "do something" (p. 111). The changes in the body resulting from an internal or external signal or trigger lead to an emotion and some kind of emotional response (Badenoch, 2008, p. 30). Porges refers to this perception of the bodily self as *interoception* (2011, pp. 80–81).

According to Porges, "Homeostasis reflects the regulation of the physiological conditions within the body [and] response strategies reflect the stage when internal needs become less important than external needs" (2011, p. 80). The appraisal of the state of the body via interoception will likely result in an emotion that may—via transfer of affect (Schore, 2003b, p. 262) and at levels beneath awareness—be perceived in a number of ways, depending on the lens applied. The transfer of affect may occur via:

- Right-hemisphere to right-hemisphere nonverbal affective transactions (Schore, 1994, 2003b, pp. 279–281);
- Limbic-system to limbic-system resonance, which may be nonconscious-to-nonconscious attunement (Schore, 2003b, pp. 279–281);
- Intersubjectivity, whereby the intersubjective position of each person in a dyad must recognize the other as an equivalent center of expression (Benjamin, 1988, as cited in Mitchell & Aron, 1999, p. 184);
- "Mutual mapping" may "cocreate dyadic amplification of state," which may make possible the "transfer of affect" between two brains (particularly between limbic systems), potentially an adaptive or maladaptive phenomena (Tronick & Weinberg, 1997, p. 75, as cited in Schore, 2003b, p. 76);
- The relational approach (Jordan, 2000) with an emphasis on connection, disconnection, and reconnection of affective states between clinician and client;
- Transference–countertransference experiences (Racker, 1968), whereby the therapist initially, at least, unconsciously experiences certain emotional states similar to the client's states.

If the physiological appraisal system must focus too much on external demands, it is possible that extreme self-protective measures, such as maladaptive defense mechanisms, may be employed. Further, the internal homeostatic process, which is supported by adaptive defense mechanisms, may well be compromised.

If the arousal-regulating interaction between two brains is attuned to internal emotional states, affect synchrony is said to have occurred; conversely, if the opposite, asynchrony, occurs, misattunement follows, eliciting a stress response in the brain (Schore, 2003b, pp. 7–12). Generally, a sufficient number of synchronous interactions will lead to an affect management style characterized as secure attachment, whereas certain types of asynchronous interactions, if too frequent, may lead to various types of insecure attachment styles.

In ideal circumstances the regulation of affect is the achievement of optimal and tolerable levels of arousal. This achievement of optimal and the tolerable levels occurs via the maintenance of autonomic balance between sympathetic ergotropic (high) and parasympathetic trophotropic (low) states of arousal (Schore, 2003a, p. 26). As noted, the divisions of the autonomic nervous system work to maintain homeostasis/balance (Johnson, 2002, p. 242). For instance, should the expression of emotion prove to be too intense, and not tolerable, gaze aversion may occur to decrease the resonance between the two brains (Panksepp, 2009) and dysregulation may follow, that is, the autonomic balance is disrupted, somehow (see Cole, Michael, & O'Donnell Teti, 1994, regarding the development of emotion regulation and dysregulation). Figure 2.2 illustrates possible strategies to address homeostatic disruption, a process that Siegel (2007) describes as going beyond a person's brain's "window of tolerance." Disrupted homeostasis can be perceived, addressed, corrected, or made worse by the "transfer-of-affect" constructs described in the bulleted list in the preceding paragraph.

Which Functions of the Limbic System Are Related to Emotions/Feelings/Affect Regulation?

Though many refer to the limbic system as a major regulator of emotions, LeDoux argues against the limbic system's existence, describing emotional systems throughout the brain, rather than located exclusively in the "limbic system" (1996, pp. 98–102, 186, 200). Ratey (2001) also describes emotions as complexly distributed throughout the brain and not "conveniently isolated" in a specific area. Despite that point, however, Ratey (2001) and others use the concept of the limbic system, consisting of various structures, as a way to explain some of the functions of the brain regarding emotion and its expression or management. Finally, Porges stresses the adaptive function of the autonomic nervous system's limbic circuitry in managing emotional states (1997, p. 65). One helpful description of the functioning of the branches

---

FIGURE 2.2.
Types of Affect Regulation in Response to External or Internal Event

---

Event (either internal and/or external) leads to a physical/bodily reaction, leading to representation by brain of affect/emotion/feeling

Possible outcomes to events if reaction exceeds brain's "window of tolerance," all leading to some type of affect regulation:

Interactive regulation

"Borrowing" right-brain function(s) of other may lead to restoration of homeostatic states

OR

Autoregulation in autonomous contexts

Indicates history of appropriate interactive regulation that has developed into capacity for self-regulation without use of problematic defenses/behaviors

OR

Types of autoregulation that are problematic:

Behaviors of other causes pain (worst case: abuse) leading to SNS activation and then the PNS counterregulation (may overcompensate via toxic defenses, e.g., dissociation)

Right brain of other not available for interactive regulation (worst case: neglect) leading to PNS states of low arousal (including vegetative vagal; see Chapter 4) and problematic autoregulation

---

of the autonomic nervous system is as *coupled* or *uncoupled*. This means that the excitatory and inhibitory branches either work together (coupled) or one branch is dominant (uncoupled) in the management of the intensity of affects (Schore, 2003a, pp. 5–35).

This chapter focuses on selected primary limbic structures that register and manage emotion, particularly the intensity of the emotion. According to Cozolino, the orbital (behind the eyes) area of the prefrontal cortex is considered the apex of the limbic system (2002, pp. 180–181) because it (1) mediates data about the external and internal experiences; (2) has an inhibitory role in autonomic nervous system functioning, leading to affect regulation; and (3) plays a role in reading facial expressions. The limbic system is active in our experience of motivation, emotions, and mood (Buelow et al., 2000, p. 153), and it plays a role in aggression, memory, stress responsiveness, maternal behavior, some aspects of sexual behavior, some aspects of hunger and satiation, circadian rhythms, and certain types of learning (Sapolsky, 2005, pp. 36–37).

The ways in which these functions are manifested affect the manner of emotional expression (e.g., the degree of accuracy in reading facial expression regarding danger may lead to over- or underreaction). In the clinical treatment literature, historically, the regulator of emotions has been considered to be the defense mechanisms (Clark, 1991; Vaillant, 1992; Strean, as cited in Edward & Sanville, 1996, p. 10). Current understanding of the autonomic nervous system, with its dense interconnections to the limbic system, may give clinicians a more complex conception of the self-protective experience (i.e., defense mechanisms) the brain is attempting to implement. For example, in the history of Cori (Chapter 1), her family seemed to have been able to manage difficult emotional upheavals (i.e., the loss of Cori's father when Cori was in elementary school). Each family member seemed to function adequately, the family was integrated into the supportive aspects of the community, such as the church, and all members seemed to be productive and to take pleasure in one another's company.

From the discussion of the functioning of the autonomic nervous system in Chapter 1, it could be speculated that Cori's family created a milieu for the development of homeostatically balanced brains and internal bodily processes of its family members. As noted previously, *homeostatically balanced* means that the excitatory and inhibitory branches of the autonomic nervous system work in harmony. Neither the excitatory (sympathetic branch) nor the inhibitory (parasympathetic branch) should be exclusively designated for managing emotion (McCabe & Schneiderman, as cited in Schore, 2003a, p. 28; Izard et al., 1991; Cassidy, 1994; Lewis & Miller, 1990; Cicchetti & Toth, 1991; King, as cited in Schore 2003a, p. 29). A harmoniously balanced autonomic nervous system responds to a situation as a function of the intensity of affective expression that would be considered appropriately within normal limits. For example, with the trauma of multiple losses following Hurricanes Katrina and Rita, Cori's family members' affect management capacities were surely altered by the traumatic stressors. As the supportive structures of their former apparently normal lifestyle were stripped away abruptly, even the family support that the internal affect management systems had provided may have been severely compromised. Cori begins the session (this chapter) with recently noticed affect management strategies (which may have been her way to cope with the family upheavals) possibly resulting in poor school performance. How the autonomic nervous system functioning may delicately shift according to context (interaction with the clinician) is illustrated in the clinical session with Cori.

Defense Mechanisms

The next section provides a brief overview of defense mechanisms, including definitions by various theoreticians and researchers and the functions that followed from those slightly differing definitions. Additionally reviewed are seminal concepts related to defense mechanisms, including clinical opinions regarding the degree of conscious, unconscious, and nonconscious aspects associated with defensive operations, as well as ways to categorize them (e.g., hierarchically, along the line of degree of adaptation; degree of awareness of self-protective behaviors; or flexibility versus rigidity in use of a defense).

What Are Defense Mechanisms?

Defense mechanisms are modulators of emotional arousal. Today, the contributions of the study of the brain and its functions have led the mental health field to understand the ways in which affects are managed from an interpersonal neurobiological perspective. Learning about the structures of the brain that manage levels of arousal contributes to an additional way of understanding self-protective behaviors from the perspective of regulation (Schore, 1994, 2003a, pp. 71–86; Cozolino, 2002, pp. 48–51, 164, 307). Intense affects, which potentially can traumatically disorganize the self system, are seen as inviting kinds of defensive maneuvers which, if used repeatedly, can come to characterize the way in which emotions are managed (i.e., states become traits; Perry et al., 1995). McWilliams made the point that "virtually any psychological process can be used defensively," which fairly represents current thinking in that defenses exist in many forms (2004, pp. 117–119). Conventional labels and definitions of defense mechanisms can be utilized to make informed speculations about clinical interactions (see Tables 2.1, 2.2, and 2.3 on pp. 43–48).

Defense mechanisms manage difficult-to-bear affects. Rothschild (2000, p. 90) and Vaillant (1977) have a similar view, which is that defenses can be conceptualized as a previously adaptive maneuver that may become maladaptive. The *Diagnostic and Statistical Manual of Mental Disorders*—Fourth Edition–Text Revised (DSM IV-TR) defines a defense mechanism as an "automatic psychological process that protects the individual against anxiety and from awareness of internal or external stressors or dangers . . . and may be either maladaptive or adaptive, depending on their severity, their inflexibility, and the context in which they occur" (American Psychiatric Association, 2000, p. 821).

Nesse and Lloyd describe the function of defense mechanisms as helping to regulate internal states by reducing anxiety and shame while decreasing awareness of depressing and demoralizing realities (as cited in Cozolino, 2002,

p. 164). Schore defines defense mechanisms as forms of emotion-regulation strategies for avoiding, minimizing, or converting affects that are too difficult to tolerate (Schore, 2003a, p. 280; Schore, 2003b, pp. 85–91, 280–281).

How Conscious Are Defense Mechanisms?
Freud first introduced the concept of a defense mechanism, identifying it as repression whose "function [is] rejecting and keeping something out of consciousness" (1915/1959b, p. 86). By 1915, when his paper on the defense mechanism of repression was offered, Freud had already introduced the concept of the *unconscious* into an intellectual culture that valued the *conscious* mind. So it is today, as well, with the emphasis on cognition (conscious/left hemisphere) over affect (unconscious/right hemisphere) (Schore, 2003b, pp. xvi–xix; Cozolino, 2006, pp. 26, 341), with the conscious mind–brain having been the dominant focus since the 1960s.

Meichenbaum and Gilmore (1984), in trying to bridge the gap between the behaviorist (conscious/cognitive) and the psychodynamic (unconscious/affective), examined the interface between cognitive and affective functioning, using as an example the depressive process. Interestingly, neither the term *defense* nor *unconscious* was used, although the lack of awareness of the depressive process was described. This lack of awareness, which occurs by means of various defensive, self-protective maneuvers, is the unconscious experience as opposed to a conscious process that assumes awareness (Cozolino, 2006, p. 341). The self-protective measures are generally located in the lower right hemisphere and not conscious (Schore 2003a, p. 280; Schore, 2003b, pp. 280–281), with a few exceptions (i.e., some of the more "adaptive" defenses; Vaillant, 1977). In the psychodynamic literature, the unconscious is generally depicted as equivalent to affects and various issues with affect management that are out of conscious awareness (Arlow, 1977; Basch, 1975; Brenner, 1974; Green, 1977; Mahler, 1966; Novey, 1959; Rapaport, 1953; Ross, 1975; Schmale, 1964; Schur, 1965; Stolorow & Lachmann, 1975; Zetzel, 1949; Winnicott, 1963).

In the past decade, Schore (2003a, 2003b) has begun using the term *nonconscious*, referring back to Bowlby's mid-20th-century description of the internal working model of self and other as if this model were referring to nonconscious processes (Schore 2003b, p. xvi). Schore (2003b) describes the original use of the term *unconscious* to describe a seething emotional current filled with silenced memories. The recent use of *nonconscious* by Schore (2003b) describes active mental structures that are relational and may communicate with the nonconscious brain of another; there is no awareness or deliberate control posited with nonconscious processes.

As the autonomic nervous system is responsible for regulating levels of arousal and is not under conscious control (Schore, 2003a, 2003b), the defense mechanisms are thereby not conscious (for related information, see the research of Semrud-Clikeman, Fine, & Zhu, 2011, and Gainotti, 2012, regarding unconscious processing of emotion and social interaction). Again, Vaillant (1977) does suggest some more adaptive defenses that have a conscious component; see Table 2.1 for examples. The processes involved with perceiving and regulating bodily driven affective states occur at "the physiological bottom of the mind," a phrase that captures the out-of-consciousness aspect of physiological experiences (Jackson, as cited in Schore, 2003b, p. 230) that are registered in the brain as affects.

The regulation of bodily driven affective states is accomplished by the interconnection among the structures of the limbic system ("orbitofrontal–insula, medial frontal anterior cingulate, and amygdala systems"), which are also interconnected with brain stem monoaminergic and hypothalamic neuroendocrine nuclei (Schore, 2003b, p. 230). These structures in the brain register both external (exteroceptive) and internal (interoceptive) environment and all connect to the autonomic nervous system (Neafsey, 1990). (Note: For discussion of recent relevant research on how defense mechanisms coordinate and interconnect neuronally across several brain regions, see Northoff, 2010; and Northoff, Bermpohl, Schoeneich, & Boeker, 2007). Environmental experiences largely determine whether the autonomic nervous system preferentially engages the PNS (low arousal), the SNS (high arousal), or both PNS and SNS simultaneously, or achieves a balance between the two branches.

How Are Defenses Categorized?

Since first described by Freud in 1915/1959b, defense mechanisms have been organized into a variety of schemas. Anna Freud (1936) initiated the tradition of categorizing defenses hierarchically (Schamess, as cited in Berzoff, Flanagan, & Hertz, 1996, p. 85), departing from her father's conceptualization of repression as the primary defensive function. Concurrent in time with Anna Freud was Heinz Hartmann (1958) who contributed the idea that the individual adapts to the environment, either by changing the external environment (alloplastic) or by changing his or her inner landscape (autoplastic). The autoplastic adaptations are surely, in part, defensive operations utilized to cope with less than "average expectable environments" (Schamess, as cited in Berzoff et al., 1996, pp. 95–97, referring to Hartmann's [1939] oft-repeated phrase).

Like others, Vaillant (1977) and McWilliams (2004) described the defensive operations in a hierarchical fashion. Vaillant used a schematic table to identify four "levels" of adaptive mechanisms that are pathological, immature, neurotic, or mature (1977, p. 80). McWilliams (2004) also selected several "higher-order defensive processes" and several presumably lower-order ones, termed "character defenses." In an earlier discussion, McWilliams described defensive reactions as being employed as a function of either the situation or personal inclination (1999, pp. 90–92). This means that any defense might be used situationally (i.e., contextually) as appropriate, but for some, there is a characteristic (personal inclination) use of particular defenses. Elsewhere, McWilliams used the term automatic in relation to the preferential, reflexive use of defenses, which seems synonymous with "personal inclination" (1994, pp. 95–100).

The DSM-IV-TR (American Psychiatric Association, 2000, pp. 808–809) also hierarchically ranks defensive levels as a function of degree of adaptation and degree of awareness of difficult experiences (high adaptive level, mental inhibitions, minor image-distorting level, disavowal level, major image-distorting level, action level, and level of defensive dysregulation). Social work educators Sheafor and Horejsi simply define and list common defense mechanisms, with the caveat most contributors make, which is that clinicians must take care to explore the underlying forces that invite the employment of emotionally self-protective behaviors (2008, pp. 163–166, 261–262).

Conte and Plutchik's 1995 collection of papers by major contributors in the theory and measurement of ego defenses addresses important issues such as whether defenses are "adaptive or maladaptive, flexible or rigid, problem-solving oriented, or forms of self deception" (p. ix). Additionally, they note the disagreement in the mental health field regarding whether some or all defenses should be considered pathological, how defenses should be defined and labeled, whether a hierarchical range regarding levels of maturity should be determined, and finally, just how many exist (Conte & Plutchick, 1995, p. ix). For example, Semrud-Clikeman et al. (2011) sort defense mechanisms as "cognitively oriented" versus "emotionally driven" (p. 142), and Northoff (2010) discusses a "region-based versus mechanism-based approach" to the locations of defensive functioning in the brain. As this chapter examines the ways in which the limbic system is related to defense mechanisms, it emphasizes arousal considerations when attempting to understand the choice of certain defensive operations (Schore, 2003b, pp. 58–107; Cozolino, 2002).

The Role of the Autonomic Nervous System in Defense Mechanisms

The quality of the reciprocal regulation of affect between child and caregiver is critical in developing internal defenses that manage the level of arousal tolerated ("window of tolerance," Siegel, 2007) in the child's brain and later in life, as well (Schore, 2003b, p. 165). Reciprocal regulation is accomplished, in part, by mirror neurons that provide direct internal experience and therefore understanding of another person's acts and intentions, thereby creating a bridge, in effect, between two brains (Siegel, 2007). This bridging between two brains occurs rapidly: Neurons processing fear may take 120–160 milliseconds (ms) (Kawasaki et al., 2001); the amygdala takes 14 ms to react to visual information (Keysers, Xiao, Földiák, & Perret, 2001); and bringing sensations to conscious awareness can take from 400 to 500 ms (Keysers et al., 2001). Perceiving others' affective states rapidly facilitates the "meeting and matching" of emotional states (Bebee & Lachmann, 1988).

Kohut's concept of the *selfobject* (1971) and Bowlby's concept of the *internal working model* (1988) capture the resulting internalized experience of the brain (particularly the right hemisphere; Schore, 2003b, p. xv), which, in part, determines the way affect is managed. Likewise, the concepts of internalized representations of self and other (Kernberg, 1980), RIGs (Stern, 1985), and secure attachment (Bowlby, 1988) all essentially describe affect management strategies.

Certain early experiences are more likely to lead to the development of active/energizing, up-arousing, excitatory defenses (sympathetic branch)—for example, a chronically overstimulating environment, including one involving abuse. Conversely, some experiences are more likely to lead to passive and inhibitory reactions that lower arousal (parasympathetic)—for example, an understimulating, even neglectful, environment. The third case is the situation where the environment is chaotically unpredictable (e.g., abuse *and* neglect), where no habitual strategy for affect management is possible to acquire, and hence the behavioral response is erratic and unpredictable, as well.

Too frequent mismatches in reciprocal regulation (from caregiver toward the infant/child) of affect may lead to dysregulation and ultimately to the subsequent acquisition of problematic defenses. In contrast, "frequent enough" synchronous experiences leading to attunement set the stage for the development of homeostatic (balanced) defenses (i.e., a flexible employment of defensive maneuvers, according to context). Always the reminder, the context in which a defense is utilized determines whether or not the defense is problematic (Vaillant, 1977; McWilliams, 1999).

What is the significance to psychological treatment of learning about the arousal systems in the body? A clinical focus on arousal management will reveal patterned ways the brain typically manages, for example, certain emotions, emotional intensity, and/or valence of emotions. Assessing these patterns leads to clinical speculations about past environmental influences in affect management, childhood and adult attachment styles, and experience-dependent psychiatric diagnoses, and will inform the theoretical treatment orientation to best clinically address the problematic arousal management pattern. A focus on typical ways that each client manages emotions will generally uncover defense mechanisms that have been used to protect the client emotionally. Applying biological information about the autonomic nervous system's arousal function to definitions of defense mechanisms from various sources leads to a systematic sorting out of defenses that seem primarily to manage excitatory or inhibitory affects or emotions. Additionally, there are defenses that do not have an extreme quality to them. There are also people who do not manifest a predictable use of defenses whose behavior is erratic and chaotic.

To review in some detail, defenses can broadly be divided into four types of arousal strategies:

1. Homeostatically balanced defenses, using the parasympathetic or sympathetic branches as appropriate for the situation.
2. The parasympathetically driven defenses that attempt to decrease the level of stimulation because the brain cannot easily manage the higher levels of stimulation.
3. The sympathetically driven defenses that attempt to increase the level of stimulation, as the brain cannot easily manage the lower levels of simulation.
4. Disorganized defenses and behaviors that seem to be without a predictable strategy; meaning, either parasympathetic or sympathetic branch is engaged in a way not generally appropriate for a situation (Schore, 2003a, 192–196).

A most important point, also made in Chapter 1, is that when defenses are utilized in an automatic and characteristic manner, one consequence may be to compensate for the more vulnerable branch of the autonomic nervous system. What this means in practical terms is the underutilized branch may be avoided in a predictable fashion. The defensive maneuvers that are utilized automatically are not conscious. For example, a personality prone to acting out and regression (i.e., the more aroused, sympathetically driven behaviors) may avoid affects that are sad, despairing, depressed, and generally in a lower range of arousal. Over time, the brain may become trained to respond to most situations with an automatic reaction of higher levels of arousal. This would certainly be inappropriate if a situation would normally call for a lower level of affective expression. This pattern may follow the Hebbian principle that "neurons that fire together wire together" (Hebb, 1949). With multiple repetitions, neural circuitry may become dedicated to activation of either high or low levels of arousal; the opposite arousal branch may, thereby, become less likely to be activated.

I speculate that many defenses are nonconscious in operation. Nonconscious implies that the active relational mental structures located in the right hemisphere may communicate with the nonconscious brain of another (Schore, 2003b, pp. xiv–xix). This process may underlie defenses that are interpersonal, such as passive–aggressiveness, hypochondriasis, or projective identification.

As can be seen in Tables 2.1, 2.2, and 2.3, a conventional description of defense mechanisms proceeds fairly logically by whether there is an increase or decrease of stimulation provided by the defense or a balance between the two. The list of defense mechanisms is not exhaustive, but it is intended to be fairly representative. Also, the effort to identify defenses by level of affect managed has been attempted retrospectively. Consequently, there is room for disagreement both from current practitioners and from the clinicians who coined the terms initially. There is very little systematic discussion of the arousal management provided by defenses by most clinical literature that discusses defensive maneuvers.

To summarize, the best possible developmental scenario is that the child experiences sufficient, appropriate interactive/dyadic affective regulation with a reliable other over time such that an effective management strategy is imprinted in the neural circuitry, allowing the child, and later the adult, to cope autonomously, by relying on internal resources, when a reliable other is not available in a moment of need for emotional regulation. The effective management of affects is the hallmark of a homeostatically balanced autonomic nervous system. The environment may present problems to a person, but the self-protective strategy/defense, ideally, would not itself create problems. Only when inflexible, rigid, and automatic maneuvers are employed would the defenses be considered "maladaptive" (Vaillant, 1977) or to be "character defenses" (McWilliams, 1994).

Should maladaptive defenses be routinely, predictably, and preferentially used in order to regulate arousal (as in preferentially using the same arousal strategy, unconsciously), there is often considerable cost to personality development and to the person's ability to adapt to life in general (Vaillant, 1977). There are situations where both branches of the autonomic nervous system (Schore, 2003a, pp. 160–167) are active at the same time, and other situations where a parasympathetically dominated behavior may involve both branches of the vagal system (Schore, 2003a, p. 167; Porges, 2011).

The material in Tables 2.1, 2.2, and 2.3 is intended to link the concept of level of arousal with the function of the particular defense. For example:

- Table 2.1: arousal level appropriate to the situation (homeostatic)
- Table 2.2: a decrease in arousal creating avoidance or numbness
- Table 2.3: an increase in arousal expressing active or excessive behaviors or internal reactions.

In Tables 2.2 and 2.3 the words or phrases that describe the level of arousal are underlined.

An asterisk indicates a defense mechanism that is interpersonal and nonconscious in nature, as opposed to most defense mechanisms, which are intrapsychic (within the personality of the individual) in nature. Of course, the intrapsychic defenses can have interpersonal aspects, in that others may notice or be affected by their manifestation. However, the interpersonal interaction is not the original aim.

TABLE 2.1.
Homeostatically Balanced Defenses

Description:
Defenses that may be managed by either sympathetic (excitatory) or parasympathetic (inhibitory) branches, depending on the context, and for which the level of arousal is appropriate to the situation.

Affiliation*
dealing with emotional conflict or stressors by turning to others for help or support (American Psychiatric Association, 2000, p. 811)

Altruism*
vicarious but constructive service to others

Anticipation
realistic planning

Humor
expression of affects without personal discomfort or poor effect upon others, in contrast to wit, which is more aggressive

Self-assertion
expressing feelings and thoughts directly in way that is not coercive or manipulative (American Psychiatric Association, 2000, p. 813)

Internalization
a shift in functioning promoting flexibility in handling internal and interpersonal states (Rutan, Stone, & Shay, 2007, pp. 84–85)

continued on following page

TABLE 2.1. continued
Self-observation
reflecting on own thoughts, feelings, motivation, and behavior and responding appropriately (American Psychiatric Association, 2000, p. 813)

Sublimation
channeling potentially maladapative feelings or impulses into socially acceptable behavior, rather than damming up or diverting them, leading to modestly satisfying results (American Psychiatric Association, 2000, p. 813)

Suppression
decision to postpone focus on conflict or situation; intentionally avoiding thinking about disturbing problems, wishes, feeling, or experiences (American Psychiatric Association, 2000, p. 813).

Note. From Vaillant (1977, pp. 383–386) unless otherwise noted.
*A defense mechanism that is interpersonal and generally nonconscious in nature.

TABLE 2.2.
Defenses That May Be Managed by Parasympathetic Nervous System

Description:
Defenses that attempt to <u>decrease</u> the levels of stimulation/arousal and thereby are likely affected by the parasympathetic branch of the autonomic nervous system.

Asceticism
gratification derived from <u>renunciation</u> of pleasure

Autistic fantasy
daydreaming as <u>substitute for relationships, action, or problem-solving</u> (American Psychiatric Association, 2000, p. 811)

Blocking
<u>inhibition</u> of thoughts and impulses

Controlling
managing external events as <u>substitute for</u> (<u>avoidance of</u>) emotionally managing internal experience

Denial
<u>minimizing</u> experience by lack of awareness

continued on following page

TABLE 2.2. continued

Displacement

solving conflict by assigning impulse to different person/situation than original one (<u>avoiding</u>)

Dissociation

drastic modification of personal identity to <u>avoid</u> emotional distress; dissociation involves a <u>numbing</u> of responsivity (Schore, 2003a, pp. 217–219); dealing with emotional conflict or internal or external stressors via a breakdown in consciousness, memory, perception of self or environment, and/or sensory–motor behavior (American Psychiatric Association, 2000, p. 811)

Inhibition

renouncing certain functions to avoid anxiety from various sources of conflict

Intellectualization

<u>thinking about rather than feeling affect</u> to defend against anxiety from unacceptable impulses; excessive use of abstract thinking, making generalizations to <u>control or minimize</u> disturbing feelings (American Psychiatric Association, 2000, p. 812)

Introjection

<u>diminishes</u> anxiety over ambivalence regarding separation from loved one or anxiety over feared other; isolation of affect or splitting affect from content, resulting in un<u>awareness</u> of either idea or affect

Obsessiveness

<u>avoiding</u> anxiety by neutralizing or <u>minimizing</u> affects without distorting external reality (Conte & Plutchik, 1995, p. 286); attempting to <u>ignore</u> or <u>suppress</u> thoughts, impulses, or images or to neutralize them with some other thought or action (Rosen, as cited in Kaslow, 1996, p. 244)

Passive–aggression*

a <u>passive</u> set of behaviors; indirectly and unassertively expressing aggression toward others (American Psychiatric Association, 2000, p. 812)

Repression

moving from conscious awareness of an idea or affect to <u>avoid</u> anxiety

Schizoid fantasy

fantasy and <u>autistic retreat</u> to resolve conflict

Note. From Vaillant (1977, pp. 383–386) unless otherwise noted. Underlines signify words or phrases that indicate arousal levels.

*A defense mechanism that is interpersonal and generally nonconscious in nature.

TABLE 2.3.
Defenses That May Be Managed by Sympathetic Nervous System

Description:

Defenses that actively <u>increase the levels</u> of stimulation/arousal and thereby are likely affected by the sympathetic segment of the autonomic nervous system.

Acting out/regression

<u>direct expression of impulses</u> that reflect unawareness of wishes or affect that accompany them; regression—breakdown of functioning, <u>moving</u> back to earlier developmental stage (Kernberg, 1979)

Delusions & hallucinations

positive symptoms (<u>active</u>) psychotic conditions (American Psychiatric Association, 2000, pp. 821, 823)

Derealization

an <u>alteration</u> in the perception or experience of the external world so that it seems strange or unreal (American Psychiatric Association, 2000, p. 822)

Devaluation

<u>inflated</u> sense of self maintained by degrading representations of others (Kernberg, 1976, p. 17)

Distortion

<u>employing</u> sustained feelings of delusional superiority or entitlement

Externalization

<u>actively</u> experiencing parts of one's own personality in the external world

Help-rejecting complaining*

<u>repetitiously requesting</u> help in a way that disguises covert feelings of hostility or reproach, which are then expressed by rejecting the help offered (American Psychiatric Association, 2000, p. 811)

Hypochrondriasis*

transformation of reproach toward others into self-reproach, with effort to draw attention to physical complaints

Identification

<u>assuming</u> the actions of another (Loewald, 1973); incorporation and introjection are considered primitive forms of identification, similar to imitation (Blanck & Blanck, 1986, pp. 22–23)

Identification with the aggressor

<u>identifies</u> not with the person of the aggressor, but with the aggression (A. Freud, 1939, p. 112)

continued on following page

TABLE 2.3. continued
Idealization
attributing exaggerated positive qualities to others (American Psychiatric Association, 2000, p. 812)

Mania
flight from internal reality to external reality; denial of depression (Winnicott, 1963, p. 132)

Omnipotence
feeling or acting as if one possesses special powers or abilities and is superior to others (American Psychiatric Association, 2000, p. 812)

Projective identification
an interpersonal set of behaviors in which conflict or ambivalence is managed by experiencing the most unacceptable side as being a quality of an other; pressure is exerted on the other to identify with the assigned quality so that the person with the conflict can remain unconscious regarding the quality as being about him or her as well (Schore, 2003a, 2003b)

Projection*
attributing qualities of the self to another (American Psychiatric Association, 2000, p. 812); can become quite active and result in, for example, quite prejudiced behaviors, rejection of closeness through suspiciousness, hypervigilance to danger, and injustice-collecting

Psychotic denial
refusing to acknowledge and negating what is seen, heard

Rationalization
expressing the opposite of the impulse

Reaction formation
substituting behavior, thoughts, feelings that are opposite to own unacceptable thoughts and feelings) (American Psychiatric Association, 2000, p. 812)

Repression
removes disturbing wishes, thoughts, or experiences from conscious awareness; however, the feeling may remain conscious (American Psychiatric Association, 2000, p. 813)

Sexualization
assigning an object or function with sexual significance to not feel anxiety over prohibited impulses

continued on following page

TABLE 2.3. continued
Splitting

mixed feelings <u>cannot be experienced simultaneously</u> (American Psychiatric Association, 2000, p. 813); cannot synthesize good and bad introjects; no unified sense of self (Freed, 1980, p. 550)

Somatic reactions

bodily reactions to experiences that become imprinted in neural circuitry (implicit memory system) (Rothschild, 2000, pp. 7, 43, 82)

Undoing

<u>making amends</u> symbolically for unacceptable thoughts, feelings, or actions (American Psychiatric Association, 2000, p. 813)

Note. From Vaillant (1977, pp. 383–386) unless otherwise noted. Underlines signify words or phrases that indicate arousal levels.

*A defense mechanism that is interpersonal and generally nonconscious in nature.

Case of Cori, Continued

This section focuses on the (1) information necessary to define and identify defense mechanisms; (2) ways to practice differentiating the level (high or low?) of emotional arousal each defense is attempting to manage; and (3) suggestions regarding the role of the clinician in improving clients' defensive functioning. Additionally, neurobiological phenomena may be mentioned as they are manifest in the clinical exchange.

For this case, referring to the following would be useful:

- The schematic of the nervous system with the enlarged section of the limbic system (Figures 1.0 and 2.0)
- Tables of the defenses divided into their respective up- or down-regulation of affective intensity (Tables 2.1, 2.2, and 2.3)
- Schematic of stress circuitry (Rothschild, 2000, pp. 10–11; see Figure 4.0)
- Figure with gross anatomical brain structures and their functions (see p. 65)
- Case history of Cori, presented in Chapter 1.

Case Material

Note: In the following commentary on the clinician–client interactions, neurological considerations are <u>underlined</u>.

When the clinician first met with Cori, the meeting was tense. The minute Cori walked into the room, the clinician was uncomfortable, guarded, and uncharacteristically, found that she could not easily relate to Cori. Cori was unsure about what exactly she was doing talking to a counselor.

Perhaps Cori's affect was communicated immediately to the clinician. The appraisal of others' affects takes under 300 milliseconds to register on the face of the perceiver (Kawasaki et al., 2001; Keysers et al., 2001). Cori may have then registered the clinician's affect in her own right hemisphere and then upon her own face. Both client and clinician may have been registering distress and discomfort in around 1 second of elapsed time (Schore, 2003b, p. 224).

CORI: I don't know why I was sent here (*slightly belligerent, challenging*).

This interaction seems sympathetically driven, in that there is an up-regulated, agitated level of arousal, perhaps verbal acting out or regression. There was an assumption that Cori's grades, having "dropped off," indicated a previously adequate, or at least better, level of school performance than the current academic work.

THERAPIST: (*trying for calm, matter-of-fact demeanor*) Well, your teachers are concerned about your sudden drop in grades, and that sometimes means that a student might be worried about something.

The clinician was trying for calm, matter-of-fact demeanor, perhaps attempting to deliberately choose behaviors whose effect may have been to lower the level of arousal. This may have initiated the parasympathetic branch to counterregulate the uncomfortable level of arousal (sympathetically driven) that peaked upon greeting Cori. Simultaneously, her words had a slightly upbeat, concerned, reaching-out-to-Cori tone, which was somewhat up-regulated (sympathetically driven).

CORI: People in my family don't worry too much about things these days.

Cori was mentioning one of the possible affect management strategies (i.e., ". . . don't worry too much") that people in her immediate family currently utilized to down-regulate: defenses that minimize, such as denial, suppression, repression, blocking of affect, and isolation of affect.

THERAPIST: Did they worry about things in the past, but don't right now?

Clinician was trying for attunement and affect synchrony (right-brain to right-brain and, more specifically, limbic system to limbic system resonance, which may be nonconscious-to-nonconscious attunement (Schore, 2003b, pp. 279–281), as she attempted to stay with the topic and yet gain a sense of past functioning.

CORI: Naw, not really. We're strong. Like, do you know where I got my name? (*Turns slightly in chair, sideways to clinician; has a matter-of-fact, declarative tone with first comment and slightly aroused tone of voice with the change of subject.*)

Cori may have tried to avoid affect of some kind, by turning her body away and with her dismissive tone of voice. She may have been attempting to stay down-regulated (parasympathetic branch) perhaps in order to avoid becoming overstimulated. The excited and upset state may be one that she has had to manage alone since the hurricanes, without interactive/dyadic regulation by a significant relative as in her past (see history in Chapter 1). Cori may try to avoid those excited states and seek states for which she has enough affective regulation capacity to manage—that is, the more down-regulated (parasympathetic) emotional states that may underlie the dismissive, avoiding behaviors. These states may be achieved by such defenses as blocking, inhibition, intellectualization, isolation of affect, and/or passive-aggressiveness.

THERAPIST: Where?

CORI: Coretta Scott King. (*Lifts her chin with a little jerk. Slightly proud, though, again, matter-of-fact, as she gives the origin of her name.*)

Clinician was trying to follow the abrupt change in subject, to the origin of Cori's name. Cori may have been employing the defense of controlling. Clinician felt a sense of disquiet, uncertainty, and confusion, as her last effort was to try to clarify the affect management styles of Cori's family in the past. Not only did she not get an answer, but also Cori seemed to completely change the focus. This may have led the clinician to experience a disconnection due to the abrupt transition the change of subject created.

Throughout the session so far, the clinician may have been trying to use both right and left hemispheres to track the content and emotional material from Cori. Cori may be resisting an affective connection to the clinician as that may traumatize her (Kohut, 1971; Jordan, 2000) if the clinician were to prove unreliable or disappointing, similar to ways in which Cori may have been treated in the recent past. Another speculation is that Cori may have had to experience intense emotions that may have affectively connected her to the clinician. The sympathetic branch may have been arousing Cori's affect, tone of voice, and body. Cori's effort to stay out of relationship/out of connection (Kohut, 1971; Jordan, 2000) may be failing. Cori may, against her better judgment, have been warming to the clinician (who was earnestly attempting to connect and enter into a state of attunement with which Cori has had much family experience prior to fleeing New Orleans).

THERAPIST: Oh, really? (*Does not know what to do at that moment and feels slightly anxious.*)

Anxiety, a state of higher arousal, is managed by the sympathetic branch of the autonomic nervous system.

CORI: (*Goes on hurriedly, not really noticing clinician*) Yeah, and my sister Jakki, that's with two k's. You know, she is named after President Kennedy's wife, J-a-k-q-u-a-l-i-n-e (*spelling it out*).

Cori was becoming more emotionally aroused (sympathetic branch) and less inhibited (parasympathetic branch); she may have been engaging in verbal acting out or even the manic defense.

THERAPIST: Oh, that's a pretty name (*again, does not feel connected*)

Clinician's left hemisphere may have been working hard to "make sense" of Cori's affect, verbal output, and body language. The bland reply could have been an effort to be as neutral as possible and approximate, at least verbally, a balanced autonomic nervous system—that is, display affect appropriate for the moment.

CORI: Yeah, and you know what else? My grandmother's dog was named Mary, after the mother of Jesus. (*Gazes away for a few seconds after her words came out in a rush.*)

Gaze aversion may have been an automatic response to a spike in sympathetically driven arousal (Schore, 2003b, p. 263). Averting the gaze can help calm; perhaps the looking away for a few seconds may have indicated blocking, isolation of affect, or even a brief moment of dissociation (inhibitory parasympathetic branch).

THERAPIST: (*Quiet, but has urge to ask what kind of dog was Mary.*)

Maybe, at last, some topic had presented itself about which Cori is willing to be somewhat emotional and connected— that is, the family dog, Mary. The clinician's left hemisphere may have analyzed her own previous reactions, which included blurting out whatever came to her mind, and decided to stop talking. The clinician may have had the help of her own autonomic nervous system, which was more easily balancing high and low arousal in order to be more in-between and modulated. This may have allowed her to simply be silent, and quell the urge to talk by utilizing suppression.

CORI: (*Looks at the file cabinet where some student's drawings of a dog and cat are taped on the side.*) You know, I can't remember what Mary even looked like. (*Looks slightly down and her voice is soft and a bit puzzled; seems calmer.*)

The parasympathetic would be responsible for lower affective expression; this may begin a different experience, in that the clinician's contained affect may have a calming effect on Cori. Perhaps Cori's right brain was imitating or resonating with the clinician's affective state (Panksepp, 1999).

THERAPIST: (*Still quiet, and feels better about being quiet.*)

The clinician makes a decision to continue being a <u>felt presence</u> (<u>right hemisphere</u>), and not interrupt whatever is occurring within Cori or silently between them. Both may be more homeostatically balanced at this point.

CORI: I wonder if she is still alive, maybe, you know—somebody found her when, well, after . . . (*looks suddenly withdrawn and her eyes close, as if she is sleeping*).

At this point, the agitation, driven by the <u>sympathetic branch</u>, might have been counter-regulated, such that her level of arousal may have been lowered by the <u>parasympathetic branch</u>; maybe a dissociative moment? Or at least blocking of the <u>up-regulated affective moment</u>, as Cori may be having some momentary hope that Mary, the dog, was found after all and is not dead.

THERAPIST: (*Begins to imagine Mary, the dog, lost in the storm; associates to her own dog's big eyes looking at her beseechingly, and feels a catch in her throat; thinks she should do something, does not know what to do; says nothing.*)

CORI: (*Turns her face back to therapist and says quietly, without making eye contact*) I'm sorry. Have I upset you?

Cori may have become emotionally related to the clinician for first time; <u>affect synchrony</u> may have occurred wherein the internal experiences of each is becoming similar (nonconsciously), allowing for stress recovery. <u>The clinician deliberately tried to stop left-hemisphere-driven actions</u> (e.g., verbalization, analyzing, making interpretations), which may have allowed her to use her own experiences to <u>attempt to emotionally resonate</u> (<u>primarily a right-hemisphere experience</u>) with what Cori's experience may have been and with what she was currently experiencing over the loss of the family dog, Mary. Cori, apparently <u>without actually looking</u> at the clinician, <u>seemed able to perceive</u> her clinician's upset (in which the clinician was experiencing a moment of empathy). This may indicate <u>a right-brain to right-brain nonconscious</u> connection between them in which the empathy of the clinician was matched and returned with empathy by Cori. "Have I upset you?" may indicate the use of self-observation, even affiliation, <u>as both defenses may indicate homeostatic balanced via the autonomic nervous system</u>.

THERAPIST: Well, I am upset, thinking about your dog lost like that. I have a dog, and I started to think about him. (*Stops talking and she and Cori look at each other for a few seconds. The clinician has an experience as if a slight "electric current" has passed between them, which had not happened before this interaction.*)

The clinician modeled being vulnerable. Perhaps the two resonated emotionally with one another, <u>right brain to right brain</u> (Schore, 2003b, pp. 147, 263;

Schore, 1977c). It might be speculated that a partial explanation for the "electric current" may be mirror neurons providing direct internal experience and therefore understanding of another person's acts and intentions, thereby, making a bridge between two brains (Siegel, 2007; Gallese, 2010; Fuchs et al., 2010). Experiencing the upset over the lost dog with the clinician may have led to the dyadic/interactive regulation of Cori's upsetting affects.

This exchange may have been a more familiar affective situation for Cori because she was accustomed to this type of affect regulation from her family in the recent past; perhaps she will drop the recently acquired problematic way of regulating her affects. This recent effort to down-regulate by herself (the inhibiting action by the parasympathetic branch of autonomic nervous system) may have been partially responsible for her poor academic work. Defenses that shut down affect (e.g., blocking of affect) may have dulled her brain's ability to focus and concentrate on academic work.

This material about the lost dog brings Cori close to issues of attachment, loss, and affect management that were prominent in her early losses (e.g., her father). The clinical dyad now moves more deeply into affects of separation/loss in the following exchanges.

CORI: (*Looking slightly away*) You know, Mimi cries about Mary a lot. My mother gets mad at her, though, and . . . (*trails off and looks away*).

Cori may have tried to decrease the intensity of the emotion between her and clinician; Cori may have been trying to not experience highly arousing emotions for some time, and her brain may have tried to protect itself by looking away (gaze aversion; Schore, 2003b, p. 7; Stern, 1985), thereby shutting off or decreasing the sympathetic activation, perhaps via isolation of affect, blocking of affect, or dissociation. If this effort were a more contained one to decrease the level of affect with some conscious effort, perhaps Cori was beginning to employ the defense of suppression.

THERAPIST: (*Has urge to ask if Mimi is Cori's grandmother when therapist knows quite well that Mimi is the grandmother; has urge to ask how long the family had the dog. What kind of dog was Mary? Starts to tell herself to stay with Cori in the moment, though emotional flight seems like a good idea. She sees Cori looking at her again, somewhat expectantly.*) Do *you* miss Mary a lot?

The clinician struggled to avoid employing a defensive maneuver of her own to manage her increasingly intense affect (maybe beyond the "window of tolerance"; Siegel, 2007). She fought the urge to ask distracting questions (left-hemisphere request for facts) and finally, perhaps because of the expectant look (mutual gaze invites affectively laden right-brain to right-brain resonance; Schore, 2003b, pp. 7–12), the clinician managed herself well enough to ask about Cori's missing the dog, Mary. Cori was indirectly approaching the topic missing the dog, via addressing the grandmother's feelings about Mary, instead of her own feelings about Mary; the clinician may have been trying to use the defense of suppression and/or self-observation.

CORI: (*Looks away and starts refastening some clips in her hair, then takes out and reinserts her earrings, then says matter-of-factly:*) Mary lived a good life and was really old. She had arthritis in her back legs. Probably what happened to her out there in the pasture, when Barney (stepfather) let her out to pee (*starts to chatter, not so matter-or-fact*) . . . she . . . well . . . maybeeee . . . well . . . whatever. (*Stands up, sits down again abruptly, reworks her barrette in her hair.*) Jakki and I played with Mary a lot when we were little. Before the, well, you know, the storm, not so much. We moved away, you see.

> Cori's matter-of-fact presentation (the inhibiting parasympathetic branch quickly gave way to more excited chatter (sympathetic branch). The autonomic nervous system branches may be oscillating as it up- and down-regulates, or maybe approaching simultaneous activation of both branches (e.g., stands up/ sits down, fiddles with barrettes, puts earrings in/out of ears; Schore, 2003a, p. 189).
>
> This dysregulation may have been precipitated by the clinician's offer of empathy and the emotional intimacy that may suggest, which may have been stressful for Cori, if it undermined her recently acquired distancing behaviors. Currently, Cori has many experiences within her family of members disconnecting and detaching when experiencing high affect. Cori may have been trying to manage anxiety by physical movement (slight acting out/regression), replacing the more studied, matter-of-fact manner, which may have been a failed attempt at self-containment.

THERAPIST: (*As Cori looks at the therapist, therapist makes a declarative statement, but in low-key voice*) Cori, you must miss Mary. (*Therapist finds an emotional space to be sad with Cori in that moment and feels a "click" with her.*)

> The clinician gently reached out emotionally to Cori's painful affects. This was an attempt to track right-brain to right-brain processes in that moment and "meet and match" (Beebe & Lachmann, 1988) the intensity of Cori's low affect. The clinician's effort to try to stay with Cori's level of intensity may have been rewarded with a "click" of affective resonance or attunement.

CORI: Yeah, well, you know Mimi, sometimes she is a Baptist and sometimes she is a Catholic. (*Makes this statement calmly; it is not the flat statements of early in session.*)

THERAPIST: (*Has no idea where this is going, feels incompetent, at loss for words. Says, in puzzled tone:*) What? (*Worries that she has once again lost a fragile connection.*)

The fragile attunement may have been in danger of becoming <u>asynchronous</u>.

CORI: Mimi bought us a statue of St. Francis (*casts a glance to therapist a bit challengingly*). Are you Catholic?

The challenging behavior was an <u>up-regulated, sympathetic activation</u>, perhaps a defensive maneuver (acting out?).

THERAPIST: (*really off balance now*) What?

The clinician continued to experience an increasingly <u>asynchronous</u> emotional position.

CORI: Well, you look like you don't know who St. Francis is. You know (*almost sarcastic*), the patron saint of animals?

Cori became increasingly <u>up-regulated</u> (<u>sympathetic branch</u>) via the sarcasm, engaging in verbal acting out/regression, perhaps to decrease the intimacy that was experienced only moments before.

THERAPIST: (*happy to know something; stammering*) Oh, oh, yes, I did, or . . . do know about St. Francis.

Again, Cori's abrupt change in topic pushes the clinician into a somewhat <u>dysregulated emotional space</u> wherein the <u>branches of her autonomic nervous system were beginning to oscillate back and forth between excited (stammering) and an attempt at inhibition of affect</u> (tried to appear to know a fact).

CORI: (*Tucks her chin down and looks at her shoes, reaches down and straightens her skirt which did not need straightening. Starts to cry.*) Mary used to sleep with me and Jakki. No one knows but Mimi, but I have a little dog charm under my pillow that she bought for me at the Dollar Store. (*Suddenly irritation in her voice*) I hate that Dollar Store. Back home, Mama would never let us shop there. (*Starts to imitate her mother*) Only poor people shop there. We can go to Finegold's, just like everybody else. (*Looks up at therapist*) Do you shop at the Dollar Store?

Cori's affect was wildly (for her) moving <u>from up to down regulation</u>, as she may have been assailed by sadness, nostalgia, and/or anger (to counterregulate the lower intensity affects) and at the end may have been trying to connect and resonate with the clinician. Cori may have been <u>dysregulated, off-balance, and automatically searching for a person to help re-regulate her</u>, much as she may have done most of her life in her family, before the trauma of Hurricanes Katrina and Rita.

THERAPIST: (*Beginning to think that "off-balance" was her middle name, again asks:*) What?

Clinician <u>mirrors</u> Cori's affective dysregulation.

CORI: (*impatient now*) I said, do you shop at the Dollar Store?

The sympathetic branch activated, but it may have been more in service of connecting and approaching than in being aggressive (Porges, 2004, see Chapter 4), as occurred earlier in session; perhaps more self-assertion than acting out.

THERAPIST: (*Associating to having to tell her supervisor about her one-syllable interventions, tried to get her mind to work*) Oh, well, actually, I have shopped there before.

Something about Cori's directness, without aggression, drew an ordinary response from the clinician. This may have been the clinician's meeting and matching (Beebe & Lachmann, 1988) Cori's question-and-answer approach. Again, the indirect nature of acting out (maladaptive) may have been replaced by a more direct, self-assertive approach (adaptive).

CORI: (*irritated*) No, I mean, do you shop there on a regular basis?

Cori, though irritated, for the first time seemed self-assertive (a high-level defense mechanism indicating more homeostatic balance of the autonomic nervous system) and intent on trying to communicate and stay on track (though clinician cannot tell in the moment where Cori might be trying to go with this line of questioning).

THERAPIST: (*Decides that she must not try to over-think this and be natural*) No, I don't. I don't like it there.

Maybe the clinician was matching the more balanced autonomic nervous system of Cori with her response in kind (self-observation, suppression, on part of clinician?).

CORI: (*somewhat triumphant*) There, you see! That's what I mean! That's what I told Mama but that only made her mad; later, I saw her washing dishes and she was actually crying. She doesn't do that too much. It's usually Mimi and Jakki who are the criers in the family. I try not to show Mama that I don't like the Dollar Store. She doesn't need any more upset. You know what I mean?

Cori's assertiveness was rewarded in that she got the clinician to be similar with her, both in their opinion of the Dollar Store, and more critically, in matching the emotional tone, right brain to right brain, perhaps via mirror neurons.

THERAPIST: (*Not knowing which part of Cori's statement to respond to*) Cori, I wonder if sometimes you just don't know what to do? (*Suppresses the urge to elaborate and lets the comment hang in the air between them.*)

The clinician, may have been using her left hemisphere to put her own experience into words and cognitively track Cori, and she (clinician) may have nonconsciously perceived that her own right hemisphere was dysregulated and confused emotionally. She may have intuitively assumed that Cori was creating in the clinician's brain the same confusing, dysregulated experience that she (Cori) was experiencing.

CORI: (*Big sigh that makes her shoulders go up and down*) Yeah. (*Long silence; another sigh*) Yeah, you got it.

Cori may have allowed herself to become dyadically/interactively regulated by the clinician, meaning that Cori had temporarily "borrowed" the function of the other person to re-regulate herself, which she was unable to do without resorting to the defenses that were compromising her functioning. In other words, Cori's attempt to not worry her mother and be a "crier" like her sister and grandmother had cut her off from anyone who would/could interactively regulate her affect. By not having anyone with whom to be in synchrony, to be in attunement, to be a reliable selfobject (Kohut, 1971), or to stay in relationship with her, Cori was unable to employ an effective internal working model of affect management (Bowlby, 1988) which would have kept her functional. The more she tried to manage her emotions on her own by being tough, stoic, sarcastic, challenging, and matter-of-fact, the lonelier and more prone to dysregulation she may have become.

THERAPIST: (*Now trying not to think, but allows herself to be with Cori somehow*) I know how that feels sometimes.

A simple, plain, not overthought statement, which had to emerge from a more balanced autonomic nervous system.

CORI: (*Walks over to the table with art supplies on it, generally used by the younger kids; she starts drawing for a few minutes.*)

THERAPIST: (*Sits quietly looking out the window; the silence is companionable.*)

Perhaps this exchange of two people in attunement was similar on some level to Cori's experiences with the grandmother in the house smelling of coffee, etc. There was no need for the rigid use of defenses because it is likely that the norm in earlier days was that family members either appropriately regulated themselves, or when in need of comfort or reassurance that they could not provide for themselves, they sought such from others, with the expectation that it would be easily forthcoming. The family likely used the more homeostatically balanced defenses (affiliation, humor, internalization, etc.) primarily, or, if necessary, the other defenses managed by either the sympathetic or parasympathetic branches as the context required.

CORI: (*Walks back to her chair and in a young and shy way and hands the drawing of the dog, Mary, to the therapist. Her statement is rather matter-of-fact, however.*) Here, you can put that up by that other dog drawing (*gesturing to the side of the file cabinet with a jerk of her head*). If we are going to talk about that old dog of Mimi's, you ought to know what she looks like.

> *Cori's resonance with the therapist may have indicated that Cori had finally experienced the clinician somewhat as she did the grandmother of pre-Hurricane Katrina/Rita days: calm, attuned, and understanding the ways that Cori felt. That calming interaction may have re-regulated (i.e., invited autonomic nervous system balanced defenses and behaviors) Cori and allowed her to contemplate addressing her emotions around the dog and all that Mary, the dog, symbolized.*

Discussion of Case

The session with Cori is not unlike many clinical hours spent with clients. There is nothing especially remarkable about the effort of both Cori and her therapist to find common ground for emotional connection and resonance. What is remarkable to study are the neurobiological underpinnings that may account for both the barriers to attunement and the possibility of attunement between two brains. Tracking the attunement and misattunement, however subtle their expressions, provides the opportunity to make an educated guess about the current way in which affect is managed; also, a window to the past may open up momentarily. For example, the dialogue about the Dollar Store did not seem germane to anything that had been discussed previously. As the clinician allowed her intuition (right hemisphere; Schore, 2003b, p. 280) to guide the clinician's authentic response (she did not like the store either), a bonding occurred that led to smoother, more fluid exchanges. The more genuine interactions did not require Cori's problematic defenses (e.g., acting out/regression, blocking and isolation of affect, dissociation, controlling). The lessening of tension and increasing emotional comfort may have recreated a semblance of the attuned and connected ways Cori's family had interacted before the hurricanes.

Examining clinical sessions from the neurobiological perspective offers an understanding of the brain-to-brain interactions that may have profound implications and generally are not conscious. When the level of arousal of the self-protective mechanisms that people erect is understood, a greater clarity is possible regarding the role the clinician's brain and personality must play. For example, in several instances, Cori was controlling of the topics of the session. At the end, similar behavior (initiating the drawing of Mary, the dog) took on a more adaptive form of defense (self-assertion) against anxiety. Something in the intervening time period invited a more balanced yet still self-protective measure. It is important to consider that Cori's right hemisphere was eventually in synchrony and resonance (e.g., via mirror neurons:

Siegel, 2007; Gallese, 2010; Fuchs, et al., 2010), if even for a few moments, with the clinician's in a familiar manner. This may have permitted Cori's brain to employ more adaptive defenses.

Predicting the arousal management systems that the client may characteristically employ may allow the clinician to know (however intuitively) which of the branches of the autonomic nervous system may be less sturdy and therefore may require strengthening via reparative interactions with the clinician's arousal system. So much of clinical work is repetitive and often discouraging. Appreciating the value of many repetitions of arousal management while interacting with the brain of another encourages patience for the possibility that the dyadic regulation of affect may eventually become imprinted in the brain of the client—who may then manage his or her own affects without resorting to problematic behaviors and defenses.

This type of case examination, though long, has the potential to make increasingly automatic the consideration of the underlying psychobiological processes that are responsible for the intensity of affect. The reflexive registration of the up or down regulation of affect creates opportunities for the clinician to appreciate his or her own brain's tracking and resonating (or not) with the client, such that the strengths and vulnerabilities in the toleration of affect are clarified, as are the defensive maneuvers employed by clients and clinicians alike.

Sample Worksheet for Identifying Defense Mechanisms in Clinical Practice Material

Worksheet 2.1, for identifying defense mechanisms, can be used on a variety of materials: cases under supervision, clinicians' cases treated from any theoretical orientation, cases in clinical literature, excerpts from fiction literature, biographies, television shows of many kinds, commercial movies, and teaching films on clinical interviews. A sample blank worksheet is provided in the Appendix; a filled-in sample worksheet, illustrating how defensive maneuvers can be examined, appears below.

The following material examines an excerpt from the previously discussed case of Cori. A defense mechanism, acting out, is erected by Cori to defend from difficult affects. The neurobiological underpinnings of the interactions are broken down into some of their component parts. One reason for identifying the purpose and function of self-protective behaviors is to consider how the brain-to-brain contact within the therapeutic alliance may improve the functioning of the brain of the client, though many repetitions may be required. Increasing tolerance for difficult affects and decreasing reliance on rigid, perhaps, toxic defensive behaviors are goals for most therapeutic approaches. Through the therapeutic alliance the client could potentially strengthen a branch of the autonomic nervous system that has characteristically been underutilized.

The old concept of borrowing the ego function of the worker (Kaufman, 1963, pp. 196–198) captures the process by which a brain, for example, that has developed an automatic penchant for high arousal to most situations encountered, may actually be calmed, neurobiologically, by another brain. The resonance between the aroused brain and the calm brain not only has a temporary soothing effect, but also may have a long-term effect. The interactive/dyadic shift in arousal may become inscribed in the brain as a challenge to the lop-sided automatic reaction—for example, to use the same branch of the autonomic nervous system in response to almost any situation. New neural structures created in response to the dyadic regulation give the aroused brain, in this instance, a chance to not only calm down in the moment, but the co-created affective tolerance may have a chance to become permanent, particularly if repeated.

Identification of the purpose and function of defense mechanisms, though always a speculative endeavor, is a necessary part of identifying the affect management strategies employed by clients. The clinician may thereby be better informed about the specific types of interventions needed. Retrospectively, the clinician may gain clarity on the ways that his or her own brain assisted in automatically re-regulating the dysregulated experience of the client. Given enough repetitions, the existing neural circuitry may be enhanced and strengthened and new neural circuitry may be created to manage affects in an improved manner.

Sample Worksheet 2.1.
Identifying Defense Mechanisms

The following analysis is based on the first few exchanges between Cori and the clinician in their first session (see case study above in this chapter).

Example of self-protective (defended) behavior
that is focus of clinical attention:

Cori's initial challenging and belligerent tone of voice could be seen as self-protective, as could her behavior a few exchanges later, when she abruptly changes the subject, asking, "Like, do you know where

I got my name?" in a slightly aroused tone of voice. Noteworthy: Cori brings into the discussion the low affect management styles her family uses to deal with emotions (e.g., "People in my family don't worry too much about things these days"). So in the first few exchanges she goes back and forth between her own slightly aroused state and mentioning her family's ways of lowering arousal.

Defense and definition of defense:

The challenging tone of voice and abrupt change of subject could be thought of as mild form of verbally acting out. (Acting out is defined as a direct expression of impulses to remain unaware of the wishes or affects that accompany them.)

Speculation about anxiety or experience that defense seeks to manage:

Clinically, it could be speculated that the defense of acting out verbally was nonconsciously intended to protect Cori from the anxiety she may have felt from being called into the school counselor's office and as a way to deal with the unknown—that is, to present a strong front, unafraid. Of course, she has experienced trauma in the recent past with the multiple losses, and those losses surely have had an effect on her coping, though their specific contribution to this encounter is unknown.

Coping styles of defense (Conte & Plutchick, 1995):

Avoid (withdraw from)

Minimize (reduce): Acting out may have helped Cori minimize her uncomfortable level of arousal, i.e., the anxiety.

Substitute (doing unrelated pleasurable activities to solve a problem)

Help-seeking (by retreating to immature behaviors)

Replacement (improving weaknesses)

Mapping (getting information before acting)

Blaming (attributing cause to someone else)

Reversal (doing opposite of feeling state)

Is defense more active, high arousal or more passive, lower arousal?

Acting out verbally is somewhat arousing in this example; it may *express an impulse to fight (challenging, belligerence) or flee (changing the subject to origin of her name)* (Both fight and flight are amygdalar driven behaviors; see Chapter 3 for details.)

Part of the autonomic nervous system that manages the level of stimulation that accounts for the level of arousal in the brain: sympathetic or parasympathetic?

The higher level of arousal of the verbally acting-out behaviors (challenging, belligerent, abruptly changing the subject) may be accounted for by the action of the SNS of autonomic nervous system.

Or is the defense homeostatically regulated, with the SNS and PNS coupled together and functioning as a team?

N/A for this exchange between Cori and me.

Or are both the PNS and SNS active simultaneously?

N/A for this exchange between Cori and me.

Or is the PNS using avoidance of others to manage affects and achieve subdued, frozen, submissive, passive, even dissociative manner?

This may be what some of the family members are either seen by Cori as trying to do (i.e., go for low affective arousal . . . be strong, don't worry), or they are actually quite subdued and low in their affective expressions.

Or is PNS managing affect by using (borrowing) another's regulation, though the affect is in low arousal range?

In the case material, there is the impression that Cori is on her own to manage her emotional life, as opposed to the family's historical experience of closeness; additionally, her community experiences before Katrina and Rita seemed quite supportive.

Is the defense flexible or rigid? Support your answer.

If Cori's earlier experience of being able to depend on family and community can be reconstructed, that may allow her to be less distant and tough; however, if she is left to manage herself because her family is preoccupied with adjusting to the new environment and all the reasons why that is so, she may develop affect management strategies (defenses) that are more down-regulated and appear more autonomous than she had exhibited pre-hurricanes.

Is defense problem-solving oriented or a form of self-deception? Support your answer.

At the time of the interview, it seems both; she solves the problem of being unable to be dependent on her family, as she could before the hurricanes , and she can deceive herself that she is just fine taking care of herself.

Does the defense require the person to adapt to environment, or is it an attempt to change the external environment (Hartmann, 1939/1958)? Explain.

The acting-out defense in this instance seems to change Cori internally; perhaps her relationships may begin to adapt to her "new" tough exterior and begin to ignore her or leave her alone, etc., but for this time period, it seems likely that the primary reason for the defense is her need to be active (fight–flight).

Which part (SNS or PNS) of the autonomic nervous system is less sturdy and needs to be strengthened?

From the history, it might be speculated that until Katrina and its aftermath, Cori might have been homeostatically balanced in her autonomic nervous system functioning. However, currently, circumstances may be inviting a less vulnerable set of coping strategies, and she has adopted a more soldier-like emotional presentation. Overuse of the acting-out defense mechanism could lead to a preference for the more highly aroused public face (sympathetic), with less likelihood of using the decreased arousal system (parasympathetic).

Which part of the brain of the clinician may help strengthen the above part of the autonomic nervous system? Explain the dyadic experience between the client and clinician that has the potential of improving (stimulating) affective/emotional tolerance.

The clinician needs to allow her sympathetic branch to resonate with Cori's via moment-to-moment tracking, so that, as the session unfolds, the girl may be able to experience the lower affects (sadness, loss, regret, etc.) via the clinician's parasympathetic branch attunement to the emotions underneath the arousing defense of acting out. The hope would be that Cori could be empathically in connection with another person as she allowed herself to experience less bearable emotions. Using the less utilized (recently, at least) parasympathetic would strengthen her capacity to bear lower, painful feelings. Hopefully, this experience would, in turn, decrease the need for certain defenses that could become maladaptive, such as acting out.

Is the defense adaptive or maladaptive? Explain.

As with many defensive maneuvers, a behavior used to cope with a stressful situation can become maladaptive over time if used too rigidly, frequently, or with no reflexive (nonconscious) consideration for context. However, for this time period, being "tougher" may temporarily serve Cori well, given the stressors of loss of home, family, beloved pet, school, friends, and self-esteem.

CHAPTER 3
Threat Management and the Amygdala

FIGURE 3.0.
The Amygdala and the Limbic System

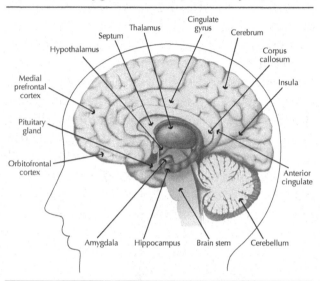

This chapter addresses both obvious as well as subtle reactions to various levels of emotional and/or physical threat originating from the environment. Additionally, a sense of threat may come from a person's own thoughts or feelings and thus be purely internal. Though the entire personality may become involved in addressing and managing perceived threat, the focus here is on a small but important structure in the lower limbic system, the amygdala, which plays a large role in the perception and management of threat. A comparison of the amygdala with selected brain structures (e.g., upper limbic system and the cortex) that also manage threat includes the following areas: levels of consciousness, modes of social engagement, bodily and emotional states, and memory systems. The early-maturing structures have different effects on external behavior and internal experience, depending on the interactions with the environment. These same structures (1) have separate ways to store and process affect-related meanings of threat responses, ambiguity, and aggression; (2) have different degrees of implicit memory and self states; and (3) are differentially engaged as a function of the different attachment styles.

Overview of the Amygdala: Location and Description

It is a surprising fact that a small almond-shaped structure in the brain, the amygdala, may have such a big effect on personality functioning. It is located within the limbic system, beneath the temporal lobes on each side of the brain (Brody, 1992, p. 92). Under certain circumstances, the amygdala, particularly the right amygdala, becomes the primary manager of neural networks involved with fear responses, facial recognition, attachment, and arousal (Whalen & Phelps, 2009; Schore, 2003a, 2003b) and has a key role in aggression and sexual arousal in males (Saplosky, 2005, p. 139). The left amygdala is responsive to verbalizations more than is the right and is not so involved in arousal management issues as is the right (Schore, personal communication, 2011). As the permanent "manager" of these functions, however, the amygdala is not a desirable developmental outcome. Why not? The short answer is that what begins as an advantage at birth and in early childhood can become a disadvantage as the personality develops. (For details on right- and left-amygdalar functions, see Cozolino, 2006, p. 181; Schore, 2003a, pp. 239, 256–258, 294; Schore, 2003b, pp. 82, 225–227; and for details on amygdalar function in primates, including humans, see Whalen & Phelps, 2009, pp. 2–106.) Because the amygdala is active at birth, it confers protection on the infant by providing rapid responses to safety and danger, thereby helping to ensure survival— certainly an advantage. However, developing an overly sensitive and chronic emergency response system could be a disadvantage. The amygdala errs on the side of caution; it "behaves first and thinks later." In situations of danger, this fast-track reaction has high survivability. However, too much stress or trauma (cumulative relationship trauma or other types of trauma) may have two related outcomes:

1. May cause an overreliance on the amygdala to respond to threat.
2. May cause an underdevelopment of other, more slowly maturing structures (limbic and higher cortical) that are also designed to manage threat and stress, but at a more deliberate pace.

Under conditions of stress and trauma, important upper right-brain functions that either never develop or develop poorly include the following:

1. The ability to discriminate among levels of threat.
2. The capacity to fine-tune responses appropriate to the situation.

Ideally, perception of threat and emotional–behavioral control are gradually taken up by the upper structures in the right hemisphere. As the developing brain is influenced by mature and healthy brains, more complex and sophisticated brain structures in the upper right hemisphere come to fulfill functions ensuring emotional and behavioral control, leaving the amygdala with the important but hopefully relatively infrequent task of signaling an alarm for immediate action to danger.

A stressful environment may maintain a pressure on the rapid response system in the brain, thereby making the arousal system in the personality either chronically overreactive or underreactive or some erratic combination. The personality can eventually become patterned by the level of arousal that is mobilized to meet most situations and can remain dominated by amygdalar functions that respond to the most minimal hint of threat, leading to chronic over/under/erratic reacting. The amygdala is connected to and influenced by a number of structures, all of which have arousal management functions (see Table 3.1 for details).

In situations of threat, immediate reactivity of the amygdala can override the slower, more thoughtful responses managed by the upper right-brain structures, which, if the threat is real, helps with survival. However, if the upper right-brain structures are chronically eclipsed by amygdalar reactivity and there is no real threat, serious clinical symptoms will manifest. In contrast, in the best-case scenario, the brain matures and the amygdala functions helpfully as a safety–danger early warning system, leaving the upper right and left brain to plan, anticipate, and, in general, carefully orchestrate behavioral responses.

Relationships Among Relevant Structures: Hierarchical and Separable Functions

What are hierarchical and separable functions and why are they important to clinical work? The term *hierarchical functions* means that from lower to higher cortical structures, there are differences in the levels or intensity of experiences laid down in neural circuitry (e.g., the lower structures can be quite unmodulated and intense, as in the flashbacks occurring in the amygdala, in contrast to well-functioning higher cortical structures, which have memories that can be consciously retrieved in a deliberate manner). *Separable functioning* means that each layer of the brain has distinctively separate functions (e.g., the amygdala may react more rapidly to perceived or real threat, whereas structures within the upper right cortex, if appropriately developed, are designed to consider whether to inhibit or express impulses, before doing so).

If traumatic and stressful memories are primarily stored in the lower structures, then the automatic and reflexive ways in which lower structures

TABLE 3.1
Structures Affecting and Interacting with the Amygdala

- Anterior cingulate (involved with emotional and somatic experience; Cozolino, 2006, p. 77)
- Orbitofrontal areas of the prefrontal cortex and frontal areas of the temporal lobes (mature management of emotions; Cozolino, 2002, pp. 179–180)
- Direct connections to the ANS (regulation of arousal levels in body; Cozolino, 2002, p. 181)
- Sapolsky would add the septum (inhibits amygdala) as part of the limbic system; puts the "brake" on aggression as generated by the amygdala (2005, p. 110)
- Hippocampus (explicit, retrievable memory, can be made conscious; Cozolino, 2002)
- Frontal cortex inhibits amygdala (Sapolsky, 2005, p. 104)
- Insula involved in resonating with somatic and emotional states of others (Damasio, 1999; Craig, as cited in Buchanan, Tranel, & Adolphs, 2009, p. 305; Blakeslee, 2007)
- Hypothalamic–pituitary–adrenal (HPA) axis (stress response system). (Rothschild, 2000)

operate will dominate. Difficult, traumatic experiences, if they occur too early in the development of the brain, happen too often, and/or are too traumatic, will compromise the development of upper cortical structures. Additionally, should stress or trauma occur, ideally, the developing brain structures will have the experience of another, more mature brain to help manage the emotional responses. The "scaffolding" provided by a mature brain gives the higher cortical structures opportunities to slowly mature. Many repetitions of interactive affect management will strengthen developing neural circuitry, such that the young brain will eventually have conscious choices available with which to manage affects. Of course, an infant will not be making conscious choices because consciousness develops later than the capacity to "download," so to speak, the functional capacities of the caretaking other.

However, should there be insufficient dyadic regulation of affect enough of the time to allow for the proper development of higher cortical structures (which are more deliberate and not as reflexive as the lower structures), the default structure may become the amygdala. The amygdala can even become enlarged with overuse (Sapolsky, 2005, p. 109). Other structures may not develop well, particularly the hippocampus (another important memory structure located higher in the right limbic region of the right hemisphere). Images and urges that invite immature and reactive behaviors in the lower brain structures can begin to characterize a person's habitual responses. The ability to consciously recall and summarize experiences can be compromised (these memories would be retrieved from the hippocampus). Instead, traumatic experiences may be relived via enactments or flashbacks (these memories are activated by the amygdala; Cozolino, 2002, p. 97). Such experiences cannot become available to the conscious mind for review and processing.

From the "bottom up" of the social–emotional brain located in the right hemisphere are three levels of the limbic system in ascending order: "amygdala, anterior cingulate, and insula-orbitofrontal" levels, according to Schore (2003b, p. 234), with Cozolino adding the frontal portions of the temporal lobes as the highest level of the limbic system (2002, pp. 179–180). If the brain matures normally, these structures remain interconnected and associated as somatic (bodily) and affective (emotional) self states are processed with increasing complexity (Barbas, 1995). The implication is that more socially attuned, appropriate ways of interacting with the environment will be the rule in personality functioning, not the exception.

Hierarchical Functions

Hierarchical considerations include a review of levels of consciousness, modes of social engagement, somatic and emotional self states, and memory systems, which are all addressed in this section.

Levels of Consciousness

Different states of consciousness influence behavior as well as inner felt experience, possibly by evoking quite different responses. To reiterate essential points already discussed: The unconscious fast-reacting urges of the amygdala (fight, flight, freeze, submit, and sexual responses in males; Sapolsky, 2005) are utilized in the case of actual danger of some sort. Otherwise, the slower and more measured process involved in choosing how to react, managed by the comparatively more conscious anterior cingulate and orbitofrontal cortex, will generally prevail. The conscious left hemisphere will also be involved in the deliberate choosing of responses, but it is slower than the right hemisphere to react to internal and external sources of threat (Schore, 2003a, 2003b).

If the more unconscious structure (amygdala) determines reactions, then the processing will utilize more extreme behavioral solutions to an immediate situation (high/low arousal, active/passive response, danger/no danger assessment). For survival reasons, the motto is "Act now and sort things out later." The amygdala is "loosely adjacent to the hypothalamic and autonomic structures" (Schore, 2003b, p. 234), which are part of the arousal system and drive the "act now" effects. The anterior cingulate and orbitofrontal cortex (both more slowly maturing than the amygdala, not fully functional at birth, and dependent on the environment for shaping functioning) will have a more complicated manner of considering the degree of threat and immediacy of response necessary. For more detailed explanation of the stress management that occurs in the hypothalamic and autonomic interface (HPA axis, or hypo-thalamic–pituitary–adrenal axis; see Chapter 2 on defense mechanisms, and Rothschild, 2000, pp. 3–14).

Modes of Social Engagement

The developing anterior cingulate and the orbitofrontal cortex are quite sensitive to interactions with the environment as they mature postnatally, unlike the amygdala, which is functional at birth. The potential effect of stress and trauma could be a brain that favors the processing paths of overly developed lower structures (e.g., amygdala) over higher cortical structures. The dominance of the amygdala can overshadow proper development of other structures that manage emotions. Without the necessary influence of better-developed brains over time, the amygdala-dominated brain is left to regulate itself with crude hyper- or hyporeactive primitive reactions (Sapolsky, 2005, p. 110).

However, there is ample evidence that repetitive contact with a person or persons with better brain development can start or restart development of higher cortical structures leading to actual change in neural functioning (Schore, 1994, 2003a, 2003b). The goal would be to decrease dominance of amygdalar reactivity. The key is to increase interactions with others who have less inappropriate hypo-/hyperreactivity, so that regulation of one brain by another can occur. Multiple repetitions of regulated dyadic interactions can eventually create neural structures for self-regulation. Eventually, the amyg-dalar-driven brain functioning will decrease and the upper cortical functions will proceed autonomously, or if necessary, can recruit another brain temporarily to assist with functioning. In the case study in this chapter, there are many good examples of Mr. Ryan going back and forth between amyg-dalar dominance (outbursts or immediate depressive moments) and using his doctor to manage his affects in the moment.

Somatic and Emotional Self States

There are five domains of self-experience, as theorized by Wallin (2007, pp.

61–70), which seem to map onto the hierarchical structuring of conscious-ness and reactivity. These domains of self-experience, if all goes well, seem to be distributed, over time, from the subcortical areas (particularly the amyg-dala) to the higher cortical structures, both in the upper right hemisphere and the left hemisphere. Each of these five domains is described by Wallin as undergirded neurobiologically by an increasingly complex maturation of emotional and behavioral systems (see Benes, 1989, for the cortical–hippo-campal connections). These self states include the following:

1. The somatic self—infant's developing physiology shapes bodily self's responsiveness to experience (p. 62).
2. The emotional self—bodily sensations take the form of emotions and spark action tendencies (p. 63).
3. The representational self—grounded in emotional experience, often of a highly charged nature (p. 65).
4. The reflective self—the experience of others who have "our mind in mind" makes possible awareness of internal experience (p. 67).
5. The mindful self—the conscious awareness of experience (pp. 67–68).

As described by Wallin, the unconscious somatic (bodily) self, the emotional self, and the representational self are inscribed early in life in what is likely the amygdala and elaborated upon in what is likely the higher cortical struc-tures as development proceeds. The reflective and mindful selves result from interactions with the milieu as life proceeds beyond infancy and early child-hood, and experience is potentially accessible to consciousness (p. 67).

As early bodily sensations, which may later also become emotions, are experienced repeatedly, the neuronal circuitry may begin to associate care-taker actions with safety or danger, an amygdalar function. These states can, in time, become traits (Schore, 2003a, p. 198), meaning that the subcor-tical structures can become habituated to the subtlest of environmental cues regarding the degree of safety or danger. Again, should the early somatic, emotional, and representational self states become overly sensitized to regis-tering fear, the development of the other self states (e.g., reflective self, mindful self) may become compromised in many ways, in particular, to become dissociated experiences.

Memory Systems

Both the amygdala and hippocampus function as memory systems, but they process different types of memory. The hippocampus stores what are consid-ered to be more conscious memories, and the amygdala stores less conscious memories. Sherry and Schacter (as cited in Cozolino, 2002, p. 97) concluded that the hippocampus more finely discriminates among data coming from the external environment, whereas the amygdala generalizes from that same data. Because the amygdala is operational at birth (whereas the hippocampus takes into late adolescence to mature: Benes, as cited in Cozolino, 2002, p. 95), amygdalar reactivity to small indications of safety and danger early in life contribute to our survivablility capabilities. Decreased hippocampal volume has been reported in depressed clients, suggesting one possible effect of a compromised development (Sheline, Wang, Gado, Csernansky, & Vannier, as cited in Cozolino, 2002, p. 98), as has amygdalar volume (Jacobs & Nadal, as cited in Cozolino, 2002, p. 97). Perhaps in this instance, it is the underuse of either memory system that results in decreased volume. Another study has found that with compromised development, there is a decrease in hippocampal volume and an *increase* in amygdalar volume (Sapolsky, 2005).

As the brain matures, the hippocampus, with its ability to "remember" and sort through past situations, comparing them (Eichenbaum, as cited in Cozolino, 2002, p. 95), hopefully can become the regulator of reactions to stimuli, leaving to the amygdala the task of responding to genuine danger with fight, flight, freeze, or submission as an immediate option, given the amygdala's direct connection with the ANS (Cozolino, 2002, p. 181). Obviously, if the child's brain has been over- or understimulated, the gradual acquisition of a capacity to engage in more complex processing of events by the hippocampus may be compromised, leaving the brain somewhat at the mercy of automatic hypo- or hyperreactivity of the amygdala.

According to some (van der Kolk & Greenberg, 1987; LeDoux, Romanski, & Xagoraris, 1989), the amygdala is the origin of the experience of the "flashback"— the instantaneous reexperiencing of past traumatic events as if those events were actually occurring in the present moment. The hippocampus would not be the memory system involved in flashbacks. Additionally, past fears and phobias are also amygdalar-driven (Jacobs & Nadal, as cited in Cozolino, 2002, p. 97). The stimulus–response pairing of any event with anxiety or fear is learned at the amygdalar level (Cozolino, 2002, p. 242). Further, the amygdala broadly determines the emotional significance of threatening stimuli (Morgan & LeDoux, 1995, p. 687).

To briefly review hierarchical functions: The amygdala (low subcortical structure) has the least consciousness wherein the earliest experiences, including somatic (bodily) states as well as traumatic states, are stored. As stated elsewhere, the amygdala stores implicit memory and is the most reactive to internal and external events. These memories are not accessible via conscious effort, but tend to surface in the nonverbal action realm (Wallin, 2007, pp. 259–306). This is in contrast to some higher cortical structures, such as the hippocampus and upper right cortex, which are the location of explicit memory. These structures, when properly developed, are less reactive than the amygdala and have the capacity for thoughtful consideration of behavioral options, regulation of affect, and the representation of self and other experiences.

Separable Functions

Related to the hierarchical considerations noted above are issues of separable functioning (Schore, 2003b, p. 234). Separable functions include storing and processing affect-related meanings to threat response, ambiguity, and aggression; differing degrees of implicit memory and self states; and differential engagement as a function of the different attachment styles. Separable functioning means that each of the layers of the right hemisphere may produce distinct styles of thinking, feeling, or behaving, depending upon how the environment has impacted those structures (e.g., duration of stress, amount and timing of stress/trauma, as well as relationship to the person who is the source of the stress). Some clinical implications of separable functioning may give clinicians a way to assess the following:

- Development (the more primitive, crude and impulsive a reaction, the greater the likelihood that lower cortical structures are responsible)
- The flexibility or rigidity of memory functions
- Global reactions versus reactions to the particulars of the current situation
- Different degrees of consciousness
- Quite different experiences of the self (traits, behaviors, ways of thinking and coping with emotions)

Several structures in the brain process experiences differently from one another. Those structures include (from the bottom up) the amygdala, the anterior cingulate, and the insula-orbitofrontal and frontal portions of the temporal lobes (Cozolino, 2002, pp. 179–180; Schore, 2003b, p. 234). Some of the experiences that are processed differently include affective, cognitive, and behavioral functions that have been affected by the state in which they were initially experienced. For example, self states and somatic states located in the lowest section of the right hemisphere can be blocked from passing upward to the higher structures for processing; these states likely would be those that had an intolerable level of arousal (either too high or too low) and might remain dissociated, unconscious, and inaccessible to awareness.

Stored Models of Processing Affect-Related Meanings

The brain preserves the memories of emotions or affects in various locations, depending on the degree of threat, the developmental level of various brain structures, and the resilience conferred on the brain via the attachment style. To repeat, the attachment style involves a learned psychophysiological way in which affects are managed that is imprinted in the neurocircuitry.

Threat Response and Ambiguity

Whalen (1998) suggests that the amygdalar response serves to clarify a potential threat response (p. 290). The amygdala recognizes and responds to socially salient stimuli, but what in the social environment constitutes a "socially salient stimuli?" Sander, Grafman, and Zalla (2003) described the human amygdala as an evolved system for relevance detection. It is suggested that "it is *ambiguity* or *relevance* to which the amygdala is sensitive" (Buchanan et al., as cited in Whalen & Phelps, 2009, p. 289; emphasis in original). Buchanan et al. further note: "Stimuli that predict threat some of the time, as in a partial reinforcement schedule, produce greater amygdala-dependent conditioned responses than do those that consistently predict threat" (2009, pp. 289–290). The activation of the amygdala while negotiating the social milieu is a measure of the amygdala's role in deciphering ambiguity: "The unpredictable nature of social interactions is what influences amygdala function" (Buchanan et al., 2009, p. 290). When making "sense of ambiguous situations, subcortical circuits are more likely to guide conscious awareness" (Cozolino, 2002, p. 94). Suslow et al. found that the right (but not the left) amygdala has a role in the "detection and consolidation of memory for marginally perceptible threatening facial expression" (2006, p. 243). McGaugh similarly found that "the amygdala modulates the consolidation of long-term memories of emotionally arousing experiences" (as cited in Knapska et al., 2006, p. 3858). There is speculation that the amygdala modulates visual attentional processing in the visual cortices (Anderson & Phelps, 2001; Vuilleumier, Richardson, Armony, Driver, & Dolan, 2004) at the earliest processing times—*before the cortical information has even reached the amygdala*. Other studies have also presented evidence for the amygdala's faster response to visual information as compared to the cortex (Amaral, Price, Pitkanen, & Carmichael, 1992; Johnson, 2005). Viewing fearful faces (presumably a threat condition), adolescent subjects who were high-risk for major depressive disorder showed greater amygdalar and nucleus accumbens (also involved in emotional regulation; Farmer, 2009, p. 33) activation than did those in the low-risk group (Monk et al., 2008).

Aggression

The amygdala is a limbic structure with a key role in the processing of aggression and fear, as well as sexual arousal in males (Sapolsky, 2005, 139). As stated several times elsewhere and worth repeating, the amygdala sends inputs to the frontal cortex to perform an action, not particularly thought out well (Sapolsky, 2005, p. 114). Several areas should be mentioned briefly in relation to how compromised amygdalar functioning influences the manifestation of aggression; psychopathy; the experience of posttraumatic stress disorder (PTSD); the expression of borderline personality traits; and the production of the neurohormones testosterone, estrogen, and progesterone.

Psychopathy in individuals seems to stem from a chronic state of low affect and underreactivity to social cues (controlled by the parasympathetic branch), but over-reactivity to their own frustration (resulting from extreme arousal by the sympathetic branch). In contrast, the high-arousal symptoms of PTSD and/or the expression of borderline personality traits may result from excessive pruning of the parasympathetic branch, with the result of an overreactive sympathetic branch. In none of the cases described above is the orbitofrontal cortex functioning adequately in one of its major roles: the regulation of affect, particularly the inhibition of impulses. This is a result of the "overpruning of orbitofrontal and anterior cingulate connections with the amygdala" (Schore, 2003a, p. 298).

According to Blair (2004) and Schore (2003a, pp. 291–295) there are two kinds of rage expressions: cold predatory *and* hot reactive. With psychopathy, the hallmark of underreactivity leads to being less influenced by others' emotions. Reduced amygdalar volume and reduced amygdalar activation occur in psychopaths when they are exposed to emotional cues (Blair, as cited in Allen, Fonagy, & Bateman, 2008, p. 143). Schore attributes the dissociative response, if extended into periods of hypoarousal via the parasympathetic branch, as responsible for the pruning of orbitofrontal connections into the subcortical autonomic arousal system (including the hypothalamus), thereby fixing the psychopath's autonomic nervous system at low arousal rates (2003a, pp. 300–301). Hence the cold rage reactions.

Although reactive rage expressions (Schore, 2003a, p. 300) characterize the aggressive behavior of people with borderline personality traits or PTSD, the part of the brain responsible is different from that in psychopaths. Borderline personality organization may result from excessive cell death during critical periods of development in the connections between the hypothalamus and the sympathetic branch, such that affective instability results. The lack of connectivity between the prefrontal cortex and the amygdala will arrest the development of the inhibitory function of the "corticolimbic limbic-hypo-thalamic connectivity" (Schore, 2003a, p. 300).

In psychopathy, "reactive" aggression has a different basis from that of nonpsychopaths (e.g., traumatized persons; Raine, Meloy, et al., 1998). Psychopaths do, however, express reactive aggression on occasion because they are likely to continue with unrewarding strategies that invite frustration. This is because the prefrontal cortex of the psychopath does not learn from experience; this impairment leads to an inability to stop behaviors that had previously been unrewarding. This is in contrast to predatory stalking behaviors, which primarily characterize psychopaths' style of functioning, but have little or no emotional reactivity (Schore, 2003a, pp. 298–303).

According to Sapolsky, the role of alcohol, testosterone, and crowding in the elicitation of aggression has been overrated (2005, p. 115). Testosterone does not activate amygdalar neurons, but it does further activate already activated neurons (Sapolsky, 2005, p. 120). The correlation between aggression and testosterone levels is that aggression elevates testosterone levels, not the reverse (Sapolsky, 2005, p. 120). The ratio between estrogen and progesterone is relevant for female aggression in that fluctuating levels around menstruation and parturition have been tied to aggressive or fiercely protective behaviors (Saplosky, 2005, p. 121).

Degrees of Implicit Memory and Self State

Reading facial expressions is a vital function of the amygdala, the location of implicit memory and early self states. Clearly reading the face of the care-taker is a critical survival function, according to Cozolino, who speculates that fear may the strongest early emotion and the one emotion necessary to distinguish safety from danger (2002, p. 243). As the brain of the infant becomes increasingly specialized via development of the amygdala in gathering survival information from the face of the caretaker, the amygdala organizes neural circuitry to memorialize such information into states of the self. The inhibitory effect of the more deliberate hippocampal memory system is not available/ matured in infancy and childhood, and if the caretaker does not modulate stressful stimuli, the result may be memories that influence behaviors by "favoring" dreaded states, beliefs, fears, phobias, and so on, at unconscious levels (i.e., states become traits; Perry et al., 1995). In such situations, there is no upper cortical involvement and therefore no conscious (explicit) memory (Cozolino, 2002, p. 245).

Wondering if the amygdala contributes something vital to social cognition, Buchanan et al. suggested that "by modulating social cognition at the earliest times as well as at later times . . . the amygdala may be particularly well positioned to contribute what is the hallmark of social cognition: modulating all of cognition" (2009, p. 312). Buchanan et al. also noted that attention, perception, memory, decision making, and emotional reaction are involved in cognition and are amygdalar functions, as well (2009, p. 312).

Bowlby (1988) described attachment templates or schemas beginning at birth and continuing throughout life that involve memories of interpersonal interactions, which, especially if repeated enough, can lead to expectations of others' behaviors and predictions of how others might react. Significantly, the amygdala is one of the structures that register such interactions (termed *implicit cognitions*) between the infant and others, and these interactions lead to different types of attachment, as noted previously, depending on the quality of the interactions. Knapska et al. (2006) studied the transfer of emotional information between people and found that the amygdala was activated. Lemche et al. stated that "a key role of the amygdala [is] in mediating autonomic activity associated with human attachment insecurity" (2006, p. 623)—a comment that correlates the arousal system (ANS) with attachment strategy.

Implications of Attachment Style as Equivalent to Affect Management Category

Attachment styles are, in effect, also affect management strategies. Three types of insecure attachment styles have been identified as forming in childhood, often beginning in infancy, in addition to the secure (ideal) style. Later in adulthood, according to many researchers, the possibilities for attachment styles include secure, earned secure, and several adult variations of the insecure styles of childhood. Each of the insecure styles of attachment in adulthood correlates fairly well with certain disordered personality organizations. Siegel summarizes in chart form the four adult attachment classifications used extensively by child development researchers (secure/autonomous, dismissing, preoccupied, and unresolved/disorganized) in correspondence with childhood attachment classifications (secure, avoidant, resistant or ambivalent, and disorganized; 1999, p. 74). However, other researchers have broken down the adult classifications more finely, and in Chapter 5, I use those descriptions to speculate about the underlying arousal functions of the autonomic nervous system and the likely clinical diagnoses.

The amygdala, seat of implicit memory (not retrievable by conscious and verbal means), "modulates the consolidation of long-term memories of emotionally arousing experiences" (McGraugh, as cited in Knapska, 2006, p. 3858). According to Bowlby (1988) and Cozolino (2002), attachment styles are forms of implicit memory. The question arises: how to account for the flexibility of the secure attachment of childhood and adulthood? Considering one major contribution to the opposite of flexibility may be helpful. Amygdalar memories are rigid and inflexible, whether resulting from trauma or early nonverbal/para-verbal experiences. This rigidity is at the seat of the insecure attachment styles. Style implies a predictable way of managing affect and thus behavioral expression. Only secure attachment styles have flexibility in their expression.

Secure attachment begins as an implicit memory. It seems logical that a once-formed amygdalar implicit memory, which has migrated to and been consolidated in the right hippocampus and upper cortical memory systems (the more mature memory systems), would be flexible, plastic, malleable, and open to being affected by ever-changing internal and external experiences. This is unlike the memories formed by various types of trauma, which can remain stored in the lower structures of the right hemisphere (e.g., the amygdala). Implicit memories that are not traumatically induced would likely be easily available for processing and updating by higher cortical structures. Certainly, the functional affect management strategy of the securely attached would also be housed in the implicit memory system, but would not be problematic.

Amygdalar functioning can be affected in numerous ways and on several levels: by stress hormones, by neurotransmitters, and by other brain structures. Specifically:

Stress hormones
- Pain
- Fearful responses
- Uncomfortable levels/types of sensory information (Sapolsky, 2005, p. 109)

Neurotransmitters
- Anticipation of pleasure, via dopamine, which fuels the ability of the frontal lobe to inhibit impulses (Sapolsky, 2005, p. 114)
- Low serotonin levels, which are associated with impulsive aggression (Sapolsky, 2005, p. 114)

Structure
- The septum, which puts the "brake" on aggression that is generated by the amygdala (Sapolsky, 2005, p. 110)

When the amygdala is compromised, the following may occur:

- Impaired recognition of facial expressions (Cozolino, 2002, 176)
- Impaired role in making social judgments, particularly regarding the "untrustworthiness" of faces from their appearance (Buchanan et al., 2009, p. 304)
- Lack of empathy (Baron-Cohen, et al., 2000; Buchanan et al., 2009, p. 306)
- Inability to pay attention to the eye and information in the expression conveyed (Buchanan et al., 2009, 308-310)

Right-amygdalar memories of the traumatic type contribute to dissociative affect management strategies (Schore, personal communication, 2008). Insecure attachments in general are affected by lower right-brain functioning, such as the problematic capacity to compare–contrast past and present (hence, flashbacks) or the inability to carefully consider behavioral choices (hence, automatic behaviors).

The concept of object constancy, from the work of Margaret Mahler (Mahler, Pine, & Bergman, 1975), seems relevant. *Object constancy* refers to the ability of the mind to retain a mental image of the positive and helpful functions of another person who has provided, encouraged, and modeled approval, soothing comfort, encouragement, admiration, and/or behavioral control (Kramer & Akhtar, 1994, p. 27; Mahler et al., 1975, pp. 109–112; Edward & Sanville, 1996, p. 459). Given sufficient repetitions with another, the brain will take on those functions for itself and, even when under stress, we can feel self-approval, self-comfort, self-admiration, or self-control—or seek such from an appropriate other person.

The use of an internalized function of the other, if "weak," may mean that implicit memories containing insecure attachment styles, and the inherent affect management strategies that accompany them, may account for little or no object constancy. It may be that the only attachment styles that include object constancy as an attribute are the securely attached or the earned securely attached. Those with little or no capacity to be alone (meaning that, in fact, in their "alone" experiences, they feel as if no one is internally "with them") have not had the benefit of being able to rely on the appropriate provision of external supplies for their emotional stability. They have not, therefore, internalized helpful functions of others—that is, object constancy is absent.

As is clinically known, those with a traumatic past may erect a variety of defenses against depending on others. Their unsatisfying emotional regulation strategies are often perpetuated, creating situations that reenact past dissatisfying interactions. These reenactments often contain the basic template of the original interactions, which created the insecure affect regulation strategies originally. If the environment cannot reliably provide sufficient affect regulation (e.g., soothing, praising, encouraging, comforting, advising, supporting, providing behavioral control) and the brain cannot provide these functions, then the person is at the mercy of external sources of emotional stabilization. However, others cannot be 100% reliable. If the memory systems cannot provide emotional containment much of the time and the person must rely instead on outside sources of affect regulation, instability of emotional regulation can result.

In my clinical experience I have often observed behavior that I have come to think of as "reverse object constancy." It is likely a combination of acting out, projection, and/or projective identification in which a person creates in others extremely difficult emotional states in order to be remembered. He or she is fearful of being entirely forgotten without some action on his or her part. It may be a variant form of mentalization (Allen et al., 2008). Object constancy at its most functional may serve as a protective factor against the development of problematic defensive behaviors and inner experiences. As a colleague once said, "Good enough (m)othering leads to good enough defenses" (Rachel Hanss, personal communication, 2008).

Case of Mr. Ryan

Working with case material of whatever origin (cases either orally presented or in written form, movies, literature) can be enhanced by considering the neurobiological substrata. This approach is not specific to any particular treatment theory or strategy. The atheoretical nature of the exercise of considering the case of Mr. Ryan is a good example. There are likely a variety of treatment theories appropriate for Mr. Ryan's psychological issues. Knowledge of some of the neurobiology underlying encounters between or among people may inform clinical work. When considering the case of Mr. Ryan, the list of selected functions and characteristics of the amygdala in Table 3.2 is helpful because each exchange is examined in relation to (primarily) the amygdala, but also a few of the other structures and functions mentioned in this and earlier chapters.

Mr. Ryan, a fireman, and his physician have spent some time focused on his recovery from the burns he received in a work-related fire. Mr. Ryan had been awaiting his young son's heart surgery on the day of the 9/11 tragedy, and he had extreme emotions about not being able to help in the city on that day. Later at a fire call subsequent to 9/11, he made an uncharacteristically bad decision, resulting in his own severe burn injuries. In the following transcript, doctor and patient were going over the current medical situation in some detail, beginning with a good-humored, practical, and collaborative manner between them.

TABLE 3.2
Functions and Characteristics of the Amygdala

- Plays key role in aggression, fear, and sexual arousal in males (Sapolsky, 2005, p. 139)
- Rapidly processes information, internally and externally generated, but crudely so, compared to later-maturing corticolimbic areas (Schore, 2003a, p. 236)
- Clarifies a potential threat response (Whalen, 1998)
- Greater amygdalar-dependent conditioned responses with partial reinforcement schedule than consistent threat response (Lloyd & Kling, 1991)
- Generalizes about data coming from external environment; does not as finely discriminate (like the hippocampus) (Sherry & Schacter, as cited in Cozolino, 2002, p. 97)
- Recognizes and responds to socially salient stimuli (Buchanan et al., 2009, p. 289)
- Sensitive to ambiguity or relevance (Buchanan et al., 2009, pp. 289–290)
- Predictions and expectation of behaviors of others (Cozolino, 2002, p. 94)
- Pays attention to information conveyed by the eyes (especially fear) (Buchanan et al., 2009, pp. 308–310; Vuilleumier et al., 2004)
- May modulate visual attentional processing in visual cortices before the cortical information has even reached the amygdala (Anderson & Phelps, 2001; Vuilleumier et al., 2004)
- Role in making social judgments, particularly regarding trustworthiness of faces (Buchanan et al., 2009, p. 304)
- May not only contribute something vital to social cognition, but perhaps to the modulation of all cognition (Buchanan et al., 2009, p. 312; Bowlby, 1988)
- Detection and consolidation of memory for marginally perceptible threatening facial expressions (Suslow et al., 2006, p. 1)

continued on next page

TABLE 3.2 continued

- Determines the emotional significance of threatening stimuli (Morgan & LeDoux, 1995, p. 687)

- Modulates consolidation of long-term memories of emotionally arousing experiences (flashbacks, phobias, past fears; McGaugh, as cited in Knapska et al., 2006, p. 3858; Jacobs & Nadal, as cited in Cozolino, 2002, pp. 97, 242; van der Kolk & Greenberg, 1987; LeDoux et al., 1989); the stimulus–response pairing of any event with anxiety or fear (Cozolino, 2002, p. 242); transfer of emotional information between people (amygdala to amygdala; Knapska et al., 2006, pp. 3858–3862)

- Links visual representation of face and bodily experience of emotional response to that face plus presumed emotional state of that other person (Adolphs, as cited in Buchanan et al., 2009, p. 305), leading to empathy (Buchanan et al., 2009, pp. 305–306) or "theory of mind" (attributing internal mental states, intentions, desires, and emotions to others; Baron-Cohen et al., 2000; Fine et al., 2001)

- Responds to genuine danger with signals to fight, flee, freeze, or submit as behavioral options to be instituted instantly (e.g., immediate approach–avoidance) (Cozolino, 2002, pp. 176, 181; Ogden, Minton, & Pain, 2006, pp. 4–5)

- Not a conscious processor of experiences (implicit) (Bowlby, 1969; Cozolino, 2002, p. 245)

- Role in attachment behaviors; mediates autonomic activity, particularly associated with attachment insecurity (Knapska et al., 2006, pp. 3858–3862; Lemche et al., 2006, p. 623)

DR. HAYSE: Tell me how you have been doing since last week. How is the flexibility of the new skin?

MR. RYAN: Well, I sure am not as flexible as I was, but when I don't do the treatment, I feel it.

DR. HAYSE: How often do you go to the physical therapist?

MR. RYAN: OK, OK, I missed the last two times I was supposed to go; but, Jesus, that therapist hurts me sometimes.

DR. HAYSE: Let's get back to that later. I think you know that the skin will improve with the PT treatment. Now, going on, I notice that your blood pressure was better last week than today, but it is still close to normal today. Your weight is good . . . and your other vitals are OK. How are you sleeping?

MR. RYAN: Sometimes good enough, sometimes not.

> *The encounter between the doctor and the patient at this point seems trusting, with no indication of a potential threat. The conversation is concrete and structured, not vague or ambiguous, which would <u>activate the amygdala</u>. The transfer of emotional information between the two appears a matter-of-fact exchange of medical information; the history of this doctor–patient relationship would predict that Mr. Ryan could anticipate/expect a bearable level of arousal.*

DR. HAYSE: Tell me about your moodiness, Mr. Ryan—how's that going? I've had some thoughts about ways to address that.

MR. RYAN: OK, Doc, I'm all ears. I hope you don't have some idea of using this psychoanalysis bullshit, because, it won't work on me, you know (*getting agitated and slightly belligerent, looking the doctor in the eyes*)?

> *The <u>amygdala may recognize and register socially salient stimuli</u>, such as being vigilant to a potential threat when the doctor brings up Mr. Ryan's "moodiness." <u>The amygdala tends to generalize with faint/vague data, and, because it also mediates the autonomic threat response, it can signal to fight, flee, freeze, submit, or be sexual</u> (especially in males).*
> *The patient is somewhat self-assertive, perhaps aggressive; looks directly into the doctor's eyes; and makes an assumption about the presumed motivation and emotional state of the doctor (perhaps assuming that the doctor was taking an authoritative stance with him?).*

DR. HAYSE: You know, Norris—do you mind if I call you by your first name?

> *The doctor approaches the patient on a first-name basis perhaps to counteract the defensive <u>aggression stirred up</u>; aggression is particularly registered in the amygdala.*

MR. RYAN: Uh, no, I guess. I call *you* by your first name—that would be *Doctor*, right (*wryly and with a grin*)? No, it's OK. Really. As much time as I spend talking to you and all the rest (*stops for a second and stares over the shoulder of Dr. Hayse*), it's fine. (*He then shakes himself a little, shifts around on the chair.*) Are you goin' to start actin' like a psychiatrist on me, now (*patient's voice began a bit loud, got more uninhibited and more aroused by end of statements*)?

> *The patient oscillates from a "fight" response (interrupting and taking control of the exchange) to perhaps a passive–aggressive acceptance with, "No, really, it's OK," and then to trying to talk himself into more trusting stance toward*

the doctor. The effort seems to fail, as indicated by his bodily reaction (shaking himself, shifting in chair) and ends with another challenge to his doctor, suggesting some sense of perceived danger at however low a level.

DR. HAYSE: Well, actually, Norris, I really do need to talk to you about your problems with your mood. Your wife called me again; she is still worried about you (*trying for an even and conciliatory tone of voice, even though he looks away*).

It is likely that the doctor's ANS <u>is more homeostatically balanced and coupled than the patient's</u>, with a hippocampal memory system that is finely discriminating, <u>able to consider quickly, but not too automatically reactive</u>—meaning that the doctor is not responding as if there were danger and is, in fact, trying to remain calm in the face of patient's obvious upset.

MR. RYAN: AWWW, noooo, women are worrying all the time—you gotta know that, yourself, right (*looks away*)?

The amygdala is now dealing with ambiguous data: the doctor's conciliatory tone, combined with looking away, so that the patient cannot glean information from the face and especially the eyes. Here the patient attempts to affiliate, which reflects a high-level adaptive, homeostatically balanced defense mechanism. Perhaps he is trying to calm down the agitation that may be stirred up by a distrust of what the doctor intends to recommend.

DR. HAYSE: Well, sometimes they are right, you know? (*trying for firm, but friendly tone; looks back at patient, a little authoritatively, but still role-congruent*).

The doctor's <u>amygdala may be quite sensitive to relevant information</u> coming from patient—that is, patient upset. The patient is trying to work with him in some moments, and/or maybe the doctor is trying to capitalize on past good will between them.

MR. RYAN: There you go again, listening to somebody besides me. I told you that I am OK. You are beginnin' to sound like my old man, always contradicting me on what I know about myself (*stopping again, looking out the window, shrugging his shoulders, looking down at his shoes*).

<u>The patient goes from hyperaroused</u> (verbally acting out in aggressive manner) <u>to hypoaroused</u> (dissociative? isolation of affect? blocking of affect? suppression?), <u>which can be initiated by the amygdala's deep connections to the ANS</u> (sympathetic = excitatory; parasympathetic = inhibitory). Mr. Ryan's <u>amygdalar memories</u> of his bossy father, while looking directly at the doctor (who embodies another level of authority) perhaps may be too stimulating, <u>so the amygdala may modulate visual attention by looking away.</u>

DR. HAYSE: Well, you remember when your father talked to us about your drinking too much; he was right about that, too, wasn't he? (*taking similar voice-of-authority tone as previous comment*).

MR. RYAN: See, what did I say? You're talking to my wife and my father and not me! You know, that's one of the reasons I joined emergency service, because no one can second-guess you. You have to make split-second decisions, and no time to consult a God-damned committee (*getting more agitated; starts pacing, starts to say something several times, stops, and then sits down hard on the chair*).

> *Again, there may be vascillation between the two branches of ANS: the SNS (excitatory) and the PNS (inhibitory). Mr. Ryan may have an ingrained (experience-dependent affect management style) preference for situations that invite reactivity (split-second decisions) over more hippocampal, upper limbic/cortex influenced situations that allow for a slower, more considered decision-making process (no time to consult a "God-damned committee").*

DR. HAYSE: Norris, why don't we just talk about this a little bit? You really do need to slow way down on the drinking, and you need to take the Lexapro I prescribed for you for your bad moods, nervousness, and sleeping problems. Your wife told me you were not taking the pills, is that right?

> *The doctor might be patiently, yet unconsciously, trying to engage in mutual affect regulation via his upper cortex and limbic region, suppressing his own more impulsive, reactive amygdalar responses. In so doing, a limbic-to limbic-system contact between the two of them may occur, such that the patient may calm down. In fact, he is deflated to an alarming degree, as can be seen below.*

MR. RYAN: (*Slumps down into his seat, and looks away from the doctor. The doctor is so concerned that he goes around his desk and sits in a chair closer to his patient.*)

> *The doctor's apparently empathic response, mediated by brain structures, helps the patient manage his affect by providing calming behavior; the doctor may have become alarmed by the suddenly low level of affect in his patient (PNS = inhibited behavior).*

DR. HAYSE: Norris, we need to talk about this. Can you look at me? Let us get back on track here. Norris, you are making me nervous here with how nonresponsive you are. This reminds me of how you were when you were first came into the burn unit. (*Finally, the doctor reaches over and touches Mr. Ryan on his badly scarred arm.*) Norris, I am sorry, I can see that I have really driven you far away; can you came back to this conversation and let's try this again?

The doctor seems to be trying to somewhat raise the level of the patient's affect by asking him to look in his eyes, where important information (socially salient data) may be registered—such as, for example, his confidence that the patient can get through this situation. The doctor may be trying to transfer emotional information between them, particularly (perhaps) that there is safety, not danger. On a nonconscious level, the doctor's linking together the visual representation on his own face of calm and confidence and his bodily experience of a calmer emotional response may invite the patient's body and emotional system to respond similarly.

MR. RYAN: (*at almost a whisper, head down on his chest*) Look, Doc, I am ruined. My life is over; my wife and my dad are out of it when it comes to knowing how f****d up I am. They need to just leave me alone—I can take care of myself.

The apparent withdrawal by the patient in this moment is managed by the parasympathetic branch (PNS) of the ANS. His amygdala may be signaling an inhibitory freeze or submit response (types of dissociative responses, managed by the reptilian vagal system; details can be found in Chapter 4).

DR. HAYSE: Mr. Ryan, I respect what you have done with your life. You know that I think you have punished yourself for not dying in one of those towers, too. You have, in some way, joined those men with your injuries. But you have to live for your son and wife and all the rest who love you. Personally, I feel sick about the extent of these burns; but we can better manage your psychological response. I am going out on a limb here, but you need medicine, counseling, and you need to let us help you. I am not sure how much of what I am saying you can hear right now.

Again, the doctor is trying to make emotional contact using both sides of his brain (left/logical and right/emotional) by being self-revealing and delivering a coach-like pep talk full of both encouragement and blunt truths. The doctor may be trying to overcorrect to compensate for the PNS-dominated low affect of the patient, which seems to have alarmed the doctor. The doctor is trying to dyadically regulate Mr. Ryan's affective state, which seems impenetrable at this moment. It is worrisome if Mr. Ryan's ANS remains uncoupled so that PNS-dominated behaviors become the norm.

MR. RYAN: OK, OK, OK, Doc. You made your point (*resigned but not angry*). I can see that you are trying to help, but where do my ideas come in here?

Mr. Ryan is exhibiting low affect; perhaps unconsciously he is trying for the mammalian response, which is characterized by low affect but capable of being engaged by another—in contrast to a severely withdrawn state, which is not responsive to approach (see Chapter 4 for reptilian versus mammalian responses to threat).

DR. HAYSE: Well, I hate to sound like an AA slogan, but being a drunk is just a short-term solution that will become a long-term problem, so let's get some ideas from all of us, you included, and see where to go from here, OK?

The upper limbic system and right cortex moderate strivings to be reasonable and encouraging. Mr. Ryan may now be able to invoke the attachment engagement systems of his wife and son for emotional regulation. He may be slightly more willing to follow the lead of his doctor, who mentioned his family. Perhaps the mature right-brain memory systems (e.g., hippocampus) are being utilized so that Mr. Ryan can resonate with the doctor's reasonableness. Although it is unknown which original attachment (affect regulation) strategies developed, we could guess that they might have had some elements of the excitatory insecure regulation because of Mr. Ryan's tendency toward impulsivity. With very little data and in wake of the 9/11 trauma, as well as subsequent traumas, it is difficult to determine for certain the original affect management strategies.

MR. RYAN: (*looking subdued and beaten*) OK, why don't we meet with the wife next time, OK?

Mr. Ryan may not be manifesting a reasonable stance so much as a subdued and submissive emotional posture to the doctor. The rather defeated manner may reflect the amygdala's signaling for this reaction. Some literature describes the submission response as involving both the PNS and SNS simultaneously; the external behavior shows low affect, but the internal experience is stimulated by the act of holding back action (Schore, 2003a, 2003b; Ogden et al., 2006).

DR. HAYSE: Look here, Norris, I can tell that you are down about almost everything and basically can't stand the thought of getting help. We cannot make new skin for you, but—and not to sound like a broken record—it doesn't have to be like it is right now. And next time should be this week; you are a man of action, so let's get with it here.

The doctor may be attempting an emotional transfer of information, using "look here," and he sensitively calls upon an important self state, "a man of action," as he tries to use his own arousal to ratchet up the patient's arousal. Dr. Hayse may instinctively (right amygdala) know that his patient's past fears and somewhat phobic response to returning to the fire station need vigorous addressing, in the spirit of the patient's previous (to his injury) assertive behaviors. The amygdala modulates social cognitions, and perhaps all cognitions.

MR. RYAN: Look, I know you guys are probably right—no, not probably— you *are* all right. Its just that, well, I never had to deal with everything so f*****d up; I used to be able to fix anything, no matter what, and take chances and things always turned out.

The hippocampal memory system (mature, long-term, not reactive, allows for consideration of options, unlike amygdalar memory system) *may be accessed temporarily by the patient because the doctor took on the function of remembering the patient's former self. Mr. Ryan begins lamenting circumstances, rather than his being terrible. Even though Mr. Ryan may have unconsciously tried to join his fellow fire fighters by getting himself injured due to a judgment lapse, Dr. Hayse is trying to focus him on the larger picture. This is an upper limbic and cortical function, instead of a less matured, amygdalar, reactive, self-blaming, and narrow explanation for current circumstances.*

DR. HAYSE: Well, you might look at this as the biggest challenge of your whole life and taking a chance on letting us help you; you might be taking the biggest risk here. Plus, you also were a team player—and this is just a different sort of team.

Dr. Hayse offers a homeostatically regulated view of the patient; again, the doctor recalls what the patient was like before the traumas, as in his previous comments.

MR. RYAN: Ahhhh, there you go again, Doc. You always do have a way to get people moving, don't cha? All of us patients know that you never give up. So, OK, this week it is, to meet with my wife, but don't think I like this one bit (*more upbeat than earlier in the interview*).

Mr. Ryan's limbic regions may be better able to modulate emotionally arousing experiences at the end of the interview. Perhaps by resonating with Dr. Hayse's more appropriately aroused emotions of hope and confidence, Mr. Ryan can both use support from others as well as return to a version of his team player and risk-taking self. This might be understood as an amygdala-to-amygdala transfer of emotional information and an upper-right-brain to upper-right-brain as well as left-brain to left-brain contact *(Schore, 2003b, pp. 279–281).*

Discussion of Case

As can be seen in the case of Mr. Ryan, such exchanges between people may be fraught with physiological responses to psychological and emotional experiences. In Mr. Ryan's situation, his safety–danger radar was easily stimulated by mere hints of challenge, criticism, or confrontation. When Dr. Hayse actually did confront Mr. Ryan regarding his drinking and medication noncompliance, it is speculated that Mr. Ryan's overly sensitive amygdala may have begun to override the matter-of-fact tone of the interpersonal interactions. In the first part of the interview, interactions perceived as safe by the sensitive amygdala allowed for the upper limbic system and higher cortical functions of the right brain to react in a modulated manner—for example, via bantering verbal exchanges (left brain).

As the interview progressed and Mr. Ryan became stressed, un/nonconscious mechanisms began to dominate, resulting in extreme over- and under-stimulation of his responses. His ability to put the brake (septum and other higher cortical structures involved in stopping an action) on either aggressive or submissive actions was compromised. It was not until Dr. Hayse approached emotionally and actually physically touched Mr. Ryan's scarred forearm that Mr. Ryan began to be affected by the dyadic re-regulation of his emotions. The physician's brain was responding to the abrupt inhibition of Mr. Ryan's behavior by nonconsciously attempting to, in effect, "loan" his patient his own more stabilized affect management capacities. These capacities included Dr. Hayse's clear thinking; he recognized that Mr. Ryan was a team player who was accustomed to hard challenges (a reframe of Mr. Ryan's self-assessment as "f****d up"); and holding out hope to combat the despair. All of these interventions required the physician to utilize the integrated functioning of the left and right hemispheres of his own brain.

What we cannot know is whether Mr. Ryan's emotional lability and volatility have resulted solely from recent traumas such as the severe burns and resulting physical and psychological stressors, the terrible events of 9/11, and his son's heart surgery. Additionally, Mr. Ryan's tenure as a firefighter may have also sensitized the personal emergency response system in his brain. Or, we may speculate about the existence of a preexisting affect management strategy from childhood that would have created an overly reactive personality style, exacerbated by the recent trauma. Time may tell, if Mr. Ryan takes advantage of prescribed medication, refrains from alcohol abuse, seeks psychotherapy, and continues to improve medically. What is clear is that psychotherapies that take into account his reactive amygdalar function may make an excellent contribution to improving his psychological functioning.

CHAPTER 4

Therapeutic Engagement Issues and the Vagal System

Figure 4.0.
Dynamic Patterns of Regulated and Dysregulated Autonomic Arousal

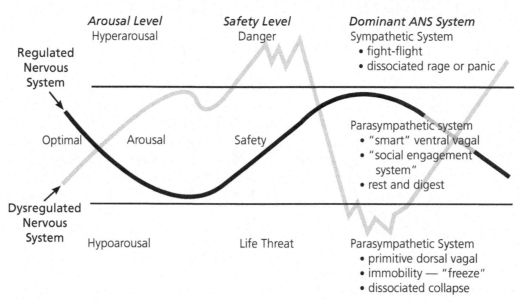

(J. Wheatley-Crosby, based on Porges, 1997, as adapted in Fosha, Siegel, and Solomon, 2009)

This chapter contains an overview of the polyvagal theory, as proposed by Stephen W. Porges. The vagal system, including its location and the brain structures closely involved with the vagus nerve, is examined as well as potential problems that may occur when the vagal system is compromised. Porges's concept of the term *neuroception*, which he coined, is discussed. Neuroception—ways that perception engages and affects neural regulation—is involved in the following behaviors: social engagement, mobilization of fight–flight, play and foreplay, immobilization due to life threat, and immobilization without fear (Porges, as cited in Fosha et al., 2009, p. 53).

Overview of the Polyvagal Theory and the Vagal System

The polyvagal theory (Porges, 2001, 2003, 2004, 2007, 2011) challenges the long-held description of the autonomic nervous system as a stress management system that only balances the functions of the two main branches of the sympathetic nervous system (excitatory) and the parasympathetic nervous system (inhibitory), as described in Chapter 2. Porges suggests that, although most organs are affected by both the sympathetic and parasympathetic nervous systems, often overlooked when describing autonomic nervous system functioning is a description of the role of vagal circuitry in adaptive reactions to stress (2011, pp. 262–263):

> Functionally, in humans the older vagal circuit is involved in adaptive reactions characterized by immobilization and decreases in metabolic output, while the newer vagal circuit is involved in regulating the calm states that promote both spontaneous social engagement behaviors and health, growth, and restoration. (Porges, as cited in Fosha et al., 2009, p. 36)

In other words, the evolutionarily older vagal branch "shuts down" behavior in the face of life threat, so much so that social interaction is not possible. The evolutionarily newer vagal branch, while also inhibiting behaviors, preserves the capacity to socially interact. However, "if the vagal brake is not efficiently working (doesn't get removed in response to various features in the environment or during specific interactions), the 'reactivity' may appear to be blunted" (Porges, personal communication, March 15, 2012).

Over the course of time, animals, including human beings, build new brain functions and neural mechanisms, while often preserving older ones. Depending on the situation, any of the neural mechanisms can be activated. The vagal system is involved in social engagement, mobilization, and immobilization. In the case of accumulated stress or trauma, perhaps some of the neural structures may become overused. The autonomic nervous system is one of those systems; how the autonomic nervous system reacts to stress and other challenges is affected by the layering of the new functions upon the old. Stress and trauma may compromise this hierarchical process of moving from the newest (evolutionarily) layer to each succeeding older circuit to manage stress. Brain structures (e.g., the amygdala) that have become oversensitized to danger may overinterpret events in favor of assuming danger when most brains would not. These oversensitized brains may, in fact, too quickly engage the dorsal vagal system (the older circuitry), resulting in a severely inhibited (PNS) unresponsive state.

In the face of stress, the brain will first utilize a newer circuit (in this case, the myelinated vagus, also called the *ventral vagal* or *mammalian response*) to meet a challenge in a calm manner (parasympathetic branch of autonomic nervous system), overriding the older circuits (Porges, 2011, pp. 159–164; Schore, as cited in Fosha et al., 2009, pp. 120–121). Porges describes the mechanisms of the vagal in the following way (paraphrased from Porges, as cited in Fosha et al., 2009, pp. 27–54): The myelinated (ventral) vagal influence can be withdrawn, leaving the SNS activated. If the ventral vagal cannot manage the stress, the second oldest circuitry responsible for stress management will be automatically engaged: the SNS. A failure in that strategy (i.e., the SNS's excitatory functions of fight or flight) will also automatically invite the default circuitry, the unmyelinated (dorsal) vagus, which is the oldest circuit. Also managed by the PNS, the older dorsal vagal will essentially "freeze" or immobilize behavior (in a "reptilian" fashion), making social interaction impossible, and therefore thwarting the possibility that another person might assist with the stress management of the situation. According to Porges, it is possible that an additional immobilization experience may occur. "Outbursts and rage (high sympathetic excitation with a total removal of the vagal brake) that people often exhibit in situations in which they will not be injured (e.g., temper tantrums) may trigger a rebound that might be characterized by 'immobilization without fear.' . . . This may be a calmness recruiting the old vagal circuit, and this maladaptive behavior may be a mechanism to calm!" (personal communication, March 15, 2012; emphasis per Porges).

The detection of, and reaction to, both safety and danger are mediated by a feedback loop between the brain and the central nervous system's connections to peripheral organs (Porges, 2009, p. 27). The peripheral organs are those outside the brain, including the skin, the largest organ of the body. According to Porges:

> The primary parasympathetic influence to peripheral organs is conveyed through the vagus, a cranial nerve that exits the brain and innervates the gastrointentinal tract, respiratory tract, heart and abdominal viscera. The vagus can be conceptualized as a tube or conduit containing several sensory and motor fibers originating or terminating in different areas of the brainstem. For example, the vagal motor pathways that regulate the lower gut originate in the dorsal nucleus of the vagus; the vagal pathways that regulate the heart and lungs originate in the nucleus ambiguous; and the vagal pathways sending sensory information from the gut terminate in the nucleus of the solitary tract. (as cited in Fosha et al., 2009, p. 35)

In his polyvagal theory Porges (as cited in Fosha et al., 2009) identifies three response systems:

1. Cranial nerves to regulate the face and to mediate calm autonomic and behavioral states
2. Sympathetic adrenal system to increase metabolic output
3. An inhibitory vagal system to decrease metabolic output and promote freezing and defecation.

The heart–face–brain communication is a good example of mutually influenced affective processes (Porges, 2009, pp. 28–29). Also, facial muscles affect the state of the brain, which in turn affects the viscera (Gellhorn, 1964). Porges makes the case that, in place of the excitatory SNS and thus the adrenal system being activated in reaction to stress, rather the "vagal brake" is released (as cited in Fosha et al., 2009, pp. 36–38). This release of the vagal brake promotes temporary mobilization and arousal; this is a better "first responder" plan to stress than activating the SNS. Porges states that the organismic cost of high excitation is at least temporarily avoided (as cited in Fosha et al., 2009, pp. 36–38). An additional consideration is the following: "A nervous system that has experienced noncontingent interactions, abuse, and trauma may go into a conservative defense mode even when the features of the person are dangerous, which could be the result of removing the vagal brake in inappropriate situations with 'faulty neuroception'" (Porges, personal communication, March 15, 2012).

What Can Affect the Vagus Nerve?

One key idea is that mutual gaze affects the heart via the vagal nerve. In evolutionary terms, the development of autonomic regulation made possible the signaling of other brains regarding safety–danger while simultaneously mobilizing via deactivation of the vagal brake. This increased ability to "multitask," so to speak, permitted energy conservation (by not activating the SNS and HPA axis—i.e., the mammalian stress response; Tarulla & Gunnar, 2006, p. 1). This integration of functions of the heart–face–brain intimately involves the data that are conveyed by mutual gaze.

Face-to-face transactions between caretaker and infant set the stage for the quality of signaling that will occur regarding all manner of information, such as safety–danger, playfulness, and the presence or absence of acceptance, rejection, pleasure, curiosity, and interest. The significance of face-to-face interaction has become increasingly clear with the contributions of Stern (1977, 1985); Beebe and Lachmann (1994); Leucken and Lemery (2004); Tronick (1989, 2007); and Trevarthen (1993a), all of whom focus on the meaning and the microregulation of arousal between caregiver and infant.

The social engagement behaviors studied by Porges (2011) have demonstrated the relationship between the vagal regulation of the heart and social engagement behaviors such as affect regulation, spontaneous social behavior, social awareness, affect expressivity, prosody, and language development.

One potential problem of a compromised vagal system is a greater dependence on the SNS for activation, leading to physical and mental health risks. Should the ventral vagus be compromised, the social engagement system would be severely affected. A compromised social engagement may be the result of differences in behavioral state regulation and a loss of neural regulation to the muscles of the face, mediating the flat affective expression often observed in several clinical disorders. The removal of the regulatory influence of the ventral vagus on the heart potentiates (i.e., disinhibits) the expression of the two phylogenetically older neural systems: the SNS and the dorsal vagus. Porges explains:

> If the vagal brake is not functioning, there is the potential for greater dependence on the sympathetic excitation of the cardiovascular system. This dependence on sympathetic excitation to regulate (i.e., cardiac output) may create health risks (e.g., hypertension) and lead to difficulties in modulating behavioral state (i.e., rage, panic, aggression). . . . The vagal brake contributes to the modulation of cardiac output by decreasing or increasing the inhibitory vagal control of the heart to influence rate and thereby adjust metabolic resources to support either mobilization or social engagement behaviors. (as cited in Fosha et al., 2009, p. 41)

In addition, Porges described certain psychiatric disorders that can have specific deficits in both the "somatomotor (e.g., poor gaze, low facial affect, lack of prosody, difficulties in mastication) and visceromotor (difficulties in autonomic regulation resulting in cardiopulmonary and digestive problems) components of the Social Engagement System . . . having a similar depressed social engagement system" resulting in "poor affect regulation, poor affect recognition, and poor physiological state regulation" (as cited in Fosha et al., 2009, p. 46).

Neuroception

Feature detectors and *defensive circuits* are nonconscious, noncognitive risk evaluation processes that determine whether or not to turn on the social engagement system. The term *neuroception* was introduced by Porges in 2003 to capture these nonconscious and noncognitive experiences in the brain, which process "sensory information from the environment and from the viscera, continuously evaluating risk" (Porges, as cited in Fosha et al., 2009, p. 45). It is suggested that neuroception may involve "feature detectors" in the brain responsible for assessing voices, hand gestures, and facial expressions, thereby providing data with which to distinguish between safety and danger and consequently influencing limbic reactivity (especially the amygdala).

If the brain cannot reliably assess safe versus dangerous conditions/situations and mistakes safety for danger or mistakes danger for safety, then it is likely that defensive circuits will be activated and the social engagement system will not be activated. According to Porges, the social engagement system is activated "only when these defensive circuits are inhibited" (as cited in Fosha et al., 2009, p. 46). The implication of this process is that over- or underreactivity of the defensive system determines whether the behavior is adaptive and contextually driven or maladaptive. Additionally, the body's physiology will also determine how responsive an individual may be to safety versus danger in the milieu. For example, a friendly overture may not be met with engagement if the body is in "freeze" mode. A different example (of sudden state change) occurred when I was driving with my 3-month-old granddaughter in the back seat with her mother beside her. The baby was looking at her mother and was content. Suddenly the baby started crying, very distressed. Her mother did her best to comfort her, but could not pick her up as we were on the highway and she had to remain in the infant seat for safety reasons. A few miles later, the baby instantly stopped crying when her mother took off her oversized sunglasses and looked at her baby, holding her gaze. We speculated that the blocked view of the mother's upper face, which contains information about safety–danger via mutual gaze, created a frightening situation for which the still-developing feature detectors in the baby's brain had no soothing data to process. In the absence of such information, the baby signaled distress in the only way she could: by painful crying.

Some areas of the periaqueductal gray (PAG) "regulate flight, fight, or freeze behaviors and the autonomic states that support these behaviors" (Porges, as cited in Fosha et al., 2009, p. 46). In fact, excitation of the ventrolateral periaqueductal gray (vlPAG) "evokes a passive reaction of immobility, a drop in blood pressure, and a slowing of heart rate . . . which evokes an opioid-mediated analgesia that might adaptively raise pain thresholds and promote the dissociated states that are frequently reported by trauma victims," also known as freeze behaviors (Porges, as cited in Fosha et al., 2009, p. 47). Fight behaviors are elicited by stimulating "rostrally within the lateral and dorsolateral PAG," and flight behaviors are elicited by stimulating "caudally within the lateral PAG and dorsolateral PAG" (Porges, as cited in Fosha et al., 2009, p. 47). Additionally, the insula, which mediates bodily state, may also be involved with neuroception (Porges, as cited in Fosha et al., 2009, p. 48).

Perceiving the difference between aggression and play is critical, for obvious reasons. There are situations in which both sympathetic activation and vagal deactivation are operating simultaneously, such as in play and sexual foreplay/activity. In contrast, in aggression, the SNS fight response is activated with limited or no PNS or vagal braking occurring. According to Porges, "if face-to-face engagement occurs rapidly with the appropriate features of concern and empathy, then the physiological state that was driven by the physical contact is evaluated for intentionality and diffused with the appropriate cues between two persons' Social Engagement Systems involved in the exchange" (Porges, as cited in Fosha et al., 2009, pp. 51–52).

Discussion and Examples of Compromised Neuroception

Personality organizations contribute to physiological states that severely affect the functioning of feature detectors, neuroception, and the social engagement system. We discuss these personality organizations in greater detail in the next chapter, but for now, consider this overview. In terms of severity, the kind of anger expression varies with certain diagnoses (Schore, 2003a, pp. 298–303), which I believe can be grouped broadly along a continuum:

PTSD $\longrightarrow$ BPD $\longrightarrow$ APD $\longrightarrow$ NPD $\longrightarrow$ Psychopathy

These personality organizations vascillate between extremes of high sympathetic arousal and to extremely low parasympathetic shutdown. However, the types of anger and aggression move in this direction (from left to right):

Hot, impulsive, volatile $\longrightarrow$ to cool, cold, predatory,
anger/rage aggression   stalking, calculated aggression

Or, the short version:

SNS (fight, flight) $\longrightarrow$ PNS/vagal (calm, freeze)

The ability to determine intentionality, read social cues, and assess safety–danger by individuals with personality disorders or personalities with such tendencies, as briefly listed below, is compromised by their hypo-/hyperreactivity. which affects their defensive circuits.

• PTSD (posttraumatic stress disorder): Characterized by the reexperiencing of an extremely traumatic event (or events) accompanied by symptoms of <u>increased arousal</u> and by <u>avoidance</u> of stimuli associated with the trauma (American Psychiatric Association, 2000, p. 429).

• BPD (borderline personality disorder): Pattern of instability in interpersonal relationships, self-image, and affects and marked <u>impulsivity</u> (American Psychiatric Association, 2000, p. 685); chronic feelings of emptiness and severe <u>dissociative symptoms</u> (American Psychiatric Association, 2000, p. 710).

• NPD (narcissistic personality disorder): Pattern of grandiosity, need for admiration, and <u>lack of empathy</u> (American Psychiatric Association, 2000, p. 685) and can be interpersonally <u>exploitative</u> (American Psychiatric Association, 2000, p. 717).

• APD (antisocial personality disorder): Pattern of disregard for, and <u>violation</u> of, the rights of others (American Psychiatric Association, 20000, p. 685); <u>lack of remorse and indifference</u> to pain of others (American Psychiatric Association, 2000, p. 706).

• Psychopathy: Absence of relational capacity to bond with others coupled with inordinate amount of <u>aggression</u> (Meloy, 1988, p. 5); <u>autonomic hyporeactivity</u> and lowered CNS arousal interspersed with sensation-seeking (Meloy, pp. 30, 38)

What constitutes a threat varies according to the personality organization. If tracking the neural substrates of different types of aggression, there may be a continuum of sorts from PTSD, borderline personality disorder (BPD), to narcissistic personality disorder (NPD), to antisocial personality disorder (APD), to psychopathy. Gacano (2000) and Meloy (1988) have argued that psychopathy should not be considered the same condition as APD, citing differing physiological responses. The psychopath has a low reactivity, including attenuated startle response, which is unlike the response in people with APD, as described by each criteria for APD (activated states and behaviors that are quite aggressive—for example, impulsivity, reckless disregard for safety, irritability and aggressiveness, and so on) (see American Psychiatric Association, 2000, p. 706). However, if a psychopath is humiliated or thwarted in his or her predatory pursuits, he or she can become rageful and vengeful. Interestingly, low heart rate is found in only one psychiatric disorder, according to Schore (2003b), which is antisocial personality, known for unmodulated aggression. I have trouble reconciling the low heart rate with the criteria of the impulsive behaviors (as described by the American Psychiatric Association 2000, p. 706), unless the defense mechanisms employed to remain in the low affect state fail, and the affect (e.g., rage) becomes uncontrollable (see Chapter 3 for details on this speculation about arousal management).

Psychopathy is not, as yet, an actual diagnosis in the current volume of the American Psychiatric Association (2000), so there is a problem in trying to compare other conditions with a condition not in the standard nomenclature (although psychopathy is slated to be included in the DSM-5, due in 2013). However, I am wondering if there are at least two types of APD behaviors: one that is more like BPD and PTSD with the impulsive volatility, rage, and aggression, and a type that is more like NPD and the psychopathic personality type, with the cold, stalking, calculating, and predatory expressions of their aggression.

It may be that the extremely calloused antisocial personality organization and psychopathic personality organization have in common a type of compromised right-brain development, leading to a diminished emotional response, including expressions of anger, unless their manipulations or coercions are unsuccessful (bearing in mind that there may be some constitutional influences and /or neurological trauma contributing to this personality organization). Narcissistic personality organization could be thought of as a milder form of the low-affect reactivity and expression of both the "cooler" form of antisocial personality organization as well as the psychopathic organization. Though the narcissistic organization can express hot rage, in fact, most of the defensive maneuvers characteristic of this organization are dedicated to staying cool, aloof, at a remove from others, generally raging only when others do not do what these individuals want, and/or when they are humiliated. (See Raine et al., 2004, regarding the role of hippocampal asymmetry in unsuccessful psychopaths.)

Steuerwald and Kosson made the point that it is untrue that psychopaths are unempathic; in fact, they are quite empathic (as cited in Gacano, 2000, pp. 111–135). Porges (as cited in Fosha et al., 2009; Porges, 2011) may describe that process as "neuroception," whereas in the case of psychopaths, they easily discern what matters to others and take advantage of such information to further their own ends. What does not seem to matter to a psychopath is the other person's experience of being mistreated, or worse. On the other hand, borderline personality organization and perhaps some of the "hotter," more rageful antisocial personality organizations are hypervigilant and hyperreactive to threats of loss, abandonment, need fulfillment, or lack of connection. This may, in part, be the result of an overactive amygdala combined with the amygdala's special role in the social judgment of faces, which can bring about the misjudgment of the degree of threat (i.e., compromised neuroception).

Schore (2003a, p. 294) suggested that the imprinting of aggressive faces compromises the decoding of facial patterns (unmodulated fusiform gyri interacting with the amygdala). What likely occurs with overattribution of threat is, in part, "both a right amygdalocortical excitatory process as well as prefrontal inhibitory influences" (Peper & Karcher, as cited in Schore, 2003a, p. 294). Neuroception would therefore be tilted in the direction of a nonconscious, noncognitive, low-threshold perception of threat. In other words, the gas is on and the brake is off, as impaired judgment regarding actual threat stimulates a response that is generally inappropriate to the situation, to an outside observer. For example, I once observed a role-play demonstration in which the leader touched one of the participants on the upper shoulder as the group was circling chairs around and getting settled. The touch was light but clearly unexpected. The group member shuddered violently, making me wonder later if the person had an easily activated startle response, as the shudder was inappropriate to the situation.

Determining threat is learned early in life, as the (m)other helps the brain of the infant to appraise danger in the environment, thereby affecting survival (Schore, 2003a; Cole, 1987). In another example, recently a staff member at the university where I teach had to bring her 7-month-old child to work with her one day. As I passed the counter where Jasmine and her mother, Diana, were sitting, both looking over the counter (Jasmine, in her infant seat), I smiled and said, "Hello, Jasmine, how are you?" Jasmine looked at me with totally blank black eyes. Diana said, looking sweetly at Jasmine and then at me, "Say hello to Arlene." The baby looked at her mother intently and when she looked back at me, she gave me a huge smile that went all over her face. This seemed to be an instance where the learning of neuroception was occurring via the appraisal system between mother and infant (facilitated by mutual gaze).

One suggestion regarding how the arousal system may become compromised relates to extreme disturbances in emotion-modulating attachment experiences and little or no interactive repair. This brain does not have available (via the ministrations of another brain) a way to rebalance itself (meaning, it stays in an intolerably high or low state of arousal or some rapidly oscillating combination of high–low effect). That being the case, the brain may repeatedly enter states of toxic chemistry, leading to cell death (high levels of glutamate and cortisol can alter the development of the limbic system, responsible for arousal states—particularly harmful during growth periods of the neuronal system; Schore, 2003a, pp. 116–119). A related finding is that individuals with sociopathic behavior caused by frontal damage do not respond autonomically to social stimuli (Damasio, Tranel, & Damasio, 1990). Additionally, Schore details other possible sources of increased levels of aggression (2003a, see Chapter 9), including the following: various insults to critical periods of right-brain development, right-brain destruction in mid-pregnancy, birth insult and stress interacting and impairing later stress regulation, impaired olfactory contributions to proto-attachment communication, shaken infant syndrome, and high levels of maternal anger and "harsh touch" in infancy.

The Case of Baby Ruth

Baby Ruth is a 33-year-old man hospitalized at the Heart Hospital and under guard by prison officials at all times. He is a witness in a federal case, which is the only reason that he is receiving such excellent medical care for a heart valve problem that could have gone untreated, if left up to prison authorities. The psychiatrist has been consulted to treat Baby Ruth for any major mental illness that he might have, so that his medication can be coordinated and he can be as creditable a witness as possible.

Dr. Baca discovered that his patient had very low blood pressure and seemed unusually calm, polite, and intelligent, considering every sentence before speaking. No topic seemed to agitate him or change his expression too much. From the extensive history, Dr. Baca was told quite matter-of-factly by Baby Ruth that he had not finished the eighth grade because he had been so disruptive and played such cruel "pranks" on the "kids who rode the short bus," and that the final straw for school officials was when he set fire to the new band hall and blamed it on one of the students who was a "gimp with a limp."

Baby Ruth's calm, matter-of-fact manner could be the result of a low baseline autonomic activity, as with psychopathy, maintained by the parasympathetic nervous system or even the vagal system. His social engagement system, though calm, may in fact signal danger to a normative social engagement system, such as Dr. Baca's, because Baby Ruth's demeanor did not match the disturbing content he was relating (isolation of affect, dissociation, blocking of affect?). The goal of a social engagement system is to promote social interactions and reduce psychological distance, neither of which was invited by the disparity between affect and content in Baby Ruth's demeanor.

The other student was so mentally compromised and therefore unable to explain himself that Baby Ruth would have gotten away with the crime except that a girl finally told on him—"the bitch," he said calmly. Baby Ruth later keyed the van of the girl's grandfather with whom the girl lived, and would have been more destructive, except that he was caught by a neighbor.

Baby Ruth's type of anger and aggression was cool, cold, predatory, and calculated.

This incident set into motion a chain of events that resulted in a series of placements in foster homes. Baby Ruth was incarcerated in the juvenile justice system for increasingly more complicated crimes, including selling alcohol to middle school children and stealing cars from long-term parking at the hospital and selling them to "chop-shops" in a nearby city. Finally, just after his 18th birthday he was caught with a large amount of methamphetamine, a small amount of cocaine, and drug paraphernalia. Even for this he did not receive the maximum sentence, because of his young and innocent looks and his ability to pass polygraph tests. He told Dr. Baca that lying was nothing to him and that he never could understand what the "big deal" was.

The vengeful, calculated behavior (burning down the band hall, blaming a mentally challenged fellow student, keying the van, selling alcohol to 12- and 13-year-old students, stealing cars) seemed to be the cold, predatory, aggression more moderated by the parasympathetic nervous system and the vagal system, perhaps not to "freeze" proportions, but a quite diminished emotional response. Baby Ruth may have the low heart rate found in the more calculating of the antisocial personality organizations. He may provide a good example of the empathy (as described by Gacano, 2000) of which a psychopath is capable, in that he knew that the grandfather would be upset over his van being keyed, and he knew that a challenged student might be a logical suspect to blame for the burning of the band hall, or he would not have performed acts which were so upsetting. He did not care that they were upset; what he cared about was that he was doing what he wanted to do (enacting "cool" predatory revenge). Though these acts were aggressive, they do not have the quality of the "hot" anger (mediated by the SNS).

Baby Ruth explained to Dr. Baca that he got his name from the fact that he lived on Baby Ruth candy bars and 7-11 hot dogs and burritos when he lived with his mother and sister in a run-down trailer park. The only time that Dr. Baca saw any emotion was during a procedure that a nurse was administering, when the hospital gown fell off his back and Dr. Baca asked about the pebbly condition of the skin. For a moment, Baby Ruth seemed to flare up such that the guard moved a little closer. Then Baby Ruth casually said that his mother's boyfriend used to burn him and his sister with his cigarettes on their backs so no one at the school would ever see.

> The sudden and unexpected display of his cigarette burn scars made Baby Ruth briefly flare up with anger/rage, perhaps in response to feeling humiliated by the exposure. This is in contrast to his blithe reporting of his own cruel acts as a child and adolescent, to which he had little emotional reactivity. Perhaps he was displaying a shame/humiliation reaction, which would engage the excitatory system (sympathetic nervous system) instantly, followed by the counterregulation of the inhibitory parasympathetic nervous system (Schore, 2003b). It also may be that there was no release of the vagal brake, which would promote social interaction and engagement in a calm manner.

Baby Ruth lived next door to a "kid who took Ritalin" so Baby Ruth started learning about the symptoms. Soon he had convinced the school nurse to refer him to a doctor. His mother was not in agreement, but he bullied her into making sure that he had medication for his new diagnosis of ADHD (attention-deficit/ hyperactivity disorder). Though Baby Ruth could not read well, suggesting the possibility of a learning disorder or of ADHD, he told Dr. Baca that he had made up the ADHD symptoms.

The only reason that he stayed in school as long as he did was for the extra time and attention he received from teachers in the math and computer classes. He hacked into the school's computer system and, for a while, was a stellar student, if his report cards were any indication. For money, he changed the grades of some of the "lazy, rich fools" who were under pressure from parents to make good grades for college.

At the end of eighth grade, in the foster home where he was home-schooled, he learned about books on tape. He had been removed from his mother's home and from the regular public school system. In lieu of being mandated into an alternative school for students with serious delinquent behavior, he was placed in a foster home that did not believe in the public school system. He became obsessed with the audio tapes and listened to his foster parents' tapes for the next 2 years, then to the public library's extensive collection. He seemed to be quite educated, despite his lack of formal schooling.

> From the history of Baby Ruth's discipline, dedication to his education, and planning, anticipation, and organizational skills, it can be seen that he is not the impulsive, out-of-control APD type, nor, of course, ADHD.

Baby Ruth, despite his boyish looks and small frame, never had much trouble in the prison population, though small and young (age 21 when first incarcerated, after serving a few years for drug charges and fraud at a microchip company, where he insinuated himself into an opportunity to have access to computers); typically prisoners who are small face additional battles. He had a reputation for being sly and vicious. Though nonconfrontational by nature, he was reputed to have engineered the death of one inmate and had somehow been involved in the bizarre "suicide" of another inmate.

Baby Ruth's "dead calm" demeanor seemed to instill fear even in imprisoned criminals. Perhaps this is an example of Porges's concept of neuroception, whereby other prisoners' nonconscious/noncognitive processing of Baby Ruth as a threat was occurring outside of their awareness. Mobilization of the "fight" behavior, in the face of constant danger in prison, may have lead to his establishing himself as a danger to others (even in the prison population) to protect himself. It may be speculated that perhaps the immobilization of the life threat state—which is characterized by a reduction in metabolic output and shutdown behaviors; mediated by vagal circuit; and potentially (indeed) life-threatening (Porges, 2009, p. 53)—may have contributed to the "dead calm" demeanor that is "reptilian-like" and a signal to others that there is no mercy in this type of personality.

Baby Ruth had left a halfway house where he was paroled. He was only apprehended because he passed out at a Walmart and was rushed to the hospital, unconscious. He was in a diabetic coma for a few days. As he had several forms of identification in his wallet, the police were involved, his identity discovered, and he was arrested. However, the FBI wanted to make a deal with him for a reduced sentence because many employees of the microchip companies where he had worked had been involved in financial scams, and the authorities were having trouble getting information to make some of their cases.

A psychologist from the Criminal Profile Unit of the FBI was assigned to take some information from Mr. Ruth to help determine whether or not the government would actually try to work with him or determine whether he would also be prosecuted "to the fullest extent of the law"—as he told his father, winking and mocking the official language of one of the agents. He told his family that they could talk about his past to the "feds, those assholes," as far as they knew it.

One of the challenges to the mental health evaluation and to the justice system's use of a character style such as Baby Ruth is in his severely flawed social engagement system. Normatively, face-to-face interaction between a child and caretaker will set the stage for signaling both for information needed for survival (safety–danger) and for quality of life (curiosity, playful-ness, soothing, etc.). In Baby Ruth's case, it may have been that he was left to manage his emotional life by himself from early childhood. This may have led to a compromised capacity to find emotional comfort in others. Toxic processes (*pruning of neural circuitry* necessary for attachment-related behav-iors; Schore, 2003a, pp. 118–120) can occur in the brain of the developing child. This pruning will preserve, as in Baby Ruth's case, the poorly connected but superficially charming, manipulative, low reactivity to all but those circum-stances that have personal meaning only to him. It could also be that Baby Ruth exists in a rather chronic dissociative state, punctuated only by flashes of rage, when he is thwarted in his selfish goals. This could be the result of the activation of the vlPAG, which mediates immobility, a drop in blood pressure, and a slowing of heart rate—which in turn activate an opioid-mediated anal-gesia that might adaptively raise pain thresholds and promote the dissociated state (Porges, 2011, pp. 195–196).

The Case of Bebe

Bebe is a chemist working in the technology industry, the only female on her team. All her life she has had to contend with people underesti-mating everything about her, especially men. Many made assumptions about her intellect and potential based on her diminutive stature and strikingly beautiful looks, inherited from her mother, an immigrant from Central America who found work as a domestic and was paid in cash. Her employers were a family in South Texas who did not have to observe the laws about hiring "illegals" and so kept many families who worked for them on their large ranch over the generations.

It was assumed that Bebe would work in the business part of the ranch as her academic achievement in math and science in high school was remarkable, given that she was "just a Mexican girl from the ranch." In fact, she received "a full ride," as she said, to a major Texas university, where she earned a degree in chemical engineering, gradu-ating cum laude. She received scholarships for her doctoral work at a top-tier university where she studied chemistry, co-oping in the micro-chip industry where she works today, 10 years later. At various points in her education, her mother's employers offered to help pay for her expenses, but she flatly refused, grateful that she did not need their money. She always vowed to take nothing from them.

Bebe's mother was hurt by her "ungrateful and disrespectful" at-titude and did not understand it at all, since she felt saved by her em-ployers from the dangerous experiences in Central America that she had endured. However, her mother could give only occasional hints about what happened to her as she tried to make her way across several countries to come to America. Bebe came to her first session with the goal in mind to "do something about my passivity with certain types of men."

THERAPIST: What do you mean, "certain types of men," Dr. Villareal?

BEBE: Oh, please, call me *Bebe*. We are about the same age and that sounds way too formal, like something my mother would insist on. Unless you mind if I call you *Kaye*?

THERAPIST: That is fine with me. So, getting back to the reason for your visit . . . ?

> *It seemed that Bebe's social engagement system (promotes positive social interactions, reduces psychological distance, and promotes a sense of safety between people) was working well as the session began, though the tone of voice would be important to know, as Bebe may have been a little testy, sarcastic, etc. There is no way to know, but initially, she seemed to engage with a minimum of guardedness.*

BEBE: (*interrupting*) Yeah, right, well, the deal is, I have always had trouble with people, mostly men pushing me around, getting me to take second authorship, caving in to, well, you know, hitting on me, etc.

THERAPIST: What is "etcetera"?

BEBE: What *etc.* means is that I can*not* take up for myself, cannot be assertive, never mind aggressive—I am spineless in certain situations. Look at my mother, coming through Mexico with those coyotes, those bastards! (*looking hard at the therapist*) Do you know what coyotes are?

> *Bebe was looking hard at the therapist: Mutual gaze and face-to-face transactions set the stage for the quality of signaling safety–danger, playfulness, and a variety of kinds of emotional information. Also conveyed are levels of arousal between two people. The heart–face–brain connection is driven by vagal regulation of the heart, which affects social engagement behaviors (e.g., affect regulation, spontaneous social behavior, social awareness, affect expressivity, prosody).*
>
> *Bebe may be checking out something about the therapist, such as, does the therapist actually know something factual (cognitive knowledge)? In addition, feature detectors in the brain, responsible for assessing voices, hand gestures, and facial expressions for safety–danger, contribute to neuroception, which is the processing of sensory information both from the environment and from the body to evaluate risk. The question about "coyotes" may*

have been a sort of test helping Bebe to assess threat with the <u>nonconscious/</u> <u>noncognitive parts of her brain</u>.

THERAPIST: (*thankful and relieved that she did know; feeling that this was some sort of test*) Yes, they are paid to get people across the river into Texas or Arizona without the border patrol catching them and sending them back over the border or locking them up. But people suffer at the hands of the *coyote*; losing everything, from their money and possessions to their lives, because the *coyotes* only care about the money, if the stories are true that I've heard.

The therapist's feeling thankful and relieved may have been energized by the mobilization function of the <u>sympathetic nervous system</u>, which is activating and arousing, perhaps making the therapist more alert and vigilant to needs of the client. The clinician was thankful and relieved that she did know about coyotes, though perhaps activated by a lower affective (<u>parasympathetic</u> <u>nervous system</u>) experience. It is difficult to know if thankful and relieved are low- or high-affect experiences; it could be either.

BEBE: (*a bit sternly*) What are you writing down on that notepad?

THERAPIST: (*Thrown off balance for a second, thinking that Bebe would respond to comments sketching out her bare knowledge of coyotes; then instantly worried that she had talked too much about what little she knew regarding crossing the U.S. border*) Oh! Well, as we discussed earlier, I am taking notes, more now than in later sessions. Often, I need to write down facts, dates, etc., at the beginning as a person talks about their personal history—not so much later on.

The therapist clearly was pressured in her speech and not calm. She was a bit too talkative and <u>anxious in her behavior (all activated by the sympathetic</u> <u>nervous system, not the release of the vagal brake, which would be the</u> <u>conservation of energy)</u>. <u>Neuroception</u> may have been occurring between therapist and client with levels of arousal beginning to be matched.

BEBE: Oh. OK, I guess (*looking distracted and unfocused a bit*).

Perhaps Bebe was somewhat dissociated, having created in the therapist her own (Bebe's) perhaps <u>intolerable level of sympathetic arousal</u> (the process begin- ning with the coyote question). Once the therapist had empathically resonated with Bebe's level of arousal and had begun to experience Bebe's affects and their intensity as her own, <u>then Bebe may have "cleansed"</u> (Schore, 2003b, pp. 58–107) <u>her mind of the arousal, via projective identification and dissociation</u>.

THERAPIST: (*feeling anxious that some thread had been lost in the session*) And as I mentioned, a complete copy of this record is yours at any time, but the original is permanently kept in my files

Again, the therapist may have been emotionally aroused *(sympathetic nervous system), as she kept chattering on about the record-keeping.*

BEBE: Oh, I see (looking bored and puzzled).

Again, Bebe may have been in a state of low affect *(parasympathetic nervous system or perhaps, release of the vagal brake); maybe some kind of mild immobilization. The clinician may not have been able to tell if it was immobilization without fear or immobilization with life threat—or if it was immobilization at all and not just parasympathetic nervous system driven calm. The* "bored and puzzled look" *did not have the feel of a calm, parasympathetic nervous system activated, socially engaged state, however.*

THERAPIST: (*Making herself stop and concentrate on something of substance, trying to get back to the focus that preceded what seemed like a derailment; then deciding to focus on the derailment itself, thinking, "might as well go for it because I don't know what else to do."*) Bebe, did you notice how we got off track somehow in this discussion? Thinking back, I thought we were about to talk about your wish to be more forceful in certain situations, and somehow we got sidetracked. What was your experience (*knows that her wording was too stilted and proper a way to phrase the question*)?

A mutual regulatory system of arousal *may have been occurring, with the therapist trying to regulate her too high level of arousal to somewhat try to match Bebe's low affect (bored and puzzled).*

BEBE: (*more energetic and engaged*) Yeah, yeah. I guess I can see what you are saying. Though I have great concentration in science and at work, I swear to God (*emphatically*), sometimes in ordinary conversation, I lose it; I don't even know what was said by me *or* the other person. Once, at grad school, I made a perfect score on a ceramics exam. No one had ever ever done that before. The prof was a known asshole, just trying to get the students; rumor has it that no one has made a score like that since then, but I'm not really sure of that. Sure glad I learned that because that is what I do every day.

Bebe has become more emotionally aroused. Was the vagal brake released? Or is this sympathetic activation?

THERAPIST: (*Has no idea what she is talking about regarding the work, but decides not to ask for fear of getting off track again.*) So, Bebe, you are saying maybe that we got off track just like what can happen with social conversation, but that does not happen in your work or in your past academics?

The therapist was clearly trying to mobilize her resources, both emotionally (right brain) and intellectually (left brain). The therapist also may have been using neuroception (not consciously, however) as she was trying to detect the real underlying issue/emotion/experience the client was trying to communicate. The therapist had been knocked off track by the up-and-down nature of the arousal in the exchanges so far. As the therapist tried to manage her own affect, she may have been trying for a calmer or matter-of-fact demeanor (parasympathetic nervous system/calm/easier to engage socially). The therapist may have been trying for a homeostatically balanced level of affect to attempt to discuss the derailment, and using her left brain, decided to focus on the process, rather than the content, of the interchanges.

BEBE: Hey, you really are trying to pay attention, aren't you? Actually, looking back, that is exactly what happens; several coworkers have actually asked me if I had ADD [attention-deficit disorder]. Imagine that? Christ, despite everything, I have been on the fast track at work, no pun intended here (*laughs*); but, as you say, I cannot "track" a conversation. You know, I have never really sat down and thought about this.

Something about the therapist's intervention seemed to invite a more focused, less dissociated (if that was what it was?), more socially engaged reaction, which is somewhat playful (a hybrid state requiring features of both the state of mobilization ("arousal") and social engagement

THERAPIST: What exactly do you mean, "this"?

The therapist was trying to stay on track by asking to what Bebe's use of "this" refers. Her modulation of her own emotional/behavioral state allowed her cognitive processing to work more effectively.

BEBE: (*chattily, open in affect*) Well, you know the counselor I had in grad school was real nice, but kinda like my mother; she was encouraging and all that, but sort of, I don't know, formal. I think I was maybe too young and felt like I should, you know, maybe respect her advice about not working so hard, not needing to be so competitive, and ruining my health, etc.

The therapist was maintaining same stance as for previous comment by Bebe—that is, paying close attention to Bebe.

THERAPIST: There is that etcetera again.

Therapist was still calmly tracking Bebe (social engagement served by accurate neuroception).

BEBE: Yeah, I am beginning to think that I am saying things, but not really.

THERAPIST: Well, let's stop and think about what you just said: " . . . saying things, but not really."

This exchange seemed to make possible accurate neuroception on both parts leading to social engagement. The insula's processing of bodily state (Blakeslee, 2007), together with a proper decoding of facial patterns and information, permits an upper right-brain to right-brain connection that does not overattribute threat and accurately attributes safety in this encounter.

BEBE: " . . . saying things, but not really." Seems funny to quote myself, but when I focus on that, my mind goes back to two things. One was in high school when I took away the Rotary Club scholarship from this big jock who actually had a brain, but did not study as hard as I did. I had to thank those Rotary guys, and the jock's father was the president that year so he had to give me the award for $3,500 in front of the whole school. Was he ever pissed (*bitterly*), and he *just had* to make a reference to my being the first girl and first *Chicano* to get the scholarship. He could have at least said *Chicana*, though why say anything about my heritage, anyway? And then he said my mother's name as *Miss* Villareal, like I did not have a father or was illegitimate or something. (*Stops for a full minute, just looking at the water pitcher on the table, slightly unfocused, breathing through her mouth with kind of a whistling sound.*)

This state change may have been brought about by a memory that may have signaled the threat of imminent dangerous emotions. Bebe was vulnerable from a however brief but perhaps good connection between her and the therapist, so perhaps she trusted her enough to relate a seemingly innocuous event (the award), which, in fact, may represent a template for her presenting problem (being passive with men). Then she seemed to either release the vagal brake and experience higher affect or may have actually become sympathetically aroused (uncomfortably so?). Stopping for a full minute, perhaps becoming immobilized, she appears to move into shutdown/freeze behavior, which may be dissociative in reaction to too high and unexpected arousal (bitter, etc.).

THERAPIST: (*softly*) Bebe? Bebe? You seem to have gone inside yourself after telling about the award ceremony.

The therapist was trying to connect with Bebe, who may have become immobilized with fear as she remembered/reexperienced a traumatic event. The therapist may have been trying to "thaw" out the "freeze."

BEBE: (*Sits back in the couch and grabs a sofa pillow, holding it across her stomach and chest; sighs and looks around, as if to orient herself, surveying the room.*) Oh, yeah. The end of that story is that I forgot my notes when I went up to get the check, and just rambled on like a complete idiot; how smart did I seem then? Thank God my mother does not really understand English too well, so she did not know that I had shamed myself and her and my poor dead father. (*Looks up with an intense gaze directly in the therapist eyes.*) The *coyotes* killed my father (*begins to cry out of her left eye*).

THERAPIST: (*Trying not to be shocked about both what the client is saying and also that she is actually crying out of one eye*) What? (*Feeling like that comment was impulsively dragged out of her mouth, despite the thought that she should not act shocked or surprised.*)

> The therapist seemed very affected (immobilized?) by Bebe's reactions and rendered almost speechless herself (What? was all she could say). This is quite speculative, but perhaps Bebe's crying out her left eye was an indication of high activation of the right brain, which controls the left side, and vice versa (although there is much more mutual control of the upper face by both sides of brain per Porges (2007). Bebe gave the therapist a hard look (mutual gaze and facial muscles affect the state of the brain, which affects the viscera and heart)

BEBE: (*sarcastically*) Oh, yeah. That's what it's like to be a Mexican. You can be killed for $55 American [culturally, a common way to distinguish from the peso, i.e., Mexican currency] while your pregnant wife looks on, you can be humiliated in front of your whole school before people who have known you literally all your f****g life. They assume that a religious Catholic woman like my mother was a street whore having me by some (*starts almost chanting*) "*Miss* Villareal, *Miss* Villareal, *MISS VILLAREAL* (*loudly and angrily*). I was the only *Miss* Villareal there in the auditorium—she was *Mrs.* Villareal and her actual name is Mrs. Guadalupe Villareal Vargus, the proper Hispanic way to say her name. And we aren't Mexican anyway, we are from Costa Rica. (*As she was talking, she became increasingly upset and loud, and after the last comment she laid her head down on the pillow, which she had been clutching to her chest and abdomen, and blindly reached around for the shawl on the back of the sofa, draping it around herself clumsily, with her eyes closed and her head on the pillow, looking about 10 years old.*)

> Bebe was clearly becoming increasingly sympathetically aroused, culminating in a shutdown that was either calmer (more related parasympathetic response) or more aroused (a shutdown/freeze/immobilization/dissociation response)— or, maybe immobilization without fear.

THERAPIST: (*Thinking that she should say nothing; she had the image of being like a sentry, watching over a sleeping child; finally, she spoke softly, having the feeling that she was waking a child.*) Bebe, what is happening to you right now?

Perhaps the therapist received the projected wish to parent Bebe and treat her carefully, like a small, frightened child; neuroception may have been working well, unimpeded by the therapist's seeming lack of skill in the encounter.

BEBE: (*No answer, but turns over to get more comfortable, grabbing the shawl more tightly around her, opening her eyes and slowly looking around, again, seeming to orient herself.*) You sure earn your money, listening to this kind of stuff, don't you (*challengingly*)?

Bebe may have been "thawing" and moving from an immobilized (reptilian shutdown) state to a calmer state (orienting herself) to an aroused state to counterregulate the low state (which can create a massive reduction of metabolic resources). Her challenging statement may have been her effort to both arouse herself and arouse the therapist emotionally.

THERAPIST: You know, I feel speechless, sort of like you were after talking about what your family went through. I wondered what words could ever be right.

The clinician was trying to be more empathic (a transitory identification with the experience of an other; Horowitz, 1983) in order to stay connected to Bebe's experience (neuroception).

BEBE: (*sitting up slowly*) Yeah (*sighing*), yeah, yeah.

Again, this may have been immobilization without fear, a state associated with prosocial and positive states that involve a reduction of movement without the massive reduction of metabolic resources.

THERAPIST: Maybe the award ceremony was " . . . saying things but not really saying them . . . " I wonder what you would have said if you really could have said what you really wanted to say?

BEBE: (*laughs*) That's a good one. There is no telling, and probably for another session. I can see by the clock that it's almost time to go, and what I really want to say, oh, God, is not fit to hear. But this "tracking" thing is interesting. I'm gonna think about that one. And along that line, I haven't forgotten that I said I was reminded of two things from my past (*stops talking, seems to be waiting*).

Maybe being out of time created a sense of safety that might have promoted social engagement and positive social interactions. Bebe may have been more vulnerable and a little playful, which is a hybrid state requiring features of both state of mobilization ("arousal") and social engagement.

THERAPIST: (*tentatively*) Are you sure you want to talk about something that might be as upsetting as what you have just said, or as you just mentioned, looking at the clock, should we talk about it another time?

The clinician may have been <u>nonconsciously utilizing neuroception, leading to social engagement</u>.

BEBE: (*with a little smile*) You know, I am a great subject changer, but I swear that this is relevant. I played basketball in high school and was really fast, even though I was always—and I mean *always*—the shortest on the court. I played every game for 4 years.

THERAPIST: (*really lost, but trying to stay connected*) Basketball?

Again, Bebe indirectly, and therefore, safely, created a bit of a playful exchange with the therapist.

BEBE: (*really smiling now*) Yeah, I know exactly what it means to "run out the clock" on the opponent when your team is winning. I think that is what I do to people: I run out the clock so I don't have to fall apart like today. And, as to the other thing I don't want to talk about; let's just say it involved the old grampa who they let hang around the ranch office and what he did to me when I was 11 years old. After that, I got to be a great talker in both English and Spanish. While I was cleaning the office, I was running out the clock on that old . . . whatever . . .

With the safety of the beginning of a trusting experience with the therapist and the safety of the clock running out, Bebe hastily brought up what was surely a traumatic stalking behavior by the employer's relative. Perhaps conditions permitting a kind of <u>social engagement</u> with a small amount of trust were just beginning?

THERAPIST: Well, our clock has indeed run out. How are you right now, after all that emotion?

<u>Neuroception, empathy, and social engagement</u> may be prompting this gentle question.

BEBE: It's not the emotion, it's going away like a rag doll that worries me.

As Bebe described the dissociative experience, social engagement may have occurred.

THERAPIST: Hopefully, the "rag doll" times will not take you so far away from another person after you are so real about yourself.

The therapist was reiterating the value of social engagement and noting that the immobilization with life threat/freeze/dissociative/reptilian experience was not desirable.

BEBE: Exactly. (*Gets up, folds the shawl, and places the pillow carefully on sofa*). Now, it's like I was never here (*gives a lopsided smile with the left side of her face*). See you next week.

Is the right brain controlling the left face again? Could it be that this has been the best way for difficult experiences to be expressed—through her body?

Concluding Comments

Information about the arousal system greatly enhances clinical skill in understanding the manifestations of both the intrapsychic and interpersonal behaviors in the clinical encounter. The polyvagal theory adds such interesting information regarding the release of the vagal brake allowing an action to be taken. So instead of activating the sympathetic branch and utilizing the arousal system (sympathetic nervous system), which may need to be held in reserve, releasing the vagal brake preserves that energy. Additionally, the concept of an older "reptilian" and newer "mammalian" system of low energy is easy to remember and helps differentiate between calm (parasympathetic nervous system) and "freeze" (vagal system) states in clients. The social engagement system requires a calm parasympathetic response so that people can approach without fear. If that does not work, then the sympathetic branch will become activated and fight or flight will occur. And if the person is trapped, the immobilization (freeze) response will occur. These experiences may occur repeatedly in clinical work, yet remain unnoticed by clinician and client, so subtle might they be.

CHAPTER 5

Personality Disorders as Affect Management Strategies

This chapter examines the effects of the physiological arousal system when it becomes organized into expectable behaviors, such as personality disorders, attachment categories (also described as attachment classifications or styles), and defense mechanisms. The terms *categories, styles, traits, templates, classifications*, and *patterns* all describe stable and predictable phenomena of a particular kind. The templates examined in this chapter are those that are clearly affected by extremes in arousal. These "extremes" have either become imprinted into the neural circuitry as automatic reactions, or they trigger defense mechanisms to manage their expression—or both.

The point is that behavioral extremes can be understood to have physiological correlates. Identifying the neural substrates that are responsible for the extremes may help clinicians appreciate their own reactions to such behaviors and assess the degree of their therapeutic input—or absence thereof. The proposed features of the definition for *mental disorder* in the DSM-5 (proposed publication date 2013) are similar to those in the DSM-IV-TR (American Psychiatric Association, 2000), in that there is an emphasis on "a behavioral or psychological syndrome or pattern that occurs in an individual that reflects an underlying psychobiological dysfunction" (American Psychiatric Association, 2010). In part, the "psychobiological dysfunction" likely occurs in the autonomic nervous system, which has been co-opted for rigid, predictable, and extreme influences on behavior as well as inner experience.

Personality disorders are diagnosed, in part, by the presence of certain traits and behavior patterns, currently termed *criteria* (American Psychiatric Association, 1994, 2000). Many of the criteria involve traits that exhibit extremes in arousal (e.g., inhibiting traits, such as extreme reluctance, or arousing traits, such as exaggerated emotionality and theatricality) and are specific for each personality disorder. In the proposed DSM-5, personality disorders are assessed, in part, in terms of the degree to which 37 traits are present in the extreme. The work group responsible for empirical validation of the trait model has only a draft at the present time. However, just as in the DSM-IV-TR (2000), the majority of the proposed traits can be grossly sorted by extremes in arousal (e.g., arousing traits, such as emotional lability, anxiousness, aggression, histrionism, and impulsivity; or inhibiting traits, such as submissiveness, social withdrawal, social detachment, restricted affectivity, anhedonia, risk aversion, and dissociation proneness) (American Psychiatric Association, 2010).

Attachment categories are differentiated, in part, by the intensity of arousal that is manifested behaviorally. Defense mechanisms are designed to manage the levels of arousal. Defensive maneuvers all have in common, among other things, the fact that each can be sorted by its characteristic relationship to excitatory or inhibitory levels of arousal. Should the response to most situations be virtually the same arousal level, this inflexible reaction may become a problem. For example, with some personality styles, acting out (excitatory) or isolation of affect (inhibitory) may characterize the typical way that affects are managed.

Exceptions to the either–or of excitatory versus inhibitory arousal are the adaptive defense mechanisms of secure attachment and earned secure attachment, which are flexible in their utilization of self-protective behaviors and defenses. Another exception is the disorganized/disoriented attachment style of childhood, which erratically employs excitatory and inhibitory strategies in chaotic, unpredictable ways. In adulthood, the erratic responses can be seen in people with borderline personality organization, posttraumatic responses, and some of the dissociative conditions, to name a few (see Chapter 4).

What follows is a brief discussion of representative ways (not intended to be exhaustive) that personality disorders have been categorized over time, including the speculations regarding cause of the disordered behaviors. Attachment categories and defense mechanisms as affect regulation strategies are also addressed. What might occur or need to occur between the clinician or social service staff regarding problems with arousal is addressed. In the remainder of the chapter, the above concepts are examined through the lens of 14 case examples. Each case illustrates a childhood or adult attachment category; for adult categories, the closely related personality disorder(s), likely defense mechanisms, and what may predictably happen regarding arousal management in the treatment between the brain of the client and the brain of the clinician or social service staff are addressed.

Personalities Disorders

When considering personality disorders, various foci are applied: for example, developmental cause, models of self and other, and traits expressed in the disordered behavior. More recently, researchers have added knowledge about the effects of relationship experiences upon brain development and function, some of which may result in disordered personality functioning. Certainly, the foci are related to one another, but major theoreticians emphasize different aspects regarding different personality disorders.

Developmental Cause

The relational feminist perspective (Jordan, 2004) views personality disorders as resulting from serious disconnections in relationships, which isolate a person and thereby create suffering and limit growth and flexibility in functioning. Jordan objects to the term *personality disorder* on the grounds that stunted personality growth has sociocultural origins and should not be viewed as a character flaw originating with the person. Magnavita (2004), Masterson and Lieberman (2004), and Tatkin (2007) focus on relationships as having a particular effect on the personality. Magnavita (2004) proposes a unified model of "personality systemic," which includes a focus on reciprocal influences among the intrapsychic–biological, interpersonal–dyadic, relational triadic, and sociocultural–familial systems on personality development. Masterson organizes his theory and treatment of personality disorders around the insults to the developing sense of self of the child, with the influence of the maternal caretaker being of primary interest (Masterson & Lieberman, 2004). Tatkin (2007) explores the expression of personality traits in terms of one-person versus two-person psychological organization. A one-person psychological organization reflects a more limited degree of relational capacity than a two-person organization. Implicit in this concept regarding cause is the prior relationship history.

Models of Self and Other

Lyddon and Sherry (2001) discuss the beliefs that organize those working models of self–other internalized relationships as originally formed by childhood attachment styles. Kernberg (1980, p. 92; 1984, 228–230) addresses the internal structural characteristic of the personality: the relationship between the internalized representation of the self and internalized representation of the other and the linking affect. Kohut (1984) describes the characteristic manner in which a personality has internalized the function of the other, coining a term *selfobject* to capture that experience. Bleiberg (2001) describes ineffective and poorly responsive parenting as creating a coping strategy that does not respond to relationship opportunities with competent self and other reactions. He and others (e.g., Fonagy et al., 2004) focus on the capacity of the emerging sense of self to take the perspective of others while also reflecting on one's own state (mentalization, as it is termed) as a protective factor against developing a personality disorder.

Traits

Millon's early descriptions of personality disorders (1981) were organized around patterns of activity versus submission as influenced by the external social system and interpersonal dynamics. Linehan (1993) addresses ingrained personality traits from a cognitive–behavioral perspective.

The DSM-IV-TR (American Psychiatric Association, 2000, p. 685) describes personality disorders as an "enduring pattern of inner experience and behavior that deviates markedly from the expectation of the individual's culture, is pervasive and inflexible, has an onset in adolescence or early adulthood, is stable over time, and leads to distress or impairment." The DSM-IV-TR list of criteria for each diagnosis includes personality traits and behaviors, but does not generally speculate regarding the etiology of personality disorders. There are a few diagnoses for which cause is suggested (e.g., acute stress disorder, PTSD, reactive attachment disorder). Regardless of the speculated cause and the focus by the major theoreticians, traits can be found in every criteria set of the personality disorders in the DSM-IV and DSM-IV-TR (1994, 2000) that have at least an implicit, if not explicit, level of arousal as defining the behavior. For example, antisocial personality organization includes traits of impulsivity, irritability, and aggressiveness, all of which are excitatory. The avoidant personality organization includes traits of showing restraint in interpersonal situations and being unusually reluctant to take personal risks or become involved in any new activities—all inhibitory behavioral characteristics.

The proposed DSM-5's general definition of personality disorders is that they "represent the failure to develop a sense of self-identity and the capacity for interpersonal functioning that are adaptive in the context of the individual's cultural norms and expectations" (American Psychiatric Association, 2010). Elaborating on the interpersonal functioning are the proposed trait facets, discussed above. To reiterate, most of those proposed traits have either a high or low level of arousal. (See Table 5.1.)

Relationship Experiences Affect the Development of the Brain

Siegel describes how relationship experiences affect the neurobiology of the brain, including regulation of affect and bodily states, perception and meaning-

TABLE 5.1. Suggested Relationship between Arousal Branches of the Autonomic Nervous System and DSM Diagnostic Categories	
DSM-IV-TR (2000)	DSM-5 (proposed for 2013)
SNS-Dominated Personality Disorders	
Paranoid Personality Disorder	
Antisocial/Psychopathic Type[a]	
Antisocial Personality Disorder	
Dependent Personality Disorder	
Histrionic Personality Disorder	
PNS-Dominated Personality Disorders	
Schizoid Personality Disorder	Avoidant type
Schizotypal Personality Disorder	Schizotypal type
Narcissistic Personality Disorder	
Avoidant Personality Disorder	
Obsessive–Compulsive Personality Disorder	Obsessive–compulsive type
Depressive Personality Disorder[b]	
Passive–Aggressive Personality Disorder[b]	
Uncoupled Oscillating SNS–PNS	
Borderline Personality Disorder	Borderline type

Note. Based on criteria from the DSM-IV-TR (American Psychiatric Association, 2000) and the forthcoming DSM-5 (American Psychiatric Association, 2010). PNS = parasympathetic branch; SNS = sympathetic branch. See Appendix B for complete DSM diagnostic criteria for the disorders referenced above.

[a]The Antisocial/Psychopathic Type, depending on how this is eventually defined for the 2013 DSM-5, probably includes very inhibited and very excitatory responsiveness (see Chapters 3 and 4 for speculations regarding antisocial/psychopathic functioning).

[b]Proposed by DSM-IV-TR (American Psychiatric Association, 2000) for the next edition.

making, memory, and communication abilities (1999, p. 21). Likewise, Cozolino (2002) and Schore (1994, 2003a, 2003b) also represent current efforts to integrate how early relational experiences affect brain development, the most problematic of which can lead to compromised personality functioning.

Attachment Categories

As can be seen in descriptions of specific attachment categories in the cases examined below, the definition of each category generally involves the self–other interactions and expectations that have become memorialized in the neurocircuitry. This chapter is adding the arousal implicit in the attachment strategies, also imprinted in the neurocircuitry.

The right hemisphere of the brain is dominant for self-regulation (Schore, 2003a, p. xvii). How does this self-regulation occur? The left hemisphere is involved with conscious response, and the right hemisphere with the unconscious mind (Mlot, 1998, p. 1006). Schore has begun adding the term *nonconscious*, a right-hemisphere phenomenon, to his conceptualizations (1994, 2003a, 2003b). As discussed in Chapter 2, the nonconcious, according to Schore (2003b), involves active mental structures that communicate with other brains' nonconscious structures and are thereby relational in their effect. This is in contrast to the *unconscious*, which may contain silenced memories and emotions against which defenses are in place to prevent conscious awareness. Most defense mechanisms are unconscious, whereas the attachment styles and patterned personality organizations are nonconscious. Also patterned are the levels of arousal, some unconscious and some nonconscious.

From the earliest moments of life onward, infant brains attempt to establish a nonconscious synchronous resonation with significant caretakers. Sroufe (1996) described this experience as the interactive regulation of emotion. Should this dyadic experience be disrupted and "asynchrony" occur, without putting things right (i.e., without interactive repair), then the stage may be set for difficulties with affect management. For example, the affect management efforts inherent in the excitatory–inhibitory effects of drugs and alcohol are a clear illustration of using an external source of arousal regulation. Certainly, the addiction process is quite complex, but to the degree that the brain is using substances for mood management in an inhibitory or excitatory way and has an inherent or developed preference for that level of arousal, the clinician could logically speculate that the ability to tolerate the opposite level of arousal may need strengthening. For instance, if alcohol (inhibitory, depressant effect) is the drug of choice, perhaps the brain has difficulty managing emotions that are intense and excitatory. These arousing affects are governed by the sympathetic branch of the autonomic nervous system. When the client is sober, the clinician's properly functioning autonomic nervous system may be "loaned" to the client's brain to learn to tolerate upsetting and arousing or depressing affects. With enough interactive regulation of emotion, the client's brain will hopefully create new neural circuitry that can manage excitatory or inhibitory affects without always using substances or another person.

Why is it necessary to "put things right?" Repairing an emotional insult allows for stress recovery. It is stressful for the dependent brain to recover by itself. It can do so, but at a cost, particularly if the dependent brain has to recover by itself too many times. This may give rise to affect management strategies that later show up as a childhood attachment style with internal and/or external expression(s) of too much unmodulated arousal (ambivalent/resistant), too little unmodulated arousal (avoidant), or erratic arousal (disorganized/disoriented). The ambivalent/resistant strategy waits for the other to provide with bonding experiences. The avoidant strategy has, at some point, given up. The disorganized/disoriented strategy does not have a coherent strategy, often surprising others with its unpredictability.

Later in life, if these automatic and rigidly expressed affect management strategies do not change, particularly regarding the arousal preference, they may manifest as adult attachment strategies that are quite similar to various personality disorders, utilizing predictable defense mechanisms to manage arousal issues. Of course, under favorable circumstances the inherent neuroplasticity of the brain could rewire the neural circuitry such that an "earned secure attachment" (Pearson, Cohn, Cowan, & Cowan, 1994) could be created. These favorable circumstances (which primarily impact the right limbic system) include corrective relationship experiences such as a supportive family, stable life partners, and/or clinical treatment for relationship issues.

The right limbic system is particularly responsive to what Schore terms the "transfer of affect" (Schore, 1994, 2003a, 2003b), which describes how the brain creates a somatic and sensory representation that mimics how the face of the other would feel when a particular facial expression appears—a right-hemisphere function; surely this is empathy (Voeller, as cited in Schore, 2003b, p. 19). Of special interest is the work of Johnsen and Hugdahl (1991), who describe the right brain's holistic processing of information as it nonconsciously appraises, within 300 milliseconds, cues that are expressed facially.

Defense Mechanisms

When a disruption to emotional/bodily homeostasis occurs, securely attached individuals expect that the situation will be set right (Pipp & Harmon, 1987, p. 650). What is the implication of this expectation for defense mechanisms? It means that no emotionally/bodily defensive maneuver need be employed automatically in the securely attached (or those with earned secure attachment; Schore, 2003a, 2003b), as there is a confidence, reflected in a balanced autonomic nervous system, that the *regulation* of emotional states appropriate for the situation will occur. This regulation could include affect regulation by one's own resources or temporary regulation by another person, or some combination.

However, it is likely that the autonomic nervous system is "uncoupled" in those who are not securely attached (Schore, 2003a, 2003b, pp. 27–30). An uncoupled autonomic nervous system means that there is an automatic, nonconsicous preference in the brain and nervous system to overuse either the excitatory (sympathetic nervous system) or inhibitory (parasympathetic nervous system). A third option is possible in cases where life itself is threatened. The polyvagal system, mediated by the parasympathetic nervous system, will shut down functioning to such a low level that a dissociative state occurs, sometimes shutting down functioning completely, which can lead to actual death in extreme cases (Porges, 2011).

To repeat, ideally, in the face of stress, appropriate regulation of affect occurs either through the interplay between two brains or by oneself. Additionally, the ability to smoothly shift between appropriately taking advantage of the functions of another brain, temporarily, or to manage autonomously without resorting to toxic defenses is highly adaptive. What becomes problematic is rigidly using the same set of defense mechanisms, regardless of the situation—for example, automatically employing defense mechanisms that inhibit, distort, disavow, act out, or break with reality (American Psychiatric Association, 2000, pp. 808–809). Vaillant (1977) repeatedly made the point that anyone should be able to use any defense mechanism depending on the context. The more securely attached an individual, the more flexible the brain and nervous system in using situationally appropriate mechanisms of defense.

Primitive defense mechanisms result from early experiences between caregiver and the developing child. With enough repetition, the ways in which a child's brain learns to manage emotional experiences will become, in Bowlby's (1988) words, an "internal working model." Perry et al. described ingrained primitive emotional self-management as a condition in which "states become traits" (1995, p. 278). So at the point of a disruption to homeostasis, whether from internal sources or from the environment, with enough frequency, a "state" (e.g., of being alone after being criticized or being left alone with physical pain) can become a "trait" (habitually going into a state of low affect or high affect, or in some cases, a rapid oscillation between excitatory and inhibitory physiological states). Eventually a trait (e.g., of extreme self-dependence), which could originate from multiple experiences of being in a certain state at a time of disruption (e.g., being neglected at times of pain of some sort), may, under certain circumstances, be the best possible scenario.

Managing affect in a certain way (excitatory or inhibitory) may be the best the brain of a child can do, especially in cases of abuse or neglect or emotional instability in the milieu. Unfortunately, characteristic and patterned ways of managing affect can be engraved in the neurocircuitry and are generally unconscious and nonconscious, with the possible exceptions of the highly adaptive defenses (e.g., affiliation, self-observation, altruism), which have a conscious aspect to them.

It is not enough to simply recognize how personality disorders, attachment categories, and defense mechanisms share common physiology. There is a "so what?" aspect. If clinicians can identify the set of corrective emotional experiences needed by clients to improve their regulation of affect, appropriate interventions can be employed, such that clients may gradually be less prone to utilize defenses and behaviors that are interpersonally difficult. A "correction" may be directed toward the arousal of the brain (right hemisphere, mainly) in the clinician to counterbalance the level of arousal in the brain of the client. In most clinical situations, the clinician's brain is automatically resonating with the implicit experiences of the client, including the arousal correction needed. For example, it is a common and often subtle and unnoticed occurrence that the clinician may be in the opposite affective state (either excitatory or inhibitory) of the client. If the client is highly aroused, the clinician may be in a more inhibited state, automatically providing a counterweight for too much high affect. Or, vice versa. Very low affect can be compensated by the clinician's more aroused affect, hoping (nonconsciously, generally) that the client will match or approximate a less painfully low affective state. First, the clinician's brain will often match empathically the painful arousal state (however, briefly) and then struggle (often) to provide an alternative, or at least slight improvement, to the current affect state.

How does this change occur? According to Schore (2003a, 2003b), Rosenzweig (1996), and others, the capacity to change the functioning of the brain and nervous system remains throughout the lifespan. This neural plasticity is responsive to experiences with other brains; hence the necessity for clinicians to deeply appreciate the management of arousal in the brain and when arousal manifests (in whichever direction) in the clinical encounter. So, with many repetitions of emotional regulation in the client–clinician dyad, there exists the potential to change the client's neural circuitry toward more appropriate management of affect and, thus, behavior. Prominent among the brain structures in which these changes may occur are the orbitofrontal cortex and the limbic circuitries (Schore, 2003a, p. 31). For details on the building of such neural circuitry in response environmental experiences, see Cozolino (2002); Siegel (1999); and Schore (1994, 2003a, 2003b).

Case Examples

The following case examples illustrate the regulation of arousal via attachment categories in childhood and adulthood; the similarity between certain attachment categories and specific personality disorders; defense mechanisms that manage arousal (inhibitory or excitatory), which are typically associated with both the attachment category and the personality disorder; and a clinician's possible responses. The various concepts described in the first half of the chapter are mentioned as they are illustrated by case material. What connects many of these dynamic phenomena is the way(s) arousal is managed in the brain as well as the way(s) arousal is manifested in behavior. (See Table 5.1.)

Each case is organized in the same way, in terms of the following:

- Child or adult attachment category
- Management of arousal: whether branches of autonomic nervous system (parasympathetic nervous system, sympathetic nervous system) work together (coupled) or do not work together (uncoupled)
- Description of the attachment category, with traits, behaviors, and self–other experiences underlined
- Case material: Concepts described in first part of chapter are discussed as they relate to the material; concepts from other chapters are also referenced
- Brief discussion at end of each case; with adult cases, possible personality organizations and other clinical conditions that are similar to the attachment category are presented.

Childhood Category: Child to Parent

This section contains four case examples illustrating childhood attachment categories with commentary.

Case Example of Childhood Secure Attachment

Childhood category: Secure attachment category
Management of arousal: Homeostatically balanced between sympathetic nervous system and parasympathetic nervous system
Description of attachment category: Secure attachment

The child with a secure attachment is confident that the parent figure will be responsive, available, comforting, and protective, particularly under distressful circumstances. This assurance enables him or her to explore the environment and test his or her developing abilities, as described by the work of Ainsworth et al. (as cited in Florsheim, Henry, & Benjamin, 1996, p. 84).

The staff of "Camp Go Forward!", a summer camp for children who had lost a parent or parents, was discussing the campers in Cabin #8 in the daily meeting.

LEAD COUNSELOR: Elias is the most stable kid, probably in the whole camp, this term.

MENTAL HEALTH COUNSELOR (MH COUNSELOR #1): Why don't we go around the table and comment on observations about him?

MH COUNSELOR #2: I have been here for the past 4 years, right after his dad first died, and he is "Steady Eddy." Or maybe, "Steady Eli." (*Staff laughs.*)

MH COUNSELOR #1: What does that say about him?

MH COUNSELOR #2: I can tell you, if he was always like the last past two summers, he seems like he is always reasonable. And he has a great way to settle down trouble between the kids. Not that he is like some of those kids who try to be cheerful at all times—if something is bothering him, he will usually look for somebody to talk to. Or sometimes, he just wants to sit by you while you are doing something, but not super-glued to your leg, if you guys know what I mean.

> *Thus far in the staffing, Eli is described as a capable and confident boy. He may be able to <u>successfully regulate his emotions by himself or can easily seek others for comfort</u> (adaptive defense mechanism of self-assertion). Altruism (vicarious but constructive service to others) and identification (assuming the actions of an idealized other) may be the adaptive defense mechanisms motivating his attempts to "settle down trouble between the kids." These defense mechanisms are <u>generally unconscious</u>, but being highly adaptive in this situation, may have a <u>conscious aspect to them</u>, as well (Vaillant, 1977).*

ELI'S PRIVATE THERAPIST: Thanks for inviting me again to the meeting. Eli talks about the camp all year long. He likes it that I have been here. Question: Do you think that he is too capable or too "strong," giving the impression that he is not in need of friends or staff?

MH COUNSELOR #3: Hey, Doc. Right back at cha. Thanks for coming again. The kids like it that you join in, especially that revenge soccer game between the staff and kids. They talked about that for a long while, especially the own goal you made. (*Staff groans, as an "own goal" is soccer slang for making a goal for the opposing team, accidently.*)

ELI'S THERAPIST: I was actually working for their side the whole time and I meant to make that goal (*laughter*).

These adults appear to be the responsive, available, comforting, and protective kind who can provide the environment in which a child can experience the attunement and bonding that are necessary for the eventual development of a secure attachment. We might speculate that Eli's family life has been at least adequate, as evinced by his being able to manage his affect with or without others, but not by using behaviors that are worrisome to caregivers. The adults in this exchange are using the adaptive defense mechanisms of humor and altruism.

MH COUNSELOR #3: Anyway, to answer your question: He reminds me of the Three Bears, with the "just right" porridge. He isn't perfect or perfectionistic, either. He can get mad, especially on the soccer field, but he leaves it on the field when the game is over. He is generally a good sport at most of what he does.

This counselor is describing a <u>homeostatically balanced autonomic nervous system</u>; Eli manages the intensity of his emotions and consequent behaviors within normal expectable limits—not too high and unable to calm down, nor too low and unable to elevate his mood without resorting to inappropriate behavior. Eli may be using the adaptive defenses of sublimation (channeling impulses into positive activities) and suppression (conscious decision to postpone focus on a conflict) as he "leaves it on the field." This is a good example of a <u>coupled autonomic nervous system, meaning that the inhibitory–excitatory systems work in harmony, where one is not automatically overused regardless of the situation</u>.

MH COUNSELOR #1: OK, a couple of you look like you might like to add something. We have several more kids to talk about, so we need to stay focused on Eli.

MH COUNSELOR #4: I am new here this summer. What happened to Eli's dad, anyway?

PRIVATE THERAPIST: OK, brief background: The dad had a head injury from a wreck when Eli was only a few months old and died when Eli was almost 8. He couldn't work or drive, but for years was able to be the stay-at-home dad. It wasn't till the last that he was bedridden, so he taught Eli to play soccer and computer games and helped with homework. They recorded every World Cup Soccer game and would replay them for years afterward. Mom worked so dad could have insurance, and that was the only source of income, anyway. He was not a U.S. citizen, so disability income wasn't an option.

This history provides data to support the speculation that Eli had early years of attentive, invested parenting by the father, however physically and mentally *challenged the father may have been. Eli expects others to behave similarly, in the face of Eli's needs. Eli has internalized the "function of the other" (Gold-berg, 1996; Kohut, 1984), meaning that neurocircuitry may have developed that now permits Eli <u>to shift</u> seamlessly between taking care of himself and seeking competent others to take care of him when he may be less able to self-regulate. Eli may be using the adaptive defense mechanism of affiliation (bonding with others as a way to manage emotions).*

MH COUNSELOR #3: Ok, my turn, I met Eli's mom; I can tell that she talks to him a lot; she is a great listener, and so tiny, but I get the impression she is one fierce mom about Eli. She was worried that once again he was elected by his cabin to be the captain. She worries that he might be too serious and not get to play enough.

MH COUNSELOR #1: I can't add too much to what everyone has said. But I don't think Mom has too much to worry about; that is one active kid. He loves to play all the sports, even ones he sucks at, and he is willing to do all the craft projects, too. He can just enjoy himself. But he is not ashamed to talk about missing his dad or just refer to him.

ART THERAPIST: Turns out his dad was an engineer; when we wrapped those holiday and birthday presents for the kids to give to their deceased parents, he and this girl made an elaborate design of a bridge that led from camp to heaven. Eli got the engineer gene, for sure.

MH COUNSELOR #1: We need to talk about the next camper on the list now.

The counselor's comments about Eli's mother give the impression that she, as was the father, is a sensitive, concerned parent, worrying that Eli may be too serious and adult-like and not enough of a child, as he should be. She is able to take Eli's perspective, which may have modeled the empathy that Eli can now show other campers, when he mediates tension between the other children. <u>Eli may have internalized a self and other template for relating</u> (requiring many repetitions), <u>which, in this instance, manifests in sensitive perspective-taking, reflective self-awareness, and mentalization</u>.

From this information, there is little reason to believe that Eli has a mental disorder. (Note. Mental disorder is defined as "a clinically significant behavioral or psychological syndrome or pattern that occurs in an individual and this is associated with present distress . . . or disability . . . or with a significantly increased risk of suffering death, pain, disability, or an important loss of freedom. . . . This syndrome or pattern must not be merely an expectable and culturally sanctioned response to a particular event . . . and must currently be considered a manifestation of a behavioral, psychological, or biological dysfunction in the individual" (American Psychiatric Association, 2000, p. xxxi.) He uses adaptive defenses such as affiliation, self-assertion, altruism, identification, and suppression, all utilizing a balanced and coupled autonomic nervous system. It seems that Eli is behaving like a securely attached child, an attachment category and affect management strategy that invites others to be matter-of-fact with him most of the time. He is able to use the milieu in a therapeutic manner (Redl & Wineman,1951, 1952; Trieschmann, Whittaker, & Brendtro, 1969). Eli's right hemisphere, particularly the right limbic system, transfers affective information that signals others (nonconsciously and rapidly) to attend to him when he cannot, yet also invites the respect for him that he can generally manage his own affects appropriate for his age and stage of life (Karen, 1990). *Transfer of affect* means that the brain creates a somatic and sensory representation that mimics how the face of the other would feel when a particular facial expression appears; it is a right-hemisphere function (Perry et al., 2001; Voeller, 1986).

Case Example of Childhood Anxious-Ambivalent Attachment
Childhood category: Anxious-ambivalent (sometimes termed resistant)
Management of arousal: Sympathetically dominated behaviors
Description of attachment category: Anxious-ambivalent attachment

The child with anxious-ambivalent attachment is uncertain whether the parent will be responsive, available, or protective when needed. Anxious-resistant children tend to be clingy, greatly distressed by separation, and often fearful of their environments. This pattern is associated with inconsistency in parental availability and threats of abandonment, as described by the work of Ainsworth et al. (as cited in Florsheim et al., 1996, p. 84).

> The second-grade teacher was surprised at herself. She normally encouraged the children to be self-sufficient and independent. However, she let the new child, Ava, sit on her lap sometimes and allowed Ava to "help" her with some tasks, which kept Ava close by. She talked to her close friend in the teacher's workroom about it, who said that Ava was always going to the nurse's office after lunch, when other children went outside.
>
> Even though the teacher normally reserved the front tables for children with challenges, like hearing, vision, or behavior issues, Ava was quickly moved close to the teacher's desk. The teacher could see visible distress on Ava's face whenever the teacher moved to the back of

the room to help a student. Ava would swivel her head around and track the teacher's every movement. It was a little better when the teacher's aide was in the front of the room, but not much. Ava could become increasingly nervous and would wriggle around at the desk, sometimes not calming down even when the teacher returned.

Ava quickly became scapegoated. The other children realized that she was afraid of nearly everything, so they would take turns coming up behind her and shouting, "Boo!", laughing when Ava jumped. That bullying behavior made the teacher even more hypervigilant toward Ava's well-being, since the children were so sneaky about scaring her. What did puzzle the teacher was that, at times, Ava would stare off into space as if deeply daydreaming, and would startle violently when approached.

Ava's defense mechanisms may include externalization (actively experiencing the external world as parts of one's own personality) and regression (direct expression of impulses to remain unaware of wishes or affects that accompany them). These defenses are arousing and governed by the sympathetic branch of the autonomic nervous system. In this brief example, Ava does not seem to exhibit adaptive behaviors governed by the parasympathetic branch and the polyvagal system (see Chapter 4), which would be calming and promote less agitated social interaction. Ava acts as if she must ensure that adults attend to her, otherwise they may not (although sometimes they may, but not necessarily in a contingent response to the child's need; more in response to parent's own need to parent). Other children act out against her, despite the teacher's watchfulness. Ava may already have an internal working model of self and other in which she is quite weak and vulnerable and assumes that others may not notice her distress or may attack her for it.

In many group situations, particularly with children, this attachment style creates contagious group anxiety that can result in aggression against the vulnerable one. This group phenomenon is not only affected by Ava's behavior, but also by the right-brain to right-brain experiences (particularly the nonconscious) the children have in proximity with Ava. Her fear (amygdala driven) may affect the children so that they have to stamp it out—hence their aggression toward Ava. Ava's parasympathetic nervous system may facilitate the shutdown by the polyvagal system, wherein extreme numbness and unresponsiveness (dissociation) may occur, likely in response to the intolerable level of anxiety and arousal. Although the presentation of the anxious-ambivalent attachment style is generally quite active and aroused, the brain can be rescued from a painful level of arousal by dissociation.

There is no history in this vignette. However, if Ava generally behaves similarly in all situations, many theorists would assume ineffective and poorly responsive parenting (barring constitutional or medical causes). The teacher's response is similar to what may occur in a clinical situation, wherein the clinician's parasympathetic system would be required both to remain calm as well as to, hopefully, convey a synchronous resonance and the transfer of not only affect but also of the intensity of affect. Ava needs to have many experiences with calm and responsive others so that eventually her own parasympathetic branch of the autonomic nervous system can calm her, rather than primarily "borrowing" the calming effects of other brains.

Case Example of Childhood Anxious-Avoidant Attachment

Childhood category: Anxious-avoidant attachment category
Management of arousal: Parasympathetically dominated behaviors
Description of the attachment category: Anxious-avoidant attachment

The child who is anxiously avoidant in attachment style has no confidence that the parent will be responsive, caring, or protective and expects to be ignored or rebuffed. Such a child will attempt to live life without the love and support of others. Conflicts regarding dependency needs are hidden, as described by the work of Ainsworth et al. (1978) and Bowlby (1988) (as cited in Florsheim et al., 1996, p. 84).

THERAPIST: Hi, my name is Julie. Where's your mom or dad?

JENNY: They dropped us off and said they will be back at 5 p.m. This is Perry, my brother.

THERAPIST: Hi, Perry and Jenny. You know, before we meet, I have to get your parents to sign some papers. Do you have a cell number for them?

PERRY: Yeah, it's ###-####. That's this area code.

THERAPIST: OK, why don't you two help yourself to a diet drink and I will call them from the other room. OK?

(The therapist called the parents, who had driven a few blocks away, and asked them to return to the office. She waited with the children in the waiting room for a few minutes. The parents blustered in the door and were invited back to therapist's office. The therapist told the children that they would all be right back. The children just looked at her blankly.)

The blank looks may have been blocking (inhibition of thinking and impulses), isolation of affect (splitting affect from content, which results in not being consciously aware of either idea or affect), or a dissociative moment (numbness), all of which involve the parasympathetic branch (inhibiting) of the auto-

nomic nervous system; if truly a dissociative moment, the polyvagal system may be involved, as well.

MOTHER: My God, that was a hassle. What is the problem?

THERAPIST: (*professional and detached*) Mr. and Mrs. X, I cannot see your children for treatment unless I have the proper forms signed authorizing me to do so.

FATHER: (*irritated*) Well, I gave you my permission on the phone—that should be enough.

THERAPIST: (*matter-of-fact*) Actually, this kind of treatment is governed by laws about parental consent. I also did want to meet you and have you meet me for a little while before we all decided for the children to have therapy with me.

FATHER: (*challenging*) You mean, you are not sure about seeing them?

THERAPIST: (*continuing to be matter-of-fact*) It is always a good idea to meet the parents so you and your wife can make that decision. I need to also decide whether or not to see them, as well.

MOTHER: (*Grabbing forms from therapist*) Give me those forms so we can move this along.

> *The clinician may have been trying not to match the parents' affective states of agitation and acting out. The sympathetic branch of the clinician was trying not to match the level of arousal of the sympathetic branches of the parents' brains. The clinician may be using suppression (an adaptive, conscious defense mechanism) in her deliberate attempt to remain calm and refrain from expressing her irritation and displeasure about the parents' behavior.*

THERAPIST: I do not have a clear picture of what you want for your children.

FATHER: We were told that they need therapy, so we found you on the insurance and you are convenient, so here they are.

THERAPIST: Yes, but I need to know some of the concerns you have about them.

MOTHER: I am not concerned about them; they are quiet and make good grades; they do what they are told.

FATHER: Perry is not really "all boy" like my brother's kids. They are always playing baseball and hunting with BB guns . . .

MOTHER: For Pete's sake, your brother lives in the country! Perry would be breaking the law if he took a gun around the neighborhood, like those yahoos of your brother's.

The parents seemed to veer off topic easily, perhaps being derailed by dysregulated kinds and levels of affect; they seemed quite reactive to any hint that something is wrong with their children. Perhaps they were experiencing shame? The mother may have experienced being called back to the office as humiliating. *Neurobiologically, humiliation/shame/embarrassment may create a spike in arousal (sympathetic nervous system) to a painful level, often counter-regulated by lowered affect (parasympathetic nervous system) (Schore, 2003b, pp. 151–186).*

THERAPIST: What do you think therapy would do for your children? Do they have some symptoms, for example?

FATHER: Certainly not, they have no symptoms. Do they, Mother (*asking for agreement*)?

THERAPIST: Then why are they here? (*Both remain quiet.*)

MOTHER: My husband had a little accident and the judge made us get counseling for the kids.

THERAPIST: How does one relate to the other, I don't understand?

FATHER: I accidently put my foot on the gas instead of the brake and ran the car through the garage and into the kitchen.

THERAPIST: Why does that require the children to have therapy?

MOTHER: We have these nosy neighbors who called the cops. Then the welfare people [child protective services] came and took the kids away. So we had to promise to take them for some therapy. Completely humiliating.

THERAPIST: Why were the children taken away?

FATHER: These fundamentalist neighbors told the cops we had alcohol on our breath—and, there you have it, made them take the kids!

THERAPIST: Before I see your children, I need to have the police report and the judge's orders. There is no point in my seeing these children when I do not know the facts.

FATHER: Are you saying we are lying?

THERAPIST: No, but [I need] the whole story so I can understand what my role is.

MOTHER: (*to father*) See—I told you they are all going to want us to sign something and see the report. (*turning to therapist*) The other therapist said the same thing.

> *The session continued the affective interchange as above, with the parents provocative in their behavior and the clinician trying to remain calm and professional, just relaying or trying to get factual information. The parents' aroused behaviors had the feel of a habitual style of emotional response. Thus far, their character traits and defense mechanisms have included aggressively and passive–aggressively trying to get their way by bullying, acting out (leaving the children at the agency), lies of omission about the situation, regression (immature behavior), and rationalization (justifying). <u>All these defenses are activated by the sympathetic branch of the autonomic nervous system</u>.*

The therapist received the police and court documents. The father and mother were over the legal limit for driving under influence of alcohol. At 3:30 p.m. on a school day the father crashed through the garage. The children had to spend the night at a temporary foster home and then a few days with relatives. As a condition of the children returning home, the parents were required to seek medical assessment for any drug or alcohol conditions and appropriate treatment if there were any diagnosed, and the children were required to receive treatment from a child therapist until the judge was satisfied that the family was safe for the children. The parents wanted the children to be seen together, so the therapist decided to conduct filial therapy for at least a few sessions and to reserve the right to decide what was in the best interests of the children as the therapy proceeded.

THERAPIST: Hi, Perry and Jenny. My name is Julie and . . .

PERRY AND JENNY: (*together*) We know.

> *The children were being a bit rude, mocking, and aggressive (sympathetic nervous system).*

THERAPIST: OK. Why don't we start by asking what you have been told about being here for therapy?

PERRY AND JENNY: (*Looking at each other, they both remain silent.*)

THERAPIST: Maybe you might like me to tell you what I have been told about your being here?

PERRY AND JENNY: (*challenging*) OK.

The children's behavior may indicate a pattern of withholding in a passive–aggressive way (parasympathetic nervous system), combined with acting out (sympathetic nervous system), just as the parents displayed in the first meeting (identification with the aggressor?). The children may have been retreating into the slight safety of a twosome (the adaptive defense mechanism of affiliation may be the children's way to manage emotions through bonding, perhaps) (sympathetic nervous system).

THERAPIST: A judge ordered your parents to take you to a therapist to talk about what it is like to live with your parents and their drinking at home. Did you know that?

PERRY: Not really.

JENNY: (*nodding toward her brother*) What he says.

THERAPIST: (*trying to stay friendly*) OK. But first, could I find out something about you, like how old you are and what grade you are in?

As the next exchanges unfold, the children relax in response to the clinician's friendly way and they begin to answer the questions, but still in <u>guarded manner</u> (parasympathetic nervous system; being more open to relationship opportunities per Porges's polyvagal theory of social engagement).

PERRY: I am 11 and she is 10, but we are in the same grade.

THERAPIST: How did that happen?

JENNY: I started early, but our parents tell us all the time that they are glad we are in the same grade 'cause we will leave for college at the same time. They will get to travel and do what they want to then.

THERAPIST: What do they want to do?

JENNY: Watch TV and drink.

THERAPIST: What about traveling?

PERRY: (*disgusted*) The only place they travel is to the liquor store.

The children were perhaps distancing themselves from their parents by not seeming conflicted about "telling on them." The poorly responsive parenting may have created a sense of the self (of children) as not needing parents and sense of parents (other) as neglecting/abandoning with the linking affect as anger (Kernberg, 1980).

THERAPIST: What do you two like to do at home?

JENNY: I like, talk with my friends on the phone and computer (*quickly adding*), but only after my homework is finished.

The children may have to be alert to anything that could bring attention and possible criticism or worse to them (<u>amygdala registering safety–danger</u>).

THERAPIST: What are your parents and brother doing when you are on the phone?

JENNY: (*Shrugs shoulders.*)

PERRY: Here's what we do. Mostly our parents aren't home after school. We fix ourselves some food and go do our homework in our rooms. We don't know why they were home right after school when he ran into the garage. They are never home till after dark.

THERAPIST: They work pretty late, then, I guess?

JENNY: (*Looking at Perry, she shrugs her shoulders again.*)

PERRY: She doesn't work, goes early to the café. They meet there after his work and eat and drink for a while. He has a stressful job, you know.

THERAPIST: What does he do?

JENNY: (*looking at Perry*) Something with insurance—he does not stay in the office too much [because he] sees clients at their home. What is it, Perry? Long-time care?

PERRY: Long-*term* care, Jenny.

THERAPIST: Are you two good friends?

PERRY: Not really, she is a girl and I have my guy friends.

THERAPIST: Who shops for the food that you fix after school?

JENNY: Sometimes we go to the market on the way home from the bus. Perry has a debit card. Sometimes Mother has food for us, but she doesn't get what we like. She thinks we are grown-up enough to do the shopping and fix food.

THERAPIST: Do you cook on the stove?

PERRY: No! We are not allowed.

THERAPIST: How do you cook?

JENNY: Microwave, but not too much.

THERAPIST: Do you both have house keys?

PERRY: Yes, and we hid one from our parents under the yard art rabbits. Once we both forgot our keys and had to walk down to the café and, well, it did not turn so good. We have never done that again. Have we?

JENNY: Uh-uh (*looks at Perry*). Our friends are jealous of us. They wish their parents were never home. But they can't believe that we just do our homework. We never get into trouble.

> *The children looked at each other using their <u>right brains to holistically process information, nonconsciously appraising within a few milliseconds cues that were being expressed facially</u> (Johnsen & Hugdahl, 1991). A dispassionate (<u>parasympathetic branch, creating inhibitory affect levels</u>) detailing of the children's experience of being neglected and having to fend for themselves emerged quickly, as the clinician asked for concrete data about eating, shopping, cooking, and so on. With such self-sufficient children, trying to ask them to reveal their emotions may have been quite premature at this point and likely met with stonewalling. Or the children may have so little experience with anyone being interested in their inner world, that they may not have been able to describe their experiences, except in the most concrete of ways. There was little effort made by the children to protect the image of their parents.*

THERAPIST: What do you mean?

PERRY: Me and Jenny know how to shut out noise; we can do anything while noise is going on.

THERAPIST: What do you mean? What kind of noise?

JENNY: We taught ourselves what we wanted to hear. So we can study or go to sleep.

THERAPIST: Are you talking about loud TV from your parents?

JENNY: Not really; when they come home from the café, they are loud. We—I—we try to go by our rule to finish homework before they get home. Sometimes we are lucky and are asleep before they get home.

THERAPIST: What time do they usually come home?

PERRY: If we are unlucky, they come home around dark. We would rather they drink at the café and not at home.

THERAPIST: Why?

JENNY: Because if they drink at home they can get loud. I used to think that drinking made you lose your hearing, but now I know they just get riled up and fight about stupid s--t, I mean, stuff. Sorry.

THERAPIST: Do you ever get scared?

JENNY: When we were little, we were babies, scared of every little house noise. But now that we are in the fifth grade, we are smart. He has a bat under his bed and I got a can of mace from mother's purse. I wish we had a gun, but we don't.

Perry and Jenny are well described by the anxious-avoidant attachment style. The siblings do not expect responsive, caring, or protective responses by their parents and conceal dependency needs by their calm, self-reliant, and self-possessed emotional presentation (parasympathetic nervous system). The children may have developed defense mechanisms such as blocking of thoughts and feelings, isolation of affect, repression, and/or dissociation (all parasympathetic nervous system-activated defenses). The children, though appearing tough and self-reliant, have developed ways to inhibit difficult levels of high arousal, which is actually a fragile strategy because it is not flexible. Resilience is being able to tolerate increasing levels of difficult affect without resorting to toxic defense mechanisms (Schore, 2003a, 2003b). The children have already taught themselves to dissociate, isolate affect from cognition, and block affect, as it seems from their description of managing their parents' loud, drunken behaviors at night.

These children will benefit from relationships in which they can learn to bear previously intolerable levels of affect within a dyadic experience, safely using the emotional resources of another. Perry and Jenny will both need help in tolerating excitatory affects because they have trained themselves to be too calm and also because they may be extremely reluctant to become out of control, as they have seen their parents behave when both sober and inebriated.

The parents may utilize a central nervous system depressant, alcohol, to manage their highly aroused unbearable emotions. It may be that the parents' parasympathetic branch of the autonomic nervous system is compromised, so they import something that will substitute for the functions of the parasympathetic branch—in this case, alcohol. When sober, neither seems able to remain calm, easily becoming aggravated and agitating the other.

Case Example of Childhood Disorganized/Disoriented Attachment
Childhood category: Disorganized/disoriented ("Type D") attachment category
Management of arousal: Unbalanced (uncoupled) between the sympathetic nervous system and the parasympathetic nervous system
Description of attachment category: Disorganized/disoriented attachment

Children with a disorganized/disoriented attachment behave erratically and inconsistently, often sending opposing messages at the same time. These children may appear confused because they engage in "incomplete or undirected movements or expression," and they are often found to be victims of abuse or neglect, or their parental figure was grossly preoccupied with own problems (Main & Solomon, as cited in Florsheim et al., 1996, p. 84).

Setting: 2:45 p.m., nurses' report at psychiatric hospital

NURSE #1:   Start with Little Mary. What a day. She was admitted last night around 6 p.m. and was so out of control that Dr. Yanez ordered some sedation. She is only 8 years old, but is she strong!

NURSE #2:   Here is the situation. Even though she is 8, she was so malnourished until the age of 5 that she has not caught up with her growth; may never, in fact. She was removed from her foster home, the fourth or fifth she has been in, because she had to be restrained so many times. The foster parents just gave up; they have other kids there, too. She was actually brought here by ambulance.

NURSE #1:   If today was any example, she is totally unpredictable. In the day room, she seemed completely present, related, and connected to me when we were doing a puzzle. Then the other patient, also named Mary, walks in the room, I turn around to say hi, and the puzzle is airlifted in hundreds of pieces! That's the way it has been all day— you never know if she will be screamingly psychotic, yelling the same string of about a dozen curse words all in the same order, or if she snaps out of it, and is normal for a while. I swear, it seems like she is having a seizure, but she isn't. At least, I don't think she is.

CHARGE NURSE: (looks on chart and shakes her head) No seizure disorder diagnosed.

NURSE #3:   If she were an adult, I would wonder about PTSD; she seems to be preoccupied and stares off into space but not exactly like she is hearing voices, but who knows?

NURSE #2:   What is the diagnosis?

CHARGE NURSE: Dr. Y ordered psychological testing, as long as she is here. For now, she has "Rule Out Reactive Attachment Disorder and Disruptive Behavior Disorder, NOS." She is healthy, but the CPS [child protective services] worker said that there was a lot of abuse in her home, which is why she was removed. The parents are still in jail, so she won't be having any visitors.

NURSE #3: I don't know how she will do in the testing. There are times when she seems retarded, she make so little sense; but other times she gets a sly look to her and you know she is smart enough.

The disruptive behaviors are illustrations of the disorganized/disoriented ("Type D") attachment category (per staff description of erratic behaviors, which include sudden shifts in behaviors, from inhibitory to excitatory and back again). This attachment style (i.e., affect management style) constantly introduces chaos into relationships, making the interactive (dyadic) regulation of affect extremely difficult. Unlike the avoidant (reflexive unconscious preference for inhibiting emotions and behaviors) or the ambivalent (reflexive unconscious preference for excitatory emotions and behaviors), the disorganized/disoriented attachment category has no discernable pattern for managing affect via a dominant branch of the autonomic nervous system. Her defenses include self-protective maneuvers in the extreme in both inhibitory (parasympathetic nervous system; e.g., dissociation) and excitatory (sympathetic nervous system; e.g., acting out, regression) behaviors.

Adult Category: Adult to Adult

Adult attachment categories or styles, as described by Bartholomew and Horowitz (1991), are secure, preoccupied, dismissing, and fearful. They organize an internal working model of attachment along two dimensions: the distinction between self and others and the positive versus negative view of self and others (Lyddon & Sherry, 2001, p. 407). Though many contributors to the attachment and clinical research literature use this four-category model, other researchers have more finely grained classifications of attachment categories; these categories are detailed in a chapter by Florsheim et al. (1996, pp. 81–101). In the remainder of this chapter, the brief descriptions by Florsheim et al. (1996) of adult-to-adult attachment classifications are used as the basis of the speculations regarding the relationships among specific adult attachment classifications, personality disorders, and arousal management by the autonomic nervous system.

Within the adult categories that originate from childhood avoidant attachment, the automatic and preferred defensive maneuvers generally attempt for low affect (parasympathetic nervous system) because the management of high affect (sympathetic nervous system) is compromised. When high affect is evoked, an automatic and powerful set of defenses, leading to unfeeling states, often engages. And vice versa, meaning that within the adult categories that originate from childhood insecure-ambivalent (resistant), the automatic and preferred defensive maneuvers generally attempt for high affect (sympathetic nervous system) because the management of low affect is compromised. When low affect occurs, an automatic and powerful set of defenses leading to high arousal often engages. These are far from adaptive responses, but they are ones in which the person can move away, automatically and rapidly, from intolerable affect. For the brains of these persons, the extreme affective states (dissociation/numbness or quite aroused affect) are often preferable to even ordinary arousal.

But first, let us begin by visiting with Eli, the securely attached child in the earlier example, who is now an adult.

Case Example of Adult Secure Attachment

Adult category: Secure attachment category
Mangement of arousal: Homeostatically balanced between sympathetic nervous system and parasympathetic nervous system
Description of the attachment category: Secure attachment

The secure person has a positive view of self and others, moderate to high level of intimacy and autonomy, and a moderate to low level of dependency (as described by the work of Bartholomew & Horowitz, cited in Florsheim et al., 1996, p. 84).

> The following vignette about Eli illustrates a homeostatically balanced emotional experience that may indicate secure attachment (see earlier case example in this chapter of Eli as a child). The two branches of the autonomic nervous system, the parasympathetic (inhibits arousal) and sympathetic (excites), work together smoothly, with neither branch reflexively managing emotional experiences.

ELI: (*friendly, grinning*) Ay-yi-yi.—I'm back!

THERAPIST: (*delighted*) Good to see you! How old are you, now? About 25 or so?

ELI: Right.

THERAPIST: I was thinking that I haven't seen you since you were about 15? Or 16?

ELI: Right. We moved to Houston so I could get better soccer training.

THERAPIST: Yeah, you were ODP [Olympic Development Program] for soccer, weren't you?

ELI: Yeah. Mom was skeptical but we took a chance and left here.

The client and clinician were catching up on the past with humor, interest, and friendliness. The <u>level of arousal seems appropriate</u> for the situation, neither too excited nor too inhibited for a clinician–client relationship that lasted from Eli's 8th to 16th year. <u>The two limbic systems seem to be immediately in synchrony, perhaps effortlessly and nonconsciously.</u>

THERAPIST: How did it go?

ELI: As far as soccer went, good. I got scholarshipped to USC for academics and athletics and after undergrad, I played for a while for Portland. But I think I had enough.

THERAPIST: What happened?

ELI: You know life on the road is awful—and it's not the MLS [Major League Soccer]. The stadiums were high schools with little crowds; all that work for hardly any money. Most of the guys were hoping for scouts to see them play in these "modest" (*makes air quotes*) venues and maybe get offered a contract to play MLS. I actually had some nibbles myself, but decided that I was missing out on real life. And I wasn't a superstar.

> *Eli neither minimized nor aggrandized his accomplishments. He was simply reporting to someone with whom he has not had contact in 10 years, but someone who knew his past and could read between the lines (<u>right hemisphere is the location of empathy and intuition</u>; Voeller, as cited in Schore, 2003a, p. 35). Eli gave a balanced view of himself in a few sentences.*

THERAPIST: You are back here, what are you doing?

ELI: I'm in grad school in math. Not sure what I'll do. That's part of the reason I looked you up. I saw you on the soccer field recently. I play in the men's league, too, and seeing you across the park made me think that I needed someone beside Mom to talk to about some things.

> *Eli may have been exhibiting adaptive defense mechanisms, such as, affiliation, self-observation, and self-assertion (which were present when Eli was a child, as well). He may possess a <u>homeostatically balanced autonomic nervous system</u>.*

THERAPIST: Like what "things"?

ELI: (*laughing a little*) Like love and work! Wasn't that Freud who said that those were the top two things to worry about?

THERAPIST: I guess, looks like you have had a psych class more recently than I have (*laughs*).

ELI: Getting down to why I want to talk to you, I am having the idea that I should become an engineer, like Dad was. In fact, I sometimes go to the Engineering Science Complex on campus and walk around, knowing that he was in those same hallways. What do you think about that?

THERAPIST: I guess we have to ask a few questions about what it means to you to do that.

> *The dyad may have fallen into a <u>synchronous "groove"</u> from years of relating to one another. Eli got to the point after a few minutes of social pleasantries. He seemed confident that the clinician would be responsive, a <u>hallmark of the securely attached</u>. His self and other view seemed smoothly positive, at that point.*

ELI: Yeah, I would like that, but first let me tell you about the love thing, OK? They are related. Well, to go back, I decided to move back here because it is affordable to go to school and Mom is here now. She figured out, when I was in college, that if she worked part-time, with me in school and her in school, she was so poor that between us we qualified for lots of school loans. So she went back and got her degree and then her MBA, too. After all those years when we had no money, she has some now and good for her. She is helping me a little. I live in a little garage apartment behind her house. She travels a lot, so I mind the property for her and it works out, like everything with her.

> *As in the earlier vignette about Eli's mother (camp staff meeting), there is the impression of a sturdy and competent adult figure. From the history, the impression was that the father was a positive, loving figure as well. Again, there exists a positive view of Eli in relation to his mother (self and other). <u>The self and other configurations are located in the right hemisphere and are nonconscious</u> (Schore, 2003a, p. 280).*

THERAPIST: What about the woman?

ELI: Getting to it, getting to it! You can tell I am dragging this out, can't you (*smiling*)?

THERAPIST: Yeah.

> *Eli displayed some self-deprecating humor, teasing behaviors, and self-observation—all adaptive, <u>homeostatically balanced defense mechanisms, meaning neither reflexively high or low arousal</u>.*

ELI: Well, of course, Mom and Maida love each other; sometimes, I think they should be a couple! Kidding, just kidding. OK, where did I meet her? On the soccer field, of course.

THERAPIST: You know, it is a small world, and I think I know who she is. Her different name stuck in my mind and also, if she is who I am thinking about, I have seen her play co-ed soccer, and she is amazing.

ELI: Oh, crap. Do you know her?

THERAPIST: No, and not likely to ever play with or against her. I'm too old for that level of play. I was watching a co-ed soccer tourney recently and saw her play. Actually, I saw everyone else seem to just stand still, I should say.

ELI: So I can see you, even if you know about her?

THERAPIST: Yes, no ethical problem there. What is your situation with her?

Eli seemed to have a complicated understanding of himself, his mother, his girlfriend, and he also wondered if there was an ethical problem. He seemed to be able to process many aspects of a situation from various perspectives, illustrating mentalization, empathy, perspective-taking (Fonagy et al., 2004), and morality (Siegel, 1999), which are all components of the secure attachment strategy and a manifestation of a well-functioning orbitofrontal cortex and limbic system.

ELI: Here's the deal. She is on one of those soccer teams made up of lots of engineers that work for IBM. She is from Brazil, and I am a sucker for the south-of-the-border girls. You know Dad was from Mexico City?

THERAPIST: I remember.

ELI: She speaks English, Spanish, and Portuguese. Mom made sure that I am fluent in Spanish, so we can visit my dad's relatives. Blah, blah, I digress, anyway, here is my problem. She is perfect for me—my dream girl. And this is the first girlfriend that I mistrust myself about. I am worrying that I am swayed by "dad stuff" and have blinded myself to whatever . . .

Eli was struggling with trying to be self-aware; he was able to register that he was affected by being on the same campus as where his dad studied and that his girlfriend was from a Latin culture, as was his father. He was worrying that those factors may have made him vulnerable to judgment issues. He was seeking the brain of another whom he has known much of his life and whom he trusts. Under these perhaps stressful circumstances, he was trusting that the clinician would be reliable. Eli was willing to be appropriately dependent on one who has been dependable in the past. However, he sought a male figure for love and career issues, though not denigrating his mother at the same time. All of these qualities are indicators of an appropriately matured right hemisphere.

THERAPIST: Before you get into that, you said that work and love were related—how so?

ELI: Yes, she is going back to grad school for the math program I am in. All before we ever met. On the one hand, how great. On the other hand, is that too alike? And when we play co-ed ball, we are magic. Both seem to be in the right place to make give-and-go passes, assist goals—it's creepy. Our team always wants us to play next to each other, because of how we play, like no other players. You know what I mean?

THERAPIST: I see what you are saying. You seem to want to be careful and not be impulsive, even though she seems so right. Does she think so, too?

ELI: Yeah, we are talking about how to not rush along and be sensible. But there is a big attraction there. And no, we are not in any danger of doing something rash . . .

THERAPIST: But everyone needs someone to talk to . . .

These comments are more examples of Eli trying to be thoughtful and trying to consciously with his left hemisphere analyze and understand various aspects of his situation. This "trait" of being careful and thinking things through was once a "state" modeled by his parents and other responsible adults and peers; with enough repetition and examples, this state has now become a trait.

ELI: Yeah, and you are it for a while, if that's OK? I have some tutoring money to pay your fee. Mom offered, but she does enough.

Eli displayed appropriate dependency, a marker of a secure adult attachment style. As a graduate student, he allowed his mother to help him, but he also helped her take care of her property. He did not take her offer to pay for therapy, but rather appropriately wanted to pay for it himself, indicating the self-dependent and autonomous attributes necessary for adult life.

THERAPIST: Back to your graduate training: Why don't we keep thinking about that as we go along? It is common for people to have different understandings of such experiences as losing a father as a child. At different stages in our life the past takes on different meanings. We can wonder about the engineering versus math dilemma, but maybe Maida is the more pressing concern right now.

ELI: Makes sense to me.

From this session, there seems to be no reason to believe that Eli has a mental disorder. The clinician and Eli stayed in a moderate range of affective arousal, not too high, nor too low. The clinician may have been an important father figure, though surely many coaches were, as well, so Eli's choice to consult with his former therapist seems sensible. The defense mechanisms were adaptive—affiliation, self-observation, humor, self-assertion, anticipation (planning for possible problems in school and in his relationship with the girlfriend)—and are governed by a balance and coupled autonomic nervous system. He is easily the securely attached adult per the above description. As when he was a child, Eli is matter-of-fact, serious, yet sometimes humorous; playful interactions are the norm. Eli does not seem to be a personality with whom it is difficult to interact.

The therapeutic alliance will not be required to provide a corrective emotional experience by dyadically (interactively) managing Eli's level of arousal as a treatment goal. Eli's autonomic nervous system manages his level of arousal well enough. The therapeutic task with a securely attached person is to assist with troublesome life experiences; a person like Eli may need a mature adult who has the capacity to gracefully utilize both the left and right hemispheres to benefit Eli as he faces some adult decisions. Though the adult (a therapist, in this instance) may offer empathy, information, and advice and listen to a person like Eli describe his emotional experience, rewiring the brain's affective management strategy will generally not be the treatment focus.

The following three vignettes (Jack, Angus, and Cruz) are likely the adult version of the insecure-ambivalent (resistant) attachment categories; all are sympathetically driven. The next six vignettes (Crae, Zita, Mannie Lopes, Will, Andi, and a couple) are likely the adult version of the childhood attachment category of insecure-avoidant; all are parasympathetically driven. The final case (husband and wife) illustrates a milder version of disorganized/disoriented attachment (sympathetically driven) than did the case of Little Mary. To reiterate, these affect management strategies (or traces of those strategies embedded in the attachment categories of childhood) will likely be in evidence in the adult attachment categories.

Case Example of Compulsive Care-Seeking

Adult attachment category: Compulsive care-seeking
Management of arousal: Sympathetically dominated behaviors
Description of attachment category: Compulsive care-seeking. Speculation regarding childhood attachment category: insecure-ambivalent, sometimes termed *resistant* (Florsheim et al., 1996, p. 85)

A compulsive care seeker experiences a constant need to confirm the availability and responsiveness of attachment figures. These people have a heightened sense of vulnerability to loss, tend to define their attachment in terms of receiving care, and feel unequipped to take responsibility for themselves (as described by the research of West & Sheldon, cited in Florsheim et al., 1996, p. 85).

JACK: I never wanted to go into the military in the first place.

THERAPIST: Why did you?

JACK: (*a little agitated*) My parents, or should I say, my father, thought it would be good for me. He would always say that I was tied to my mother's apron strings, whatever in the hell that meant.

THERAPIST: Why are you seeking therapy?

JACK: (*more agitated*) My father would s**t a brick if he knew I was here. I don't want anyone to know, actually. My wife told me I should see somebody and if I did not, she is leaving and taking the baby to her parents'.

THERAPIST: See somebody about what?

JACK: (*upset and annoyed*) OK, goddammit, I sleep with the dog and not her sometimes.

THERAPIST: Why?

JACK: (deflated) It's a long story. I probably need to see a shrink, I feel so nuts.

> So far, Jack certainly seemed more sympathetically aroused as he was a bit disorganized in presenting his reason for being in the therapist's office. He may have been ashamed (the shame state is a spike in sympathetic nervous system, which can be quickly counterregulated by a parasympathetic nervous system lowering of affective charge; Schore, 2003b, pp. 151–185).

THERAPIST: (*matter-of-fact*) I am not a psychiatrist, but I can give you a referral, if that is what you are wanting.

JACK: Not really.

THERAPIST: (*calm*) Should we go on with the interview to see if we can work together on whatever your concern is?

JACK: (*Agitation decreases as begins to tell facts of his situation.*) Right. My wife is right, I can't do this by myself.

Jack's right hemisphere may have been getting into affect synchrony with the clinician, who had remained calm, but still interested, in spite of Jack's agitation. On the other hand, it should also be considered that the clinician's left hemisphere matter-of-fact demeanor and attempts to keep Jack on track regarding the reason for seeking therapy could be experienced by Jack as unempathic and more about the clinician's need to get to the "facts" than about Jack's obvious distress. Additionallly, the clinican may have unconsciously been protecting himself from the veteran's emotionality (primarily a right hemisphere experience) by remaining concrete.

THERAPIST: What worries you the most right now?

JACK: (*sheepishly "confesses"*) I can't sleep unless the dog is in the bed. It used to be I had to have the dog in the bedroom, but now, since the baby came, I have to have the dog in the bed. My wife is disgusted with me.

There may be more shame management, as in above comment.

THERAPIST: (*matter-of-fact tone*) Can you give me your idea about why you have to have the dog in the bed?

JACK: (*loudly*) Oh, Christ. OK. In the war I was one of the dog trainers in the obstacle course and teaching them to find explosives. I never was a handler, but I was on several missions where that damn dog saved us many times over. He would find explosives in doorways, even find people. Many of us hoped we would go out with one of the war dogs. We wanted to stay close as possible to the dog. Nobody wanted to admit it, but no person could make us as safe as the dogs.

THERAPIST: What was the dog's name?

JACK: Scout.

Clinician was a bit derailed by what the client said about the dog. He lost the synchrony and asked an irrelevant, left-hemisphere concrete question (dog's name?), perhaps to manage own affect. Clinically, a common response to manage affect, especially when surprised, is to become intellectual or ask for information, instead of staying with the uncomfortable affect in order to somehow deflect the arousal that the client may be trying to evoke in clinician's right hemisphere (Schore, 2003b, pp. 58–107).

THERAPIST: (*back on track*) Have you ever had an experience of safety like you have with the dog?

JACK: That's a helluva question (*gets completely still, with eyes unfocused*).

Something about the question may have elicited <u>difficult affects (sympathetic</u> <u>nervous system) that were immediately counterregulated by isolation or</u> <u>blocking of affect (parasympathetic nervous system) or dissociation (polyvagal</u> <u>system)</u>.

THERAPIST: (*nodding*)

JACK: (*a little more animated*) Actually, when we were little, our mother was a tall strong German farmer's wife. She could do anything. Well, almost (*gets quiet*).

THERAPIST: (*nodding*) Almost?

JACK: Our father was a mean drunk; when he got mad, he would throw whatever was around him. We would run from the barn to the house. Mother tried her best to stand between him and us and usually took the worst of his anger. Later, she would come sleep in our room.

THERAPIST: Sleep in your room?

JACK: Well, not really. She would lay down with us till me and my brother went to sleep. She never slept there all night.

THERAPIST: (*quietly*) And you are having a similar experience with the dog?

JACK: Maybe.

Nodding, talking softly, and staying <u>limbic-system to limbic-system present</u> with Jack may have allowed him to focus on the difficult childhood experience that seemed similar, somehow, to the present. He may have internalized self and other configurations of his parents that are different. It seems that he had an image of himself as needing protection and soothing and an image of his (m)other as doing just that. He may have projected that image onto the dog(s) that were actually responsible for survival (as was the mother, perhaps). He likely has an internalized representation of his self with his father as terrified and of his father (the other) as dangerous and the linking affect, fearful or even terrified.

THERAPIST: Are you having some kind of fear similar to when your dad would get out of control?

JACK: Maybe. But this time it's my dreams. I try not to go to sleep; I don't like what I dream.

THERAPIST: What do you dream?

JACK: It's the same thing.

THERAPIST: (*waiting*)

JACK: The dog saved our butts; the palm groves were dangerous: Anything could be there—people, booby traps, weapons caches. The dog was between us and certain death. I dream about losing the dog and then what would happen?

THERAPIST: What about now that you have to take care of a family?

JACK: I'm terrified, almost like being in Iraq. I don't think I can do it. My dad was probably right, I am just a p***y and a mama's boy, tied to her apron strings.

Although beyond the scope of this narrow discussion, clearly this veteran may have many symptoms of PTSD (see van der Kolk, 2006; van der Kolk & Greenberg, 1987; van der Kolk, McFarlane, & Weisaeth, 1998; van der Kolk & van der Hart, 1987; Young & Breslau, 2004). However, an array of investigators has discovered that severe trauma suffered in adulthood, along with its subsequent miserable symptomatology, may be rendered even worse by the preexistence of an insecure attachment style resulting from childhood maltreatment dysregulation (Charmandari, Kino, Souvatzoglou, & Chrousos, 2003; Jacobs, van Praag, & Gage, 2000; Gunnar & Quevedo, 2007; Harvard Mental Health Letter, 2005a; Schore, 2003a, pp. 234–265; Toth & Cicchetti, 1998; Tull, Jakupcak, McFadden, & Roemer, 2007; van der Kolk & Fishler, 1995; Wolfsdorf & Zlotnick, 2001). Faced with his terror of the marriage and plagued with the consequent reactivation of the traumatic world experienced in the war and as a child growing up, it is hardly surprising that Jack might turn from his now frightening wife to his trusted dog, deeply integrated in his mind with the feeling of life-saving security. We might even speculate that sleeping with his dog also sparks feelings of safety, connected with very early experiences of clinging close to his mother as she tried to guard him from his drunken father. (See Nijenhuis, van der Linden, & Spinhoven, 1998, p. 253, regarding the tendency, when overwhelmed, to return to earlier forms of coping.)

For Jack, facing the prospect of being a new father and husband may have reenlivened his very early internal working model of being incompetent to calm himself and manage without significant help. If so, Jack's autonomic nervous system is uncoupled, with the sympathetic branch being dominant (acting out via agitated and loud speech), resulting in regression (e.g., turning from his wife in favor of the dog, assuming his wife is herself not capable of nurturing him), projection, and externalization (actively experiencing the external world as parts of his own personality). When the level of arousal becomes too unbearable, his brain employs the defense of dissociation, blocking, and/or isolation of affect. Clearly, the brain of the clinician was trying to counterregulate Jack's arousal—with one clear exception: when the clinician was surprised by something Jack said, perhaps sleeping with the dog, or the details of the war, or maybe a combination of these. Jack needs and seeks the affect management function of another (dog/mother/ therapist). When he is fearful, and if he cannot contain his (right-hemispheric) affective expressions, he may well be described by the compulsive care-seeking attachment category of adulthood even with the existence of early adulthood PTSD. Certainly, careful clinical scrutiny must take place to differentiate the two.

If investigation leads to an understanding of Jack as compulsively care seeking (in addition to his later-acquired PTSD), then one could posit that his attachment/affect management strategy developed in childhood is quite similar to the traits and behaviors of dependent personality disorder (American Psychiatric Association, 2000, p. 725; see Table 5.2). However, before drawing conclusions, it would be imperative to gather more information about such areas as Jack's childhood experience with siblings and peers, and later on, his relationships with significant others, particularly his wife and fellow soldiers. As the therapy proceeds, the clinician will need to work hard to account for this client's current distress by trying to differentiate between those vulnerabilities developed in childhood and others stemming from his combat experiences.

Case Example of Compulsive Caregiving Attachment

Adult attachment category: Compulsive caregiving

Management of arousal: Sympathetically dominated attachment behaviors

Description of attachment category: Compulsive caregiving. Speculation regarding preexisting childhood attachment category: insecure-ambivalent, sometimes termed *resistant* (Florsheim et al., 1996, p. 85)

A compulsive caregiver insists on taking the caretaker role in all relationships, never allowing others to reciprocate. These people's own needs are met by caring for others, thus they insist on providing help whether it is requested or not. Attachment is associated with feelings of self-sacrifice and self-neglect (as described by the work of Bowlby, 1977, and by West & Sheldon, cited in Florsheim et al., 1996, p. 85).

ANGUS: (*emphatic*) Well, as they say in that God-forsaken Texas dirt ball town I grew up in, "The chickens have come home to roost."

THERAPIST: (*Upset, too, as Angus's usual demeanor had changed and the therapist was resonating with the level of the affect without, at this point, knowing the reason*) Angus, in all the time I have known you, I have never heard you

TABLE 5.2.
Comparing Attachment Category of Compulsive Care Seeking to DSM Dependent Personality Disorder

Compulsive Care Seeking[a]	Dependent Personality Disorder[b]
Experiences a constant need to confirm the availability and responsiveness of attachment figures	Has difficulty expressing disagreement with others due to fear of loss of support or approval
Heightened sense of vulnerability to loss	Urgently seeks another relationship as a source care and support when a close relationship ends
Tends to define his or her attachment in terms of receiving care	Goes to excessive lengths to obtain nurturance and support from others, to the point of volunteering to do things that are unpleasant
Feels unequipped to take responsibility for him- or herself	Unrealistically preoccupied with fears of being left to take care of himself or herself; needs others to assume responsibility for most major areas of his or her life; has difficulty making everyday decisions without an excessive amount of advice and reassurance from other; has difficulty initiating projects or doing things on his or her own (because of a lack of self-confidence in judgement or abilities rather than a lack of motivation or energy)

[a]Based on West & Sheldon, as cited in Kaslow, 1996, p. 85.
[b]From *The Diagnostic and Statistical Manual of Mental Disorders, Fourth Edition, Text Revised*. See Appendix B for complete DSM diagnostic criteria for the disorder referenced above.

remotely reference where you grew up. You remember that you refused to talk about your childhood in that wry way of yours.

Angus was slightly aroused emotionally (<u>sympathetic branch of autonomic nervous system</u>), indirectly referencing bad news and surprising the clinician with a glimpse of his past, however uncomplimentary. <u>The clinician may have had an increase in affective arousal, as well, in reaction to Angus's uncharacteristic expression of any emotion.</u>

ANGUS: (*clearly upset, squirming around in chair*) I have some bad news. I have converted, and I don't mean to a religion.

THERAPIST: Oh, no. Tell me.

Now both were obviously emotionally aroused. It may be helpful to the client for the clinician to <u>match the intensity of his affect and resonate</u> with it; it may make Angus feel connected and less alone with this terrible news of the AIDS diagnosis. This may have been an example of <u>state sharing</u> and perhaps a departure from his usual trait (wry way).

ANGUS: I know you and my friends have been telling me to pay as much attention to me as I do to my friends. And now, wouldn't you just know?

THERAPIST: We have all tried to convince you to work more closely with your doctors.

ANGUS: At least I know the drill from helping all my friends.

THERAPIST: Do you think that you might slow down just a bit now?

ANGUS: At the moment I feel OK, so I don't see any reason not to help out at hospice for a while longer.

THERAPIST: I know that you are appreciated for all your extras, but some of the people you help may be quite conflicted if they know your medical situation.

ANGUS: Well, I just won't tell them, then.

THERAPIST: That might work for a while, but your social world is really small and sooner than later, everyone knows everything; it is so like a big family or a small village, don't you think?

Arguing with the clinician may have been an example of acting out and maybe regression, <u>mediated by the sympathetic branch of the autonomic nervous system</u>. Angus's oppositional attitude was immediately creating <u>arousing affect (sympathetic nervous system) between them</u>; he may have projected upset and self-concern onto others, relegating to the interpersonal interaction(s) what should be an intrapsychic conflict.

This may be a good illustration of <u>projective identification (sympathetic nervous system–parasympathetic nervous system)</u>. Angus may project (sympathetic nervous system) self-concern onto others, they may identify with being concerned about him (as they really are concerned about him), then Angus may distance himself from those concerns, becoming ever more blasé (parasympathetic nervous system). The more Angus seemed to be blasé about his serious condition and displays his nonchalance about his health, the more agitated others may become, thereby keeping in others' minds the projected conflict originating within Angus. Angus seems to have a character style of *distancing himself from his needs. <u>Not only is he content with projecting his health concerns, but also with the intensity of affect he is projecting. When the other identifies with the upset (sympathetic nervous system), then Angus's brain is free to have a lower level of affect (parasympathetic nervous system)</u> (Schore, 2003b, pp. 58–107).*

ANGUS: (*quiet, looking down*) The only person who ever made any sense to me was Granny. She was the energizer bunny on that old watch commercial: "takes a licking and keeps on ticking." She used to see that on TV and laugh and say, "That's me, that's me all over."

THERAPIST: Has your health situation put you in mind of your childhood? You always resist talking about your family.

Maybe the clinician's reference to village/family penetrated Angus's usual reluctance to speak of the past; that, plus the disturbing effect of his health condition—he may have identified with Granny, so his internalized self and other relationships (Lyddon & Sherry, 2001) may be the following: self representation of Angus is tough and needless and other representation is weak, needy, vulnerable. From a feminist perspective (Jordan, 2004), the disconnection in his relationship may have formed his self-dependent character, and he may have become a much more active (sympathetic nervous system) personality than passive (parasympathetic nervous system) (Millon, 1981).

ANGUS: (*quiet and serious*) I know if I take care of myself, I can live OK for a long time; now it's just a chronic disease, not an automatic death sentence, like I say all the time to my friends. It is surprising how little comfort that is to me right now. Just empty words. Anyway, last night I had a dream. Here is a present for you—you always like dreams and I never have any, but here goes.

THERAPIST: (*laughs a little*) OK.

ANGUS: I saw myself at the hospice and some well-intentioned straight guy, a complete ass, had called my parents. There they were, and I haven't seen them in too many years to count, my father looking on with that pious look of his and my mother signing some forms. I am trying to see what she is signing, and then Bobby [his partner] comes into the doorway. The cops won't let him in because my parents have limited visitors to "family only." I scream, "What the f***? Bobby is my only family—you people got rid of me years ago!"

THERAPIST: And what do you make of this dream?

ANGUS: I guess maybe me and Bobby should do something legal about us; we have talked about one of us adopting the other to prevent my dream from happening . . . or at least doing something.

Angus seemed to have become more related and realistic about his situation. He used adaptive defense mechanisms of humor (the dream being a "present" for therapist), anticipation (planning for future), and perhaps self-assertion (adoption, etc.) These defenses are all modulated by a balanced autonomic nervous system. The clinician's matching and challenging of Angus on the seriousness of the situation in a matter-of-fact way may have invited Angus to be more serious and matter-of-fact himself.

THERAPIST: I think that if you were to take care of yourself, you might be emotionally hard on yourself. I hope we can keep talking about it so you will follow through with whatever you decide. If you quit being aware of yourself, you are likely to slip back into being Granny, the "keep on ticking . . ." whatever the jingle is.

ANGUS: (*sighs*) I am scared.

Here we see a synchronous right-brain to right-brain matching of affective states between the two and a transfer of the intensity of affect (the therapist's modulated affect "spread," in a sense, to Angus's brain).

THERAPIST: When you get scared, you usually get active—you bake something, or drive somebody somewhere, anything to not look at your own needs. Sometimes I am surprised that you have come to therapy for such a long time.

ANGUS: (*grins a little*) Well, I only come here because it makes Bobby happy; you know what a therapy maven he is.

THERAPIST: I hope you let your own therapy inoculate you against fear of neediness.

ANGUS: Good luck with that one (*grins in a softer way*).

Angus reverted a bit to his presentation of being the needless caretaker, but with less intensity, it seemed.

Angus's character style fits the description of the compulsive caregiver. He seemed to meet the general diagnostic criteria for a personality disorder (see Table 5.3). The caretaker personality disorder (Barbanell, 2006) may describe Angus and others who blindly sacrifice for others, neglecting themselves. Angus's activity level and defenses (particularly the manic defense defined as permitting a flight from inner reality to external reality, avoiding the sensation of low affect; Winnicott, 1975, pp. 129–134) requires an activated sympathetic branch of the autonomic nervous system much of the time. However, the stress Angus is under because of his recent news about his health may have punctured his usual high arousal state (sympathetic nervous system) and temporarily allowed him to have a lowered affect, speaking seriously (para-sympathetic nervous system low affect) with the clinician. Sufficient repetitions of being in synchrony with his clinician as they resonate with the lowered (nonmanic) affect may afford him new opportunities to develop resilience (i.e., the capacity to tolerate difficult arousal without resorting to problematic defenses; Schore, 2003b, p. 280). This resilience could create neural circuitry that might bear the lowered levels of affect and expand Angus's emotional range. Table 5.3 compares the attachment category of compulsive caregiving with the criteria for caretaker personality disorder.

Case Example of Adult Preoccupied Attachment

Adult attachment category: Preoccupied attachment
Management of arousal: Sympathetically dominated behaviors
Description of attachment category: Preoccupied attachment. Speculation regarding childhood attachment category: insecure-ambivalent, sometimes termed *resistant* (Florsheim et al., 1996, p. 84)

An interpersonally preoccupied person strives for self-acceptance "by gaining the acceptance of valued others" (as described by the work of Bartholomew & Horowitz, cited in Florsheim et al., 1996, p. 84). Experience is characterized by a sense of unworthiness juxtaposed against a positive view of others.

CRUZ: (*irritated*) Once again, I have been left out of the e-mail notice about the pub crawl.

THERAPIST: (*calm*) I thought you said you did not even like that particular group.

CRUZ: I don't. My running group is much more responsible; if they don't like me, they don't show it—at least, as far as I can tell.

THERAPIST: How do you know you got left off the list?

CRUZ: 'Cause one of my running friends is on the soccer list, too.

THERAPIST: How many of the running group are also on the soccer list?

CRUZ: A lot.

THERAPIST: The ones who are left off, do they play soccer?

CRUZ: Probably not. I see where you are going with this. You are going to say, "Look, Cruz, it is not personal about you, etc., etc." Right?

TABLE 5.3. Comparing Attachment Category of Compulsive Caregiving to Caretaker Personality Disorder	
Compulsive Caregiving[a]	Caretaker Personality Disorder[b]
Insists on taking the caretaker role in all relationships, never allowing others to reciprocate	Appears self-sustaining
Own needs are met by caring for others	Appears self-sustaining, counterdependent, and self-sufficient rather than independent
Insists on providing help whether it is requested or not; attachment is associated with feelings of self-sacrifice and self-neglect	Avoids self-need gratification but forms attachments by giving to others; pervasive and compulsive need to be needed; relentlessly overresponsible; conceals past trauma and current crises by focusing on others; avoids conflict, anger, and expression of displeasure to preserve contact with others

[a]Based on Bowlby, 1977; West & Sheldon, as cited in Kaslow, 1996, p. 85.
[b]Based on Barbanell, 2006, pp. 66–67.

THERAPIST: Yes, I was trying to see if it was personal, aimed only toward you, or not. I think it could go either way, with what you know. But it is important to try to understand what your reaction is to *believing* that you were deliberately left out.

The clinician was trying not to resonate with the aroused (sympathetic nervous system) affective state of Cruz; instead, she was trying to question him about the facts of the situation in a calm manner (parasympathetic nervous system). The clinician was not willing to argue in a challenging (aroused/sympathetic nervous system) manner. Cruz seemed to have a self-image of being rejected by more popular others. Previous sessions had provided material that described ineffective and poorly responsive parenting as having created a coping strategy that did not respond to relationship opportunities with competent self and other reactions.

CRUZ: My reaction? Why, pissed off, wouldn't anyone be? Wouldn't you be?

THERAPIST: What are you angry about?

CRUZ: Like I said, being left out.

THERAPIST: Yes, you did say that. When you are left out, what is your emotional experience?

CRUZ: Repeating myself. Pissed off.

THERAPIST: Since you are sensitive to others' opinions of you, I wonder if we should dig a little deeper into your hypervigilance about being included?

CRUZ: You know very well that I am not good at this "self-examination," don't you?

THERAPIST: Yes, but I also know that you are a skilled problem-solver at the lab, so I am hoping that we can apply that skill to *you* and try to understand your experiences from a deeper psychological stance.

CRUZ: That makes sense, but unlike at work where we have real data, there isn't much data with me. I don't remember much, so what can we work with?

THERAPIST: I know your memory for people experiences is not good, but how about trying to answer a few step-by-step questions about being left off the pub crawl list, and we can see what happens, OK?

CRUZ: OK, I guess.

> *Relationship experiences may have been negatively affecting Cruz's memory of selected social experiences (Siegel, 1999, p. 21). The clinician may have been functioning as selfobject (Kohut, 1984) for Cruz, providing the reality testing and data analysis function regarding social–emotional experiences that Cruz was not well able to supply for himself. Cruz was <u>aroused</u> (<u>sympathetic nervous system</u>) and used the defense mechanism of <u>help-rejecting complaining</u> (often a defense against dependency strivings).*

THERAPIST: OK. How did you find out about the pub crawl?

CRUZ: I heard two of the soccer players talking about it while we were all on the treadmill at the gym at work.

THERAPIST: And then?

CRUZ: (*slowly*) And then? And then I felt like I was swimming underwater for a minute; I actually thought I was going to pass out.

THERAPIST: How long did that last?

CRUZ: Ummmm . . . maybe a few seconds to a minute or so. I don't know.

THERAPIST: OK, stop on that. Have you ever had that swimming underwater sensation before?

CRUZ: You know how I hate talking about back then. Anyway, I can't remember too much about those times.

THERAPIST: Try to remember, have you ever had that swimmy sensation in the past?

CRUZ: Oh, yeah, all the time when I was a kid.

THERAPIST: Does any particular incident or type of incident come to mind?

CRUZ: Once, when my father came home from a trip to Mexico and he brought all the kids something and I guess he forgot about me. He said, "Oh, you can share that doll with your sister." And there I was, a boy!

THERAPIST: So you had that underwater feeling then?

CRUZ: I guess I did.

THERAPIST: Before that swimming feeling, do you have any idea what you were feeling?

CRUZ: I was excited to see what he brought me, and then I felt like the roof had fallen on my body and smashed me to the floor; then nothing.

THERAPIST: Was this an isolated incident?

CRUZ: I wish I could say that it was, but no.

> *Cruz may have experienced many disappointments and rejections throughout childhood, to which he responded with a painful arousal (sympathetic branch) followed by a low affective state (isolation of affect, dissociation), which is parasympathetically mediated. The "swimming underwater" (likely a dissociative moment) experience(s) may account for his not remembering social experiences, past or present.*

THERAPIST: Without going into the other similar situations, do you think you began to believe something about yourself based on such experiences?

CRUZ: What?

THERAPIST: How do you imagine that you explained to yourself your father's behavior about the gift?

CRUZ: Oh. Uh (*silence*) that's pretty obvious.

THERAPIST: Ummm.

CRUZ: He obviously did not think I was good enough to get a present like the other kids.

THERAPIST: From an adult perspective now, what would you think about a father that did what he did about your sharing your sister's doll?

CRUZ: I might think that he was a punk.

THERAPIST: Did you think he was a punk then?

CRUZ: Nobody did, including me. The whole town thought he was a god.

> *The clinician was trying for a left-hemisphere intervention, asking about beliefs, thoughts, what others thought, etc., which can have a parasympathetically modulating effect of promoting a dispassionate and reasonable reaction—a "cool" cognitive approach (Linehan, 1993). This approach may have indicated to Cruz that these memories can be remembered without such high arousal that he has to employ the "swimming underwater" defense.*

THERAPIST: Why was that?

CRUZ: Because, there he was a nobody Mexican kid from Matamoras who played American semi-pro baseball before he got hurt. *Beisbol* is everything down in South Texas, except for *futbol*.

THERAPIST: Looking back, can you think of a reason that was about him to explain why he slighted you?

CRUZ: The only thing I can think of is that he never, not once, came to my games. I was a good shortstop and good batter and fast. I kept looking for him, even into my senior year, thinking he might come to a game. Guess I wasn't good enough for him.

THERAPIST: Why would that explain his behavior about the doll?

CRUZ: This whole conversation is making me tired. I think you want me to say something, but all I can think about is going to bed.

THERAPIST: If you want to, we can pick up on this next session.

CRUZ: If you say so.

> *The clinician was clearly trying to help Cruz be more realistic about his father's behavior, which Cruz believed was due to something about him, Cruz. Cruz was having some success retrieving memories about his past, but rather quickly he tired of the effort. The level of affect may have been intolerable. The clinician's letting it go until next session could give the message that affects can be borne, especially within a synchronous dyadic state, and can be terminated without resorting to defenses such as dissociation (certainly a limbic-system to limbic-system experience—nonconscious and nonverbal—but potentially corrective emotionally for Cruz).*

Cruz's symptoms are quite similar to those for preoccupied attachment category and to the criteria for depressive personality disorder in DSM-IV-TR (American Psychiatric Association, 2000, p. 789). On the face of it, it seems a contradiction to suggest that Cruz was utilizing the <u>active, excitatory branch of the autonomic nervous system</u> and also that he met criteria for a depressive diagnosis under proposal for the next edition of the DSM. However, a way to reconcile the data is to note that the preoccupied attachment is active in striving for self-acceptance by "gaining the acceptance of valued others" in order to ward off the depressive experience (perhaps compensating for the history of blows to his self-esteem as a child).

Additionally, Cruz's dissociative ("underwater") defense argues for a compromised toleration of high emotionality, as does his becoming "tired" as the clinician attempts to connect past experiences with the father with Cruz's negative self-image. Both of these experiences are low in affect, for which he may have little neural circuitry to bear comfortably. The clinician needs to continue to "lend" his stronger capacity to tolerate low, depressing affect so that Cruz may experience the interactive regulation of it. To date, he may not have had many experiences with others who were willing to "sit with" his sad emotions, so he avoids them by staying upset with himself (an arousing experience). Table 5.4 compares the preoccupied attachment category with criteria for depressive personality disorder.

Case Example of Adult Lack of Interpersonal Sensitivity

Adult attachment category: Lack of interpersonal sensitivity
Management of arousal: Parasympathetically dominated behaviors
Description of attachment category: Lack of interpersonal sensitivity. Speculation regarding preexisting childhood attachment category: insecure-avoidant, sometimes termed *anxious-avoidant* (Florsheim et al., 1996, p. 84)

An interpersonally insensitive adult is unaffected by external feedback, is oblivious to the effect of his or her actions on others, tends to engage in antisocial behavior without guilt or remorse, and resents being held back by external demands (as described by the work of Pilkonis, cited in Florsheim et al., 1996, p. 85).

CRAE: (*irritable*) Like I said last week, I am not happy about leaving so many messages and not one—and I mean not one—return call. He could at least text me to let me know he didn't die. And after all the favors I did for him!

THERAPIST: What favors did you do for him?

TABLE 5.4.
**Comparing Attachment Category of Preoccupied Attachment
to Proposed DSM Depressive Personality Disorder**

Preoccupied Attachment[a]	Depressive Personality Disorder[b]
Strives for self-acceptance by gaining the acceptance of valued others	Self-concept centers around beliefs of inadequacy, worthlessness, and low self-esteem; critical, blaming, derogatory toward self
Experience is characterized by a sense of unworthiness juxtaposed against a positive view of others	Is pessimistic and prone to feeling guilty or remorseful
	Usual mood is dominated by gloominess, cheerlessness, joylessness, unhappiness; brooding and given to worry (no clear correlate with description of preoccupied attachment, but implied)

[a]Based on Bartholomew & Horowitz, as cited in Kaslow, 1996, p. 85.
[b]From *The Diagnostic and Statistical Manual of Mental Disorders, Fourth Edition, Text Revised.* See Appendix B for complete DSM diagnostic criteria for the disorder referenced above.

CRAE: Well, we went to the market and he just had to buy all these really expensive things, and I cooked them for him. Not to mention what happened afterward, you know?

THERAPIST: Do you mean sex?

CRAE: Well, naturally.

THERAPIST: Are you saying that you considered sex with him a favor?

Crae acted as if she deserved special consideration for cooking and having sex; in this dialogue there was little consideration shown for the other person. Her attitude may have been an example of a one-person psychological organization (Tatkin, 2007), in which there is a diminished capacity to consider others, versus a two-person psychological organization wherein there is more mutuality. The two-person organization is a more adaptive right-hemisphere, upper limbic system, and orbitofrontal cortex organization. The one-person harkens back to experiences early in life when the infant brain is only just registering others, nonconsciously.

CRAE: My God, I should say so; after all, he is way older than me. Even my husband can do better than that, and he is hardly ever interested anyway. I hate to change the subject, but did you get back to my lawyer about that silly court thing?

THERAPIST: No . . .

CRAE: (*interrupting*) Well, why not? After all, we have chatted for the past 2 weeks about it, and the court date is coming up real soon.

> *This exchange may be another example of one-person personality organization: Crae is impatiently treating the clinician as if he were a function or a service that she has a right to expect ("that silly court thing"). She did not exhibit much capacity for mentalization (reflecting on one's own state simultaneously with the state of the other) (Fonagy et al., 2004), instead treating the clinician as a "selfobject function" (Kohut, 1984). That function, in this case, as seen by Crae, may be to take active care of Crae's legal situation while Crae waits for someone to cater to her wishes without regard to the effect on the other.*

THERAPIST: I can't say that I have enough information to answer some of the questions.

CRAE: (*demandingly*) Like what questions?

THERAPIST: For instance, you have avoided talking about the shoplifting incident. I have been asked to give some background about you that may have made stealing the coat understandable. And—

CRAE: (*interrupts again*) Look, everyone I know has a fur jacket, at least. These animal rights people are kooks, and no one in my circle pays any attention to them. I was just talking to my friends and accidently went out the door with the coat. I said I was sorry and tried to pay for it, but those plebeians just called the police (*shaking her head slowly in disbelief*).

THERAPIST: According to your lawyer, you had the coat on underneath your raincoat, so how is that an accident?

CRAE: Well, OK, we were a little drunk after lunch drinks, so my thinking was off, OK? OK?

Crae seemed completely self-absorbed and self-referenced in her explanation (grandiose in explaining her asocial behavior), perhaps a good example of the one-person psychological organization. Crae's defense mechanisms included rationalization as she justified her behavior (trying to avoid criticism); passive–aggressiveness (avoiding clinician's questions); projection (attributing irrationality onto animal rights "kooks" in order to not reflect on her own irrationality in her reasoning about the fur jacket she took); and controlling (trying to manage the clinician's behavior regarding the evaluation for the court, and trying to control her lover's behavior by manipulatively cooking and having sex). All these defensive maneuvers were attempting to maintain low arousal (inhibitory parasympathetic nervous system), though her tone gets sharp (excitatory sympathetic nervous system) when those defenses do not work.

What did Crae need from the clinician? Her defenses were attempts to manage excitatory arousal (sympathetic nervous system). She was interpersonally a difficult personality type with whom it is challenging to be empathic, so many clinicians will have problems effectively resonating and identifying with her. Crae tried to avoid too much emotional contact with most others. Her defenses may evoke in a clinician boredom, irritation, disappointment, condemnation, etc. Most clinicians tend to be self-critical when feeling such emotions toward clients, making empathy even more unlikely.

As can be seen in Table 5.5, which compares the similarity between the adult attachment category "lack of interpersonal sensitivity" and the narcissistic personality organization, most of the traits and behaviors serve to keep the person out of intimate emotional contact with others (e.g., unaffected, oblivious, without guilt or remorse, lacks empathy). Most of the behaviors and traits in Table 5.5, which are illustrated by the session with Crae, are managed by the parasympathetic branch of the autonomic nervous system. The goal of a brain like Crae's is to control others and avoid being shamed. When shamed or humiliated, the sympathetic branch of the autonomic nervous system becomes painfully aroused, and anger or rages often are the result of not being able control others. The often quick flashes of anger result from the lack of experience in tolerating excitatory affect. The effort is to "stay cool" emotionally—hence the haughty, grandiose, and unempathic demeanor.

Case Example of Adult Obsessive-Compulsive Personality
Adult attachment category: Obsessive–compulsive personality
Management of arousal: Parasympathetically dominated behaviors
Description of attachment category: Obsessive–compulsive personality. Speculation regarding preexisting childhood attachment category: insecure-avoidant, sometimes termed *anxious-avoidant* (Florsheim et al., 1996, p. 84)

An obsessive–compulsive personality style is characterized by excessive differentiation and a rigid adherence to a vision of how things should be. Such a person regards relationships as secondary to work and productivity,

TABLE 5.5.
Comparing Attachment Category of Lack of Interpersonal Sensitivity to DSM Narcissistic Personality Disorder

Lack of Interpersonal Sensitivity[a]	Narcissistic Personality Disorder[b]
Unaffected by external feedback	Is unwilling to recognize or identify with the feelings and needs of others
Oblivious to effect of own actions on others	Lacks empathy; shows arrogant, haughty behaviors or attitudes; has a sense of entitlement; believes that he or she is "special" and unique and should associate only with other special or high-status people
Tends to engage in antisocial behavior without guilt or remorse	Is interpersonally exploitative, i.e., takes advantage of others to achieve his or her own ends
Resents being held back by external demands	Shows arrogant, haughty behaviors or attitudes; has a grandiose sense of self-importance

[a]Based on Pilkonis, as cited in Kaslow, 1996, p. 85.
[b]From *The Diagnostic and Statistical Manual of Mental Disorders, Fourth Edition, Text Revised*. See Appendix B for complete DSM diagnostic criteria for the disorder referenced above.

and prefers not to discuss problems and feeling with others (as described by the work of Pilkonis, cited in Florsheim et al., 1996, p. 85).

ZITA: I have our agenda for the session. Last week I was so upset that I had not printed out the topics, so this week I put it in my Blackberry and wrote it down on today's date (holds up phone and shakes it around in little circles). Looking at the clock, I see that I have about 12 minutes for each subject, so let's get started . . .

> *Zita had a backup plan to prevent upset (sympathetic nervous system) caused by forgetting her agenda for the session. She was employing the defenses of controlling and obsessive behavior (inhibiting function of parasympathetic branch of autonomic nervous system) by using her Blackberry.*

THERAPIST: At the risk of upsetting the schedule, I do want to ask how the sleeping medication is working for you?

> *The clinician was risking asynchrony with the client, which may have been stressful to Zita as her inhibitory defenses were challenged. The clinician was not going along with Zita's managing of the time allotted for each topic; Zita*

was using the defense of controlling behavior, which is managed by the para-sympathetic (inhibitory) branch of the autonomic nervous system.

ZITA: (*politely and patiently*) Well, fair enough. This medication makes me drowsy in the early morning, and my workout at the fitness center is like going through mud.

THERAPIST: Does it address your early morning wakefulness, though?

ZITA: It seems to, but I like to be able to think. Since our firm made some cutbacks, I am afraid of being on the hit list.

THERAPIST: How is that situation with your manager?

ZITA: She is so incompetent; no one has any respect for her, especially since she gave all of us some of her accounts to work on. The one I got from her had so many errors that not even a high school bookkeeping student could do that poorly. Wouldn't you know, now I have my pile of tax returns to do and have to correct her mess, too (*getting upset and agitated*). That is just not the way to work; and I refuse to lower the bar, like others in the firm. So I have to stay late.

THERAPIST: Zita, do you get paid for the extra time?

ZITA: Of course not.

THERAPIST: Do others stay late doing the extra work?

ZITA: No, I am the only one.

The clinician's conscious and nonconscious perceptual brain structures *were working hard to connect with Zita, it seemed. The clinician may have been* trying for interactive repair *(i.e., trying for synchrony) by interrupting Zita's rigid control at the beginning of the session. The clinician was concerned, remembering the particulars of Zita's struggles at work. Zita was cooperating with the clinician, giving her the medication information, and then became upset (perhaps she was reminded of being mistreated by her manager;* sympathetic nervous system*), veering away from her polite and patient demeanor (*parasympathetic nervous system*).*

THERAPIST: That would be stressful for most people. What kind of emotional consequences, if any, does having such high standards have for you?

*The clinician was making an empathic effort (*right-hemisphere function*).*

ZITA: Look, my family back in Poland is perfectionistic, too. My family is from that Polish town that paints by hand those dishes and bowls with the hundreds of tiny dots. One of the Mayras is my aunt; you see, they sign them on the bottom. Have you ever heard of those artists?

THERAPIST: That sounds familiar; I think I have admired them in a cooking catalogue. But what about your stress level, working all those hours?

ZITA: You know how hard it is to put that into words . . . frustrating . . . mad . . . disgusted with others' performance—that make me have to work extra.

THERAPIST: Do you think that has an effect on your sleeping?

ZITA: I guess.

THERAPIST: Can you describe how you are feeling when you are working late?

ZITA: Look, I want to get to the agenda. But OK, I sit there kind of numb sometimes.

Zita gave information about her family in Poland and wanted to get back to her agenda, which may buy her some emotional space to collect herself (parasympathetic nervous system), as the clinician was rather steadily moving into the emotional realm—which, for Zita, may have been too arousing (sympathetic nervous system).

THERAPIST: Before you are numb, can you go back to what you felt then?

ZITA: My memory is not that great.

THERAPIST: Just try. Think back to what you were doing before you went numb.

ZITA: (*quiet for a few moments*) I actually felt kind of sick all over my body, like nauseated and heavily weighted down . . . is that enough? I really do not like all that talk of emotions.

Zita may have been counterregulating the sick feeling (too much excitatory sympathetic nervous system arousal) via numbness or dissociation (parasympathetic nervous system activating the polyvagal system into inhibitory "freeze" mode).

THERAPIST: I know, but the chores that you assign to yourself and have angst over if they are not completed seem to haunt you. It really does not seem to leave time for people in your life.

ZITA: I don't feel like going out anyway. I'm too tired and have to get things ready for work. Now that our manager has dumped her sorry work on us, I really don't have time to go out. Besides, since all this overtime, I have lost weight and my clothes don't fit. I am going to have to shop, but guess it will have to be online, since I work past closing time lots of nights.

Perhaps the clinician was trying too hard to "work." Zita may have been giving signals (in her own way) to slow down (by talking about shopping, her weight).

THERAPIST: Your body is probably trying to tell you something, maybe?

ZITA: (*curious*) Like what?

The clinician was trying to stay away from a recital of injustices (defense mechanism of injustice collecting; parasympathetic nervous system) and to bring the experience to Zita's feelings and bodily experiences to promote self-reflection (self-observation is an autonomic nervous system homeostatically balanced, adaptive defense mechanism).

THERAPIST: I think that your dedication to perfect work is unrealistic, and you may be having bodily reactions, like nausea, and then the numbness might be compensating for the difficult bodily experiences. I wonder if we might work on ways for you to tolerate doing less-than-perfect work and leaving the office on time?

ZITA: That sounds great in theory, but in the past it makes me feel worse to "lower the bar," as you are suggesting.

Maybe Zita considered the clinician's speculations, but maybe they were too arousing (which Zita tried to avoid), and Zita reverted to the inhibiting defense of devaluation "sounds great in theory"). Throughout the clinical exchange there may have been a transfer of affect that dysregulated the clinician, such that the clinician began insisting on her own agenda. The clinician was not following Zita's material, perhaps knowing from past experience that Zita would obsessively detail concrete facts. The clinician may have been affected by the low affect that a boring list of grievances, etc. evoked. It is not unusual for clinicians to attempt to bring arousal to a more tolerable level; however, in this case, it may have been too much, too soon, and not empathic. The interventions (interpretations, psychoeducation, confrontation) may have been more about the clinician's level of comfort than Zita's.

Zita both met criteria for obsessive–compulsive personality disorder (Axis II) and fit the description of the adult attachment classification of obsessive–compulsive personality (see Table 5.6). However, she does not meet any criteria for obsessive–compulsive disorder (Axis I), based on the information in the session. With direct questioning about symptoms, she may, in fact,

TABLE 5.6.
Comparing Attachment Category of Obsessive–Compulsive Personality to DSM
Obsessive–Compulsive Personality Disorder

Obsessive–Compulsive Personality[a]	Obsessive–Compulsive Personality Disorder[b]
Characterized by excessive differentiation	Overconscientious, scrupulous, and inflexible about matters of morality, ethics, or values (not accounted for by cultural or religious identification)
Rigid adherence to a vision of how things should be	Preoccupied with details, rules, lists, order, organization, or schedules to the extent that the major point of the activity is lost; shows perfectionism that interferes with task completion
Regards relationships as secondary to work and productivity	Excessively devoted to work and productivity to the exclusion of leisure activities and friendships (not accounted for by obvious economic necessity)
Prefers not to discuss problems and feeling with others	Shows rigidity and stubbornness

[a]Based on Pilkonis, as cited in Kaslow, 1996, p. 85.
[b]From *The Diagnostic and Statistical Manual of Mental Disorders, Foourth Edition, Text Revised*. See Appendix B for complete DSM diagnostic criteria for the disorder referenced above.

meet some of the criteria for OCD. Whatever the case, Zita cannot modulate higher levels of arousal very well. This clinician's nonconscious inclination may have been to attempt to overcorrect for Zita's flight into low arousal. However, his interventions, and the client's response, may more clearly indicate the need for *him* to use the left hemisphere to think about, rather than counterregulate nonconsciously, right-hemisphere-driven behaviors. Ideally, Zita needs her therapist to stay closer to her concerns and perhaps be less abrupt about inserting the clinician's own agenda. Controlling the session is exactly what Zita does as her own affective management strategy. It could be that the therapeutic dyad is in a particular kind of synchrony, with the clinician overidentifying with Zita and not being able to "disidentify" with her way of managing affect and acting out by controlling the session.

Case Example of Adult Compulsive Self-Reliant Attachment

Adult attachment category: Compulsive self-reliant
Management of arousal: Parasympathetically dominated behaviors
Description of attachment category: Compulsive self-reliant. Speculation

regarding childhood attachment category: insecure-avoidant, sometimes termed *anxious-avoidant* (Florsheim et al., 1996, p. 84)

A compulsive, self-reliant person avoids turning to others for comfort, attachment support, or affection, and places a high premium on self-sufficiency. However, this form of avoidance is motivated by a counterdependent need to be self-sufficient, rather than by outright disdain for others (as described by the work of Bowlby, 1977, and by West & Sheldon, cited in Florsheim et al., 1996, p. 84).

RECEPTIONIST: United Way Family Services, may I help you?

CALLER: Well, well, I'm not sure, exactly (*long pause*). Someone suggested that I call, but maybe I should not take up your time here . . .

RECEPTIONIST: Maybe you would like to speak to our intake social worker? They can tell you about the services we offer here.

CALLER: Oh, well, oh, OK, I guess.

RECEPTIONIST: Please hold so I can connect you.

INTAKE SOCIAL WORKER: May I help you?

CALLER: I am feeling ridiculous. Someone told me to call you people, but now, I am not so sure, you know?

INTAKE SOCIAL WORKER: Sir, I would be glad to give you an idea of our services—that might help you out.

CALLER: So, OK, what do you do there?

INTAKE SOCIAL WORKER: We offer different types of counseling, like individual, marriage, family . . .

CALLER: Whoa, now, is this some kind of psychoanalysis stuff going on? Like the Woody Allen movies? I'm not crazy.

INTAKE SOCIAL WORKER: No, sir. We do not do psychoanalysis, but we do help people with parenting issues, marriage issues, personal issues such as stress management . . .

CALLER: (*interrupting again, somewhat agitated*) OK, OK, I got it. Do you have a bunch of psychiatrists there? I do not need any medication and don't believe in taking medicine when a person just needs to go to work or just get busy.

INTAKE SOCIAL WORKER: We do not have any psychiatrists or any doctors here; our staff are social workers, licensed professional counselors, marriage and family therapists, and psychologists . . .

CALLER: OK, I don't think those people see real crazy people. (*Shifts tone suddenly; now more conciliatory*) What do I have to do to see one of those?

> These exchanges, with the awkwardness, reluctance, uncertainty, and suspiciousness, are ways in which the caller reveals his mixed feelings about seeking some kind of help. As described in the above description of the compulsive self-reliant attachment classification, this is a form of avoidance motivated by counterdependent needs to be self-sufficient. Though nervous about being treated by doctors for "crazy people," he may not be disdainful about, so much as defended against, his wish to be dependent on someone. From a state of lowered affect, the more he engages with the staff, the more anxious he may become—a state that may move him into a compromised ability to manage. He may be more able to manage more distance via <u>lowered arousal</u> (<u>parasympathetic nervous system</u>).

INTAKE SOCIAL WORKER: If I could have a little information about your situation, I could put you on our waiting list—which, I'm sorry to say, is about 3 weeks out.

CALLER: (*sounding relieved*) Oh, well (*exhales loudly*), OK, well, 3 weeks would be great. What do you want to know?

> He seemed relieved to not have to immediately enter into a relationship in which he must receive help from another person (it may have seemed too upsetting to ask for help; <u>sympathetic nervous system</u>). Since he obviously cannot receive services immediately, he may not have to experience the arousal (<u>sympathetic nervous system</u>) and maybe the <u>parasympathetic branch could resume affect management, giving him more comfortable social engagement via the polyvagal system</u>.

INTAKE SOCIAL WORKER: Before I ask a few questions, I am wondering if you have some questions?

CALLER: Yeah, how much does this cost?

INTAKE SOCIAL WORKER: Being a United Way agency, we can offer a sliding fee scale, depending on income and dependents, so I will need to ask some financial questions.

CALLER: OK, go for it then.

INTAKE SOCIAL WORKER: Generally I do not start with the financial questions. I wonder if you could tell me what services . . .

CALLER: Look, just asking about the money; if I can't afford it, then there is no point in telling you a lot of personal information.

> *Maybe the caller employed another way to distance himself from arousing personal information that could stir up unwanted arousing emotions beyond his "window of tolerance" (Siegel, 2007). The financial discussion may have given him some relief from that prospect.*

INTAKE SOCIAL WORKER: OK, sir. What is your name, address, and telephone number?

CALLER: Mannie Lopes, Address***, phone******, and Lopes is spelled L-O-P-E-S—there is no z in my name (*emphatically*).

INTAKE SOCIAL WORKER: What is your monthly income and how many dependents do you have?

CALLER: I help my wife run her day-care center, ever since I got laid off. I keep the maintenance perfect.

INTAKE SOCIAL WORKER: What is your income?

CALLER: We clear about $1,800 a month.

INTAKE SOCIAL WORKER: How many dependents do you have?

CALLER: Funny you should ask, since I am a dependent now to my wife.

INTAKE SOCIAL WORKER: (*ignoring this complicated remark*) I see. How many dependents do you and your wife have, like children or elderly parents?

CALLER: Oh, yes, well my mother-in-law, Abuelita, is with us now, since her husband died . . . (*starts to cry and then continues slowly*), and she sort of tried to help out with the children, but mainly cleans up a little; her bones hurt her a lot.

INTAKE SOCIAL WORKER: I am sorry about your father-in-law. Did he pass away recently?

CALLER: Yes, last fall. In fact, that is why my wife said I should call you; I can't get over his death, and he wasn't even my father.

INTAKE SOCIAL WORKER: We do have staff here that know how to help with the death of loved ones.

CALLER: It's not that simple. I, well, anyway, OK, my wife might be right, that I just can't get over this by working all the time, even though it is good to not feel anything when I wear myself out.

Mr. Lopes's conflict about being independent versus having to count on others seemed clear. The social worker had no idea that Mr. Lopes would have such a strong reaction to the question about dependents, and the social worker did not explore the remark "now I am dependent on my wife." Perhaps the social worker's nonconscious automatic appraisal of the significance of this word was registering. The social worker may have decided that the intake call was no place for such a "hot cognition" (Schore, 2003b, p. 280), meaning, an upsetting or provocative thought or idea.

INTAKE SOCIAL WORKER: Sir, if I could ask just a few more questions, then I can put you on a wait list, OK? For example, do have any other dependents, aside from your mother-in-law?

CALLER: Yes, we have a 4-year-old daughter who has CF. Do you know what that is?

INTAKE SOCIAL WORKER: Do you mean cystic fibrosis?

CALLER: Yes, right.

INTAKE SOCIAL WORKER: Medical expenses are part of the formula for determining the fee for service. Could you estimate what that is, monthly?

CALLER: I'm not sure. We are on Cobra Insurance right now, but it will run out in a few months, and then her—*Carmelita* is her name—expenses will be on us.

INTAKE SOCIAL WORKER: I can see that your situation needs a review; I wonder if you could come in and talk to me about your expenses and so on. I would need to see Carmelita's medical bills over the past year (more or less) so we could help you with a sliding fee—oh, and a copy of your last year's income taxes.

CALLER: When do I have to come? In 3 weeks?

INTAKE SOCIAL WORKER: No, we could make an appointment sooner than that and get the paperwork out of your way.

CALLER: What about today?

INTAKE SOCIAL WORKER: What about tomorrow? Around 2 p.m.?

CALLER: OK. I hope I can find our taxes and that other stuff.

INTAKE SOCIAL WORKER: If you cannot find the information before our appointment, just call me and we can reschedule, OK?

CALLER: OK, OK (*sounds a bit resigned*), I'll try.

INTAKE SOCIAL WORKER: My name is Josh Samuel. Just ask for me tomorrow; our address is 2234 Comal Street. Do you know where that is?

CALLER: (*sounds surprised*) Oh, yeah, that's in our neighborhood (*perks up*). See you tomorrow.

Mr. Lopes vacillated between relief that the appointment was a few weeks away and wanting to be seen that day—which could be emblematic of his ambivalence over dependency, as described in the compulsive self-reliant attachment category. He both wanted to be dependent (hence, the call to agency) and he did not want to be dependent (his resistance to various suggestions of the staff).

He may have been under so much stress at the point of his call to the agency that he may not be as able to manage his vulnerability to his dependency wishes and needs, and they leaked through with some of his comments (e.g., "What about today?"; being glad that the agency was close by). His maintaining the day-care center "perfectly" is an example of the trait of reliability, of doing a good job; in his case, it may indicate that he is generally extremely self-sufficient. His recent job loss and heavy family responsibilities may have overwhelmed his usual defenses of obsessiveness (avoid anxiety by controlling behaviors), controlling (manage external events to minimize anxiety and avoid conflict), denial (wife has to insist that he needed help over grief), and perhaps inhibition (renouncing certain functions to avoid anxiety from various sources of conflict). All these defensive maneuvers are managed by the <u>parasympathetic branch of the autonomic nervous system</u>.

Barbanell (2006) has proposed a new diagnostic category: caretaker personality disorder. Mr. Lopes seems to meet most of the criteria. Table 5.7 compares the attachment category of compulsive self-reliant to the criteria Mr. Lopes meets from Barbanell's proposed caretaker personality disorder. These criteria describe behaviors that are primarily managed by the <u>parasympathetic branch of the autonomic nervous system</u>. Additional criteria for caretaker personality disorder include repression of joy, pleasure, and intimacy; guilt, emotional emptiness, loneliness, and physical exhaustion; and low self-esteem (Barbanell, 2006, pp. 66–67)—all of which (except perhaps for guilt) are low-affect states, <u>parasympathetically managed</u>. Mr. Lopes may experience the above affects, but that cannot be determined from the call to the agency. Interestingly, Barbanell, when comparing his proposed caretaker

TABLE 5.7.
Comparing Attachment Category of Compulsive Self-Reliant
to Caretaker Personality Disorder

Compulsive Self-Reliant[a]	Caretaker Personality Disorder[b]
Avoids turning to others for comfort, attachment, support, or affection	Avoids self-need gratification, but forms attachments by giving to others; pervasive and compulsive need to be needed; relentlessly overresponsible; conceals past trauma and current crises by focusing on others; avoids conflict, anger, and direct expression of displeasure to preserve contact with others
Places a high premium on self-sufficiency	Appears self-sustaining
Motivated by a counterdependent need to be self-sufficient, rather than outright disdain for others	Counterdependent; appears independent

[a] Based on Bowlby, 1977; West & Sheldon, as cited in Kaslow, 1996, p. 85.
[b] Based on Barbanell, 2006, pp. 66–67.

personality disorder to other personality disorders, suggests that the most similar seems to be obsessive–compulsive personality disorder, though there are strong similarities to the narcissistic personality disorder as well (2006).

Case Example of Fearful-Avoidant Attachment
Adult attachment category: Fearful-avoidant
Management of arousal: Parasympathetically dominated behaviors
Description of attachment category: Fearful-avoidant. Speculation regarding childhood attachment category: insecure-avoidant, sometimes termed anxious-avoidant (Florsheim et al., 1996, p. 84)

A fearful-avoidant person has a negative attachment view of self and others and anticipates betrayal, rejection, and criticism. Such a person is likely to protect him- or herself from rejection or attack by avoiding involvement with others. The fearful-avoidant adult category is described by the work of Bartholomew and Horowitz (as cited in Florsheim et al., p. 84).

WILL: You know, I don't understand why people keep calling me from work. They keep asking me to go out like we used to before I retired. It was hard enough to go to all those birthday lunches, happy hours, and cakes for every occasion we ate in the break room. And bowling, my God, if I never see another bowling alley, that will be too soon. Now I *still* have to invent excuses not to go.

THERAPIST: You know, Will, I have been worried for a while about your isolating yourself after you retired. A person can spend too much time alone. I know you really don't agree with me on that, and I hate to sound like a nag, but being by yourself in your house all the time can create problems.

WILL: Like what? I like my own company just fine.

THERAPIST: Oh, come on, Will. You sleep way too much; you know that your back situation requires some daily exercise and not hours of being in bed. What happened to going to the YMCA with your neighbors?

WILL: To tell you the truth, they were expecting too much out of me. After the gym, then they wanted to go to brunch at that organic food place, or drink coffee at their place . . . (*trails off*). And, anyway, since I retired, I have to watch my money; I just can't go out whenever I feel like it. And have you ever looked at the price of those organic foods? A dollar for a little carrot. I'm not paying that!

> Will did not seek the interactive regulation of emotion. In fact, he avoided social interaction. He may just be an introvert (may be a parasympathetically activated temperament trait), but he also may have given up on interactions with others as being gratifying.

THERAPIST: I thought you liked that couple.

WILL: They're OK and, to be fair, they help me when I have to go to Waco to help my son work on his place. They watch after my dog, if I can't take her with me.

THERAPIST: What about your [other] son here in town? Those little boys [of his] could use a grandfather with your kind of skills and interests.

WILL: Ahhh, I don't have that much to offer them, and they get wild sometimes and I just don't know what to do. My wife, God rest her soul, did all that when our kids were little. I just don't know what to do when they ask me to sit with those boys. I am afraid my daughter-in-law will just get mad if they come back and the house is a wreck, so I don't encourage that.

> He displayed a negative view of himself and expected criticism, as in the above description of the fearful-avoidant personality. He may not have had experiences with stressful interactions that were not "set right" (Pipp & Harmon, 1987, p. 650). He may have been thrown back on his own resources to

manage himself emotionally, leading to a preference for staying away from others (parasympathetic nervous system) to avoid uncomfortable arousal and to seek low arousal (parasympathetic nervous system).

THERAPIST: What about those times when you were helping your son and his family build things in the backyard all afternoon? I don't recall those little boys being any trouble; they followed you around like puppies, and you said they both seemed to have a knack for tools, they listened to your safety rules, and their parents were full of compliments for the doghouse they built.

WILL: You know, I only remember the bad times, like when they watch cartoons and tear around the living room, turning over furniture, and then I get criticized for being a bad grandfather.

THERAPIST: Do you really get criticized openly?

WILL: Sometimes, but mostly I see the upset on their faces and feel bad for days about it.

THERAPIST: Will, since your wife did most of the childrearing, you are not as much of a natural. But I will tell you, those young grandsons will not forget the doghouse and playscape they helped build with you. Let's put our heads together and think of other projects that do not involve cartoons and violent TV programs. Those tend to agitate kids anyway. You have some skills in building and repair that could create great memories for your grandchildren. And you said yourself, those boys were super tired, well behaved, and just ate supper and went to bed after such a day. Kids do not have many opportunities like that these days.

> *Clinician's right hemisphere may have been responding to the low affect and negative self-evaluation of Will by cheerleading a bit in an attempt to stimulate some positive, more sympathetically arousing affect, interest, and excitement. The clinician's nonconscious right hemisphere may find Will's level of affect intolerable, so reflexively the clinician raises the level of arousal, in the hope that Will's level of arousal may follow suit.*

WILL: All right, you keep saying all that every time I come in here. Nobody did anything with *us kids*, especially my grandpa. All us kids stayed as far away as possible; I even saw him sock my dad right in the mouth because my dad disagreed with him over how to fix something under the hood. And then Grandpa turned around and started to throw all the tools he could get a hold of at me and my cousin. I can tell you for sure, we all stayed away from him—even my own dad couldn't stand up to him. How was he going to keep that old man away from us, I ask you?

The fearful-avoidant attachment category is similar to the schizoid and avoidant personality organizations (see Table 5.8). However, Will seemed to care what others thought of him, unlike the schizoid personality disorder criterion 6: "Appears indifferent to the praise or criticism of others." Nevertheless, for each schizoid/avoidant criteria and behavior, the <u>parasympathetic branch</u> is involved in inhibition. From the mention of the danger and maybe emotional neglect Will appeared to have experienced in childhood, he might have been cautious about involvement with others, but perhaps he had not given up entirely. He had been married, had held a job long enough to retire from it, and had some engagement with his children and grandchildren.

What he needs within the therapeutic dyad is to safely experience some arousal, like play and pleasure, with others as the clinician suggests (i.e., the grandchildren). This may gently and safely address the traits of the schizoid (detachment and dampened emotions) and the avoidant (inadequate feelings, inhibited behaviors, and sensitivity to negative opinions of others) experiences (DSM-IV-TR, 2000, pp. 697 & 721, respectively).

Case Example of Dismissive Attachment

Adult attachment category: Dismissive attachment
Management of arousal: Parasympathetically dominated behaviors
Description of attachment category: Dismissive attachment. Speculation regarding preexisting childhood attachment category: insecure-avoidant, sometimes termed *avoidant* (Florsheim et al., 1996, p. 84).

A dismissive person has a positive view of self and a negative view of others and protects the self against disappointment by "avoiding close relationships and maintaining a sense of independence and invulnerability" (as described by the work of Bartholomew and Horowitz, cited in Florsheim et al., 1996, p. 84).

ANDI: Here I am again, but I'm not too sure why. Last time we talked about my family, which was a waste of time, in a way. I don't mean to be rude, but I am completely clear about who they are and what effect they have had on me.

> *Andi began with her disappointment in the clinician. She needed the clinician to <u>put things right</u>, meaning to offer an <u>opportunity for interactive repair</u> (<u>perhaps, apologize?</u>). Putting things right can lead to stress recovery. However, if no interactive/dyadic stress recovery/repair occurs, then Andi may have to manage her disappointment by herself. That might become a problem, if her affect management strategy is too extreme (too avoidant or too clinging).*

TABLE 5.8.
Comparing Attachment Category of Fearful-Avoidant Attachment to
DSM Avoidant Personality Disorder and Schizoid Personality Disorder

Fearful Avoidance[a]	Avoidant Personality Disorder[b] Schizoid Personality Disorder[c]
Negative attachment view of self and others	Avoidant PD: Unwilling to get involved with people unless certain of being liked; shows restraint within intimate relationships because of fear of being shamed or ridiculed; preoccupied with being criticized or rejected in social situations; inhibited in new interpersonal situations because of feelings of inadequacy; views self as socially inept, personally unappealing, or inferior to others
Anticipates betrayal, rejection, and criticism	Avoidant PD: Unusually reluctant to take personal risks to engage in any new activities because may prove embarrassing Schizoid PD: Appears indifferent to the praise or criticism of others
Likely to protect him- or herself from rejection or attack by avoiding involvement with others	Avoidant PD: Avoids occupational activities that involve significant interpersonal contact because of fear of criticism, disapproval, or rejection Schizoid PD: Neither desires nor enjoys close relationships, including being part of a family; almost always chooses solitary activities; lacks close friends or confidantes other than first-degree relatives; has little, if any, interest in having sexual experiences with another person

[a]Based on Bartholomew & Horowitz, as cited in Kaslow, 1996, p. 85.
[b]From *The Diagnostic and Statistical Manual of Mental Disorders—Text Revised* (American Psychiatric Association, 2000, p. 721). Reprinted with permission.
[c]From *The Diagnostic and Statistical Manual of Mental Disorders, Fourth Edition, Text Revised.* See Appendix B for complete DSM diagnostic criteria for the disorders referenced above.

THERAPIST: That may very well be the case, Andi, but I need to know about your experience in your family, too. And, sometimes, another person's perspective or questions might shed some light on childhood experiences. In turn, some of the relationship concerns you came in here with might be better understood.

The clinician may have been trying to stay related and engaged. However, Andi's rejection of the clinician's previous attempt to learn about her past may *have indicated that she did understand it and it was not a problem, or the opposite. It could be that Andi's <u>amygdala is warning her to stay away from arousing (potentially) information</u>, for which she does not have enough sturdiness to manage without resorting to defenses and behaviors that ultimately may not serve her well.*

ANDI: Whatever. I know that intellectually, but it really seems like a stretch. What I really need is some advice and maybe some kind of plan to deal more effectively with these guys. I keep getting these guys who are too dependent, always wanting more and more.

Andi dismissed the clinician's effort (<u>the clinician's suggestion may invite too much unwanted arousal</u>). Andi had her plan or goal for her therapy. Although the clinician ethically should respect the client's right to self-determination, clinically, it should be considered that Andi did not want to depend on the clinician and would have rather depended on herself. Andi's reluctance to depend on others could be the underlying reason for her relationship problems.

THERAPIST: When they are acting dependent, what is your reaction to that?

ANDI: (*wrinkles her nose*) Dis-guuustinnnng. I like rock-climbing, kayaking, car trips, and all that, you know—guy stuff. And I am good at those sports, too. Better than some of them. But this last guy, he really upset me.

THERAPIST: Can we go back to the disgusting feeling? What is that like when you feel that way?

ANDI: What do you mean?

THERAPIST: Most emotions have a physical component to them.

ANDI: Like what?

THERAPIST: Such as a headache or tension in the shoulders.

ANDI: Oh, let me think back. OK, when I am disgusted they usually are acting all gooshy.

THERAPIST: What physical feeling do you have when they act all "gooshy"?

ANDI: I thought I answered that question.

THERAPIST: You answered by further describing his behaving as "gooshy" but not by describing what happens to your body when a guy does that.

ANDI: Oh. Maybe I don't have any physical feeling.

Andi seemed resistant to the clinician's efforts, which may have been emotion-ally uncomfortable for her as those emotions may be <u>sympathetically acti-vated</u>.

THERAPIST: Maybe not. What about trying to remember if you had similar reactions in your family when someone acted all gooshy.

ANDI: (*emphatically*) That's a good one. The only person who ever acted gooshy was the lady next door, an African lady—like, really from Africa. She used to babysit me and my sister. They were refugees from one of those wars and her son was a professor like my parents. Their English was weird and she sang all those sad African songs. But she let us sit on her big lap and . . . (*stops, seems far away*).

THERAPIST: (Long pause; therapist just waits.)

ANDI: What were you saying? I lost the thread.

By asking about Andi's emotional/bodily reactions, the clinician may have been trying to introduce a level of affective intensity that went a bit beyond what Andi may typically display or experience. <u>The right limbic system of the clinician may have been nonconsciously registering the avoidance of arousal by Andi and trying to compensate for it or correct it somewhat, hopefully to a level that Andi could tolerate. The clinician may have been nonconsciously hoping for a "transfer of affect"</u> (Schore, 2003a, pp. 11–13) <u>and a transfer of affective intensity from the clinician to Andi.</u> The clinician may have been moving too fast for Andi's ability to tolerate arousal, perhaps? If so, Andi may have become <u>slightly dissociated</u> (parasympathetic nervous system managing <u>polyvagal system to create a "freeze" response emotionally, though briefly</u>) when Andi seemed "far away."

THERAPIST: Actually, you were remembering about the African lady with her songs and big lap and you just stopped talking.

ANDI: Crap! I haven't thought about her in years (*more animated and a little pressured speech*). Can't imagine what I was thinking about. Anyway, my parents put a stop to her babysitting, saying we were too old. But we were only 5 and 6, so I think they got mad about us sitting in her lap.

THERAPIST: Why was that?

ANDI: Don't know. Maybe they were trying to protect us from some abuse or something. But, really, looking back, I think they did not want us to get used to being so cozy with her. My sister and I call our parents snowflakes (*grins, naughtily*).

THERAPIST: Snowflakes?

ANDI: Yeah, after some alternative Christmas card that said something about parents being cold and flakey. We were the only Asian kids in this stupid church that didn't celebrate birthdays or Christmas and did not believe in spoiling kids.

THERAPIST: Spoiling kids how?

ANDI: If you coddle kids too much, they will not be able to stand on their own two feet and take care of themselves. When we were home by ourselves, we had chores and lists to complete to learn how to care for ourselves.

Andi may have been somewhat stressed by the level of arousal (sympathetic nervous system) when describing those childhood experiences. Andi and her sister were "latchkey children" (taking care of themselves after school), having received the message that being self-sufficient and not dependent was expected. What must it have been like for the children to lose the cozy experience of the warm, grandmotherly figure? To describe their parents as "cold and flakey" gives a glimpse into the girls' quality of contact with their parents.

THERAPIST: Going back to what the last guy did that upset you—what was it?

ANDI: Now that you ask, he was really good at the sports I like, better than me. Like, he is really tough. But at night around a campfire, he would want to sing and talk about personal things . . . way too much, like, way too much information. And, get this, he wanted to know personal things about me.

THERAPIST: And that was disgusting to you?

ANDI: It made me want to drink, maybe smoke, get high. Strange, because I hardly do either, but I couldn't get away from him on the campout, so had the urge to use drugs.

THERAPIST: What sensation were you trying to deal with, I wonder?

ANDI: You know, since you keep asking, it was sheer panic, if you have to know.

THERAPIST: Panic was probably a physical sensation, right?

ANDI: I guess.

THERAPIST: Where in your body did you feel panic?

ANDI: Huh? I think I felt like I was going to fly into little pieces, like go into orbit. Like all jazzed up.

THERAPIST: That seems like extreme anxiety?

> *Again, the clinician was uncovering a pattern: When aroused ("sheer panic"), Andi wanted to numb herself ("get high" may be a misnomer, in that smoking marijuana, if it was that, achieves a state of low affect) with a central nervous system depressant. This may be similar to when her parasympathetic branch shut down into "freeze" earlier in this session when describing the singing, etc., of the grandmotherly lady next door.*

ANDI: Say, what exactly is the purpose of this discussion? I wanted a plan for dealing with these guys.

THERAPIST: I am thinking that if you have a plan to deal with your own reactions first, that dealing with the guys might be easier.

ANDI: Sounds like a pat answer to me.

THERAPIST: I guess basic principles can sound a little pat. However, it seems like you want a plan for not getting involved with guys who get "gooshy" rather than a plan to wonder why you have such a strong reaction to "gooshy."

ANDI: The perfect answer is for me to agree to this universal truth, but I am still skeptical.

Andi may have been employing parasympathetically activating (low affect) defense mechanisms whose functions are minimizing and avoiding: intellectualization ("I wanted a plan"); inhibition/blocking/isolation of affect/dissociation; denial (minimize experience by lack of awareness); and controlling (struggling with clinician over a "plan" vs. understanding oneself). The criteria she meets for schizoid personality disorder is quite similar to the dismissive attachment style: Both seek low arousal utilizing defenses that foster a detached state of low arousal and avoid high state of arousal.

The clinician may have been stressed by the low affect displayed by Andi; like painfully high arousal, low affect can also be painful, inviting a countertransference reaction. For example, the clinician tried to move too fast, to pick up the arousal, and to press for data about bodily substrates to some of Andi's emotional reactions. No doubt those interventions would have been, or will be, helpful, but the timing may be unempathic and more a function of the clinician's need to intervene than Andi's need to have that intervention at that particular moment. It is clear that Andi's defenses are challenged by the clinician, perhaps prematurely.

According to current practice, Andi would be diagnosed with schizoid personality disorder, but care would have to be taken to assess her over time to determine the utility of such a diagnosis. It may be as clinically useful to organize her treatment around the dismissive attachment category, because that framework takes into account the history of past relationships (Howes, 1999), unlike the DSM-IV-TR approach, which does not speculate about etiology for the personality disorders. Andi may experience a personality disorder in a general sense: That is, she seems to have formed a patterned and stable way of relating cognitively (perceives self as positive and others as negative), affectively (typically prefers low affect [nonconsciously]), interpersonally (more comfortable with predictable structure ["plan"] to minimize the "surprises" that emotions may evoke), and in terms of impulse control (overcontrolled) (American Psychiatric Association, 2000, pp. 685–690). Table 5.9 compares dismissive attachment criteria with those for schizoid personality disorder.

Case Example of Adult Angry-Withdrawn Attachment

Adult attachment category: Angry-withdrawn attachment
Management of arousal: Uncoupled and oscillating sympathetic nervous system (excitatory) and parasympathetic nervous system (inhibitory)
Adult attachment category: Angry-withdrawn attachment. Speculation regarding childhood attachment category: insecure-ambivalent, sometimes termed *resistant* (Florsheim et al., 1996, p. 85)

The person with an angry-withdrawn attachment is likely to react to responsiveness and unavailability with anger and defensiveness (as described by the work of West & Sheldon, cited in Florsheim et al., 1996, p. 85).

HUSBAND: (*aggravated*) You know, I am having my doubts about all this "history," as you call it. I just don't see the relevance to why we came here in the first place.

> *The <u>autonomic nervous system</u> (sympathetic branch) was activated in this comment.*

THERAPIST: (*lowers her voice*) Could you reiterate your goals for why you wanted to—

> *The autonomic nervous system (parasympathetic branch) was activated to promote civilized social interaction (Porges, 2007). The clinician may have been counterregulating with his parasympathetic branch (inhibitory).*

TABLE 5.9 Comparing Attachment Category of Dismissive Attachment to DSM Schizoid Personality Disorder	
Dismissive Attachment[a]	Schizoid Personality Disorder[b]
Positive view of self and a negative view of others	Appears indifferent to the praise or criticism of others
Protects the self against disappointment by "avoiding close relationships and maintaining a sense of independence and invulnerability"	Neither desires nor enjoys close relationship, including being part of a family
	Almost always chooses solitary activities; shows emotional coldness, detachment, or flattened affectivity; lacks close friends or confidantes other than first-degree relatives

[a]Based on Bartholomew & Horowitz and Main & Goldwyn, as cited in Kaslow, 1996, p. 85.
[b]From *The Diagnostic and Statistical Manual of Mental Disorders, Fourth Edition, Text Revised*. See Appendix B for complete DSM diagnostic criteria for the disorder referenced above.

HUSBAND: (*interrupting quickly*) It was, after all, her (*nods his head sharply in wife's direction*) idea anyway.

THERAPIST: Yes, that's true, but surely (*flipping through notes from earlier session*) you wanted something as well. Oh, here it is. When we first met, you said that you wanted to get along better, if only for the sake of the children and the church. I wonder if you have current thoughts on that goal?

> *The clinician tried for lower affect and a more intellectualized comment (para-sympathetic nervous system), looking for actual "facts" such as what the client actually stated originally as his goals (left hemisphere).*

HUSBAND: (*critical tone*) You said that we could have a copy of your notes at any time. Right?

THERAPIST: (*conciliatory tone*) This is true, you just have to give me a little time to copy them for you—but not to get sidetracked. You began the session by questioning the process of looking at the past relationships of both of you. I do link past relationship experience to current relationship concerns. I have personally never seen a situation where the past was completely irrelevant, especially to the couple relationship.

> *The clinician matched the husband's "state" of detailing facts, again, and took the opportunity to "teach." This may, in some way, be less agitating to*

the husband, as picked up by the nonconscious resonating of the clinician's right hemisphere, perhaps even the amygdala, responsible for assessing safety and danger. The clinician was being very careful in response to the husband's demanding behavior, as she used her left hemisphere to stay logical.

HUSBAND: The church is crystal clear about our obligations. You stay married. You take care of the children. You support the work of the church. Period. End of story.

It is difficult to tell if the clinician was trying to lower the intensity of affect by employing a more parasympathetic nervous system-dominated, left-hemisphere set of interventions or if the clinician was trying to protect herself from the aggression of the husband by becoming more "professional"—or if the husband was matching the more intellectual tone of the clinician.

THERAPIST: (*turning to wife, speaking in concerned manner*) You have been quiet today. What has been your experience of my conversation with your husband?

The clinician was trying to engage the wife in empathic manner (right hemisphere).

HUSBAND: (*talking over his wife*) That's a problem right there. You see (*a little agitated*), there she is, a bump on a log, with me and you doing all the work. Just like at home. Church-mouse (*sneering*)!

The husband's tight, cold, self-control deteriorated a bit and he was becoming dysregulated, as he was interrupting and criticizing his wife so aggressively (sympathetic branch activated).

THERAPIST: (*turning directly to wife*) I think it is time for you to have some air time, don't you think? How has it been for you to listen to this discussion today?

Perhaps the clinician was rescuing the wife from aggression here and, at the same time, ignoring the husband's outburst. The clinician may not have wanted to match the husband's state to avoid the "transfer of affect" (Schore, 1994, 2003a, 2003b), as well as the transfer of the intensity of affect, as it might be very uncomfortable.

WIFE: I never can figure him out. If I leave him alone, it upsets him and he criticizes me. If I try to talk to him or even do what I think he wants, he criticizes me. Or sometimes he just blows up. Me and the kids are on pins and needles around him. When he flies to San Jose for a week at a time, the house is so different.

The wife may be emboldened by the clinician's taking her perspective in an empathic manner (Fosha, 2000, 2010), a right-hemisphere experience.

HUSBAND: (*coolly angry*) You need a referee? Let me weigh in on this . . .

THERAPIST: I apologize for interrupting, but I would like to pursue her experience some before you comment on it. (*turning directly to him*) Are you OK with that right now?

HUSBAND: Not really. I need to set the record straight, but OK, your turn.

THERAPIST: (*directly to the husband*) There might be a difference between the facts of what happened or was said and each person's own experience of what happened. No one really knows how another person has experienced a situation until that person has described it. Some things are irreducible or can't really be challenged. So I would like to get back for a moment to your wife's experience of you and me and our discussion. (*looks at the wife*).

> *Again, the clinician was drawn into state matching with the husband; his pushy way of assuming that others will do what he wants may have pushed the clinician to try to manage his (the husband's) affects by "teaching," another left-hemisphere, conscious intervention. The clinician did set a limit with the bullying behavior, but really gently, as if the husband were fragile (which he may be).*

WIFE: I feel shook up. I hate making him mad, but it seems that everything we do makes him mad. He seems happiest when he is in his study with his cat and the TV on sports and him on the computer at the same time.

THERAPIST: What did you feel or think about his discussion of your marriage in terms of what the church expects?

WIFE: (*Starting to cry; husband moves away physically from her to edge of his side of couch.*) That made me know that I am just an obligation—that if the church did not punish divorce, he would divorce me; that he has to stay with me, but does not really want to.

> *The wife seemed capable of being vulnerable and open, even in the face of the husband's somewhat desperate attempts to curtail or control her emotionality. He has used verbal acting out (sarcasm), regression (rudely criticizing wife), and projection (blaming) in the session, all sympathetically activated defenses (per the description, the angry-withdrawn adult attachment style reacts with defensiveness to responsiveness). Generally, an angry-withdrawn personality will try to stay remote and distant (trying for parasympathetically activated behaviors leading to low levels of affect). However, when anger is evoked, the individual can lose control of him- or herself and become aggressive. The compromised functioning of the sympathetic branch is the reason*

that the husband's brain gravitated as much as possible to the parasympathetic branch, responsible for low affect.

THERAPIST: What about your wishes to stay or leave the marriage? Do you share his beliefs about marriage being an obligation that you cannot get out of?

The clinician was making a bold statement; she had challenged the husband by rephrasing the husband's rather cold and clipped description of the church's view on marriage by saying, "being an obligation you cannot get out of." Maybe the clinician was somewhat aggressive or at least assertive? Or, maybe clinician was reacting to the bullying and refusing to submit. Whatever the case, the clinician did not simply restate what the husband said, but used the wife's term, obligation, and may have provoked the next outburst below.

HUSBAND: (*jumping in*) I never said that! Technically, we could divorce, I just meant . . .

THERAPIST: (*interrupting*) If we can let you clarify your comments in a minute, I would like to see what your wife's response is to the question about her religious beliefs on marriage.

WIFE: (*looks up, a little surprised*) My beliefs? I never thought about that. Actually, I converted when we got married. My family were plain old Methodists, and not very observant at that. I was glad he had some clear convictions, since my family didn't.

The final comment of the wife gave some insight into the projective identification that might be occurring. The husband might have been projecting the capacity to be vulnerable onto the wife, who then expressed those feelings for him. She might have been projecting onto her husband cooler, more intellectual and logical ways of being, which he certainly expressed easily. They both may have identified with the projections of the other and become more and more extreme in their positions. This dynamic only makes the one mate try to pressure the other mate to keep projected material away from his or her own mind. The wife gave a small clue about why the husband's rigidity might be appealing when she referred to the "plain old Methodists" in contrast to the "clear convictions" of her husband and his religion. Projective identification uses both the sympathetic branch in order to activate the projection and the parasympathetic branch (usually dissociation) in order to maintain unawareness that the projected material is, in fact, one's own.

The husband seems well described by the attachment category of angry-withdrawn, which is likely activated by both the excitatory and inhibitory branches, respectively, of the autonomic nervous system. He almost meets criteria for both narcissistic personality disorder (generally activated by the inhibitory parasympathetic branch) and paranoid personality disorder (generally activated by the excitatory sympathetic branch), making the diagnosis of personality disorder, not otherwise specified, appropriate as he meets criteria for more than one personality disorder (see DSM-IV-TR, American Psychiatric Association, 2000).

Based on the description of the angry-withdrawn attachment disorder, the husband's reacting to responsiveness and unavailability with anger and defensiveness is challenging to anyone who may try to engage with him, such as his wife ("I never know how he will react") or the clinician. With the sometimes rapid oscillation between excitatory and inhibitory affects that the husband exhibits, the clinician finds herself reacting with difficulty to either match or counterregulate the husband's reactions (e.g., "The church is crystal clear"; talking over his wife, coolly angry: "You need a referee . . . let me weigh in on this"; and jumping in to protest, "I never said that. Technically, we could divorce, I just meant . . .").

From the session, it seems that the husband meets several criteria for narcissistic personality disorder. For example, he is "interpersonally exploitative, i.e., takes advantage of others to achieve his or her own ends . . . lacks empathy . . . and is unwilling to recognize or identify with the feelings and needs of others" (American Psychiatric Association, 2000, p. 717). Also from the session, it seems that he also meets several criteria from paranoid personality disorder: For example, he "persistently bears grudges, i.e., is unforgiving of insults, injuries, or slights" (American Psychiatric Association, 2000, p. 694). These behaviors/traits are not explicit in the description of the fearful-avoidant attachment category, but they are certainly evident in the session. Table 5.10 compares the angry-withdrawn attachment category with the criteria for narcissistic and paranoid personality disorders.

Concluding Comments

Examining clinical experiences not only for the implicit arousal systems involved in the transactions but also for what that information means in terms of what is required from the clinician has broad applications. Speculations regarding the structures that are responsible for certain levels of arousal may easily be examined to determine the similarity among the arousal management issues embedded in an attachment category, a personality-disordered character style, and the typically unconscious defenses that manifest in the session.

However, there are likely other clinical data and issues that could be included in this examples—for example, the neurotransmitters that manage level of arousal. Additionally, though beyond the scope of this book (except

TABLE 5.10.
Comparing Attachment Category of Angry-Withdrawn Attachment to DSM
Narcissistic Personality Disorder and Paranoid Personality Disorder

Angry-Withdrawn Attachment[a]	Narcissistic Personality Disorder Paranoid Personality Disorder
Person is likely to react to responsiveness and unavailibility with anger and defensiveness	**Narcissistic PD[b]** Expects to be recognized as superior without commensurate achievements; has a sense of entitlement, i.e., unreasonable expectations of especially favorable treatment or automatic compliance with his or her expectations
	Paranoid PD[b] Suspects, without sufficient basis, that others are exploiting, harming, or deceiving him or her; reads hidden demeaning or threatening meanings into benign remarks or events; perceives attacks on his or her character or reputation that are not apparent to others and is quick to react angrily or to counterattack

[a]Based on West & Sheldon, as cited in Kaslow, 1996, p. 85.
[b]From *The Diagnostic and Statistical Manual of Mental Disorders, Fourth Edition, Text Revised*. See Appendix B for complete DSM diagnostic criteria for the disorders referenced above.

for a passing mention in two cases described in this chapter), the drug of choice for those with substance abuse issues could be examined. The logic for use of a substance for affective management seems virtually the same as for rigidly using the brain of another person for mood stabilization. For example, unless a person struggles with a polysubstance issue (i.e., not particular about drugs used), as described in the earlier part of this chapter, then generally there is a preference for a substance that either excites or inhibits. As is often the case, there is a concomitant lack of interest in, or even an aversion for, the substance that has the opposite effects.

The "arousal level of choice" (of course, unconscious) gives the clinician information about which part of his or her arousal system (excitatory or inhibitory) the client might need to "borrow." The interpersonal dynamic would be the same, as illustrated in the case examples of this chapter. If the client prefers substances that are excitatory, it is likely that he or she has difficulty with low affects. Therefore, the brain, particularly the parasympathetic branch (inhibitory), of the clinician would need to be able to tolerate low affects interactively, with the brain of the client, so that new neural pathways may be created or atrophied ones strengthened (and vice versa, with the preference for substances that inhibit).

With addictions as well as with most disorders described in the DSM-IV and the DSM-IV-TR (American Psychiatric Association, 1994, 2000) and likely also the DSM-5 (proposed for 2013), there is no cause suggested to account for the lack of balanced functioning and for compromised affective management capacities. In contrast, the research that describes childhood and adult attachment categories does consider the quality of the caretaking relationship as influencing the attachment styles. The similarities between underlying physiological arousal systems for both the styles of disordered personality functioning and attachment styles examined in this chapter easily posit repetitive relationship interactions as a major contributor to the behavioral template.

The mental health treatment culture has rightfully steered away from "parent blaming" for the existence of psychiatric problems. For many decades there has been a reluctance to attribute a correlation between childhood and adolescent developmental experiences and later mental health problems. Swinging too far in the direction of silence as to the cause of certain conditions, though, runs the risk of not offering early intervention that could head off rigid and troublesome ways of interacting, some of which may eventually become diagnosable as a psychiatric disorder, particularly a personality disorder.

Additionally, being uncurious about past developmental insults and the real possibility that neural circuitry can be strengthened or created or both (through neural plasticity) ignores research that supports the idea that the correction for disturbed personality functioning is related to the original influence of repeated early experiences. At the very least, clinicians' lack of information about the neurophysiological effects on patterned behaviors may blunt their awareness and appreciation of the rewiring of the brain that may be occurring in their therapeutic work. If we are unaware of why change is occurring in the brains of our clients, via the clinical relationship (and various interventions), we will not necessarily repeat such interventions deliberately. Fortunately, the recent decade or so has made accessible to clinicians neurophysiological information that explains, or at least strongly suggests, why many interventions work (Kandel, 2005). As the neuroscience is not wed to any particular treatment school, it is likely equally explanatory regarding why certain strategies and techniques work, particularly those that focus on the elements of the treatment relationship.

PART II
Special Populations and Topics

CHAPTER 6

The Adolescent Brain
Selected Functions That Differ from the Adult Brain

This chapter reviews the session of Cori and her school counselor again. In Chapter 1 some important neurobiological influences on Cori's family and close community were addressed. In Chapter 2 Cori's session was discussed primarily in terms of synchronous affect attunement and the opposite, asynchrony; for defense mechanisms employed; and which branch of the autonomic nervous system was being utilized (the excitatory sympathetic branch or the inhibitory parasympathetic branch). Additionally, illustrations of the functions of the right and left hemisphere and mirror neurons were described. This chapter examines ways that Cori's adolescent brain functioning is different (at times) from that of an adult brain.

Selected Sociocultural, Biological, and Neurobiological Definitions of Adolescence

Descriptions of adolescence have been influenced by culture, biology, and in the last few decades, neurobiology. In preindustrial Western eras, people were defined either as quite small children or adults, with adulthood coming as early as 10 years old (Schlegel & Barry, as cited in Epstein, 2007; Goldberg, 1993). As soon as family members could work, they did, which may have helped to confer adult status on young children. In the pre-Industrial Revolution there was no concept of adolescence (Wallis, Dell, & Park, 2004), the in-between time marking the transition from childhood to adulthood. In fact, Schlegel and Barry (as cited in Epstein, 2007) found that over 50% of the world's cultures did not have a word for adolescence; additionally, in these cultures adolescents spent a great deal more time with adults than do American teens.

Freud (1914/1957) was one of those who moved thinking in the Western world toward imagining that children had inner lives different from adults, or that children even had an inner life. Freud's early career as a neurologist may have helped him be open-minded about actual brain function, as he tried to reconstruct childhood experiences from adult narratives. Freud's consideration of the child's point of view was revolutionary thinking for the end of the 19th century (Giovacchini, 1982, pp. 227–229).

Piaget (1963), a Swiss psychologist who was influential in the 20th century, may have shaped scientific views of that time period with his contention that the brain completes its development when the child reaches the age of 12 and is capable of what he termed "formal operations" thinking. However, what Piaget could not have known then was that, although the brain does reach adult size by around age 12, extensive restructuring is still occurring (Giedd, 2005). For the past century or so, Western culture has gradually defined adolescence, biologically, as beginning with the development of secondary sexual characteristics and ending around high school graduation, at 17 or 18 years of age (Harvard Mental Health Letter, 2005a; Johnson, 2003, p. 463; Spear, 2000; Steinberg & Lerner, 2005). Toward the middle of the 20th century, a sociological definition began to develop that extended the concept of adolescence from the onset of puberty until the early 20s. Neuroscientists are currently defining adolescence as ending around age 25, when the last brain structures have matured (Dahl & Spear, 2004; Giedd, 2005).

By the age of 20, most brain structures and neural circuits are established, having undergone a period of extensive change and development during the previous 10 years or so. One of the critical structures that continue to develop until the mid-20s is the corpus callosum, the "switchboard" between the left and right hemispheres of the brain (Johnson, 2003, pp. 246–247). This is a fibrous structure in the center of the skull, going from front to back. Given the opportunity, the structure becomes increasingly able to bridge the communication and coordination between the two hemispheres, achieving the ultimate dimension in consciousness (Johnson, 2003, p. 247). Ratey, agreeing with Edelman's definition of the biological theory of consciousness, states that the essence of consciousness is "the feeling we have of owning our actions and being able to develop our self-conceptions through experience over time" (2001, p. 144).

Traditional views of hemispheric functioning have assumed that the right hemisphere cannot be conscious because it does not have the language capability of the left hemisphere. However, studies of split-brain patients (in whom the bridge of the corpus callosum has been severed) calls that assumption into question. It seems that some split-brain patients do have two kinds of communication capabilities, one characteristic for each hemisphere

(Ratey, 2001, pp. 137–140). Though remaining controversial, a large body of research supports the awareness and communication capacities of the right hemisphere (Cozolino, 2006; Schore, 1994, 2003b, pp. xiv–xix). Table 6.1 provides an overview of selected right-hemisphere functions, especially the upper right cortex.

TABLE 6.1.
Selected Functions of the Upper Right Cortex

Modulates emotional experience through interpreting and labeling emotional expressions

Mediates affective shifts and state transitions

Mediates self-reflective awareness

Detects changes in emotional state and breaches of expectation

Processes feedback information

Contains the coping system that is specialized to act in contexts of uncertainty or unpredictability

Detects "somatic markers" or "gut feelings" that are experienced in response to both real and imagined events, including threatening stimuli

Plays a primary role in optimizing cautious and adaptive behavior in potentially threatening situations

Regulates autonomic responses to social stimuli

Modulates processing of pain and coping with painful stimulus

Evaluates facial expressions

Processes emotion-evoking stimuli without conscious awareness

Controls allocation of attention to possible contents of consciousness

Mediates between the internal and external environments

Mediates emotional "hunches"

Mediates cognitive–emotional interactions

Processes affect-related meanings

Associates emotions with thoughts

Mediates social adjustment, control of mood, drive and responsibility (personality traits)

Mediates processing of "self" and self-regulation

Mediates self-concept/self-esteem

Mediates attachment

Exerts highest level of control of behavior

Mediates anger appraisal

From Schore (2003a, 2003b).

Critical Functions that are Stressed During Adolescence

Some critical functions that may be stressed during adolescence include the following: emotional regulation, whether it be self-regulation in autonomous contexts or interactive regulation with the matured brain function(s) of another person; mood regulation; impulse control; judgment; moral reasoning; acquiring left-hemisphere academic skills that are enhanced by a regulated right hemisphere; and making the most of a second chance to modulate the childhood affect management strategy, as manifested in the form of one of the insecure attachment categories. Adolescents who are disengaged from families are particularly susceptible to the problems with the above-mentioned functions (Mackey, 1996).

In the United States, adolescents seem to hover for years at the crossroads between being extremely dependent for emotional regulation upon other brains (and upon the milieu, as well) and moving toward a significantly decreased need for regulation by external resources (Sroufe, 1991; Wilkinson & Walford, 2001). The compromise of such critical functions as self-control and judgment may seriously affect the parent–child connection and may make it quite difficult for adolescents to competently navigate between emotional self- and/or interactive regulation (Dougherty et al., 2003; Sroufe, Egeland, Carlson, & Collins, 2005, p. 197; Steinberg, 2004). Due to some salient aspects of the dominant Western white cultural context in the United States, adolescents often lack sufficient parental nurturance and connection (Mackey, 1996) about the time that the external structuring effects on the elementary and early middle school milieu begin to fade.

Influences that may have led to a social world that is separate from adults may include American culture's emphasis on individualism and the overvaluing of separation and autonomy (Bellah, Madsen, Sullivan, Swindler, & Tipton, 1985; Gilligan, 1987); the media's depiction of parents' role as providing material goods at the expense of nurturance (Pipher, 1994); the pressure parents may experience to withdraw from boys because of fear of being misperceived as sexually inappropriate (Silverstein & Rashbaum, 1994); and for both boys and girls, the culture's emphasis on achievement may become a substitute for nurturance and approval (Brown & Gilligan, 1992; Silverstein & Rashbaum, 1994). The preceding factors include some that have the potential to negatively influence adolescents' connections to their parents, thereby leaving adolescents' loyalties vulnerable to shifting "powerfully to the peer group, leaving little motivation for a positive response to parental control . . . and involvement" (Mackey, 1996, p. 497). Wallis (2005) describes some issues with the middle school experience that compound the problem of the early adolescent's need for stability, which had been provided by the structure of the kindergarten through eighth-grade format until the 1980s. Additional consideration should be given to the post-World War II emphasis on education extending into the 20s and economic pressure necessitating women entering the workforce in record numbers; and leaving children, even young ones, in the care of others or fending for themselves at home. Child-rearing has traditionally been a "woman's calling" (Shaw & Dallos, 2005, p. 419), now ceded over to others, not the mother. Many other obvious factors deserve mention, but are not addressed here, such as divorce (Abelshon noted in 1983 the parental abdication that may follow divorce); loss of a family member, especially a parent; health issues; poverty; and bullying.

The waning of adult influence over the last half of the 20th century or so, combined with the more recent instantaneous availability of peer influence (e.g., social networking sites; Hallowell, 2006) suggests that engagement with others with mature, stable right hemispheres may have been compromised for many adolescents, particularly those with insecure attachment histories (see Goldberg, 1993, for a discussion of normal adolescence). Mackey cautions the therapeutic community to first assess and address relationship issues in order to decrease insecurity in the parent–child experience before guiding the parents to "back off" and set firm limits—both common interventions in family therapy (1996, p. 498; Mishna, 2007). The most favorable situation for adolescent right-hemisphere development is positive synchronized interactions with the matured brain of another person, leading to appropriate affective management. On the other hand, acquisition of left-hemisphere academic skills can be developed without involving other human beings (e.g., via television, films, the Internet, books).

To reiterate information from previous chapters, current scientific findings are clear that in order to regulate emotions (one of the most critical right-hemisphere functions), human beings are dependent on mature brains to initially assist in the microregulation of their physical and emotional world. Ideally, this interactive regulation transitions back and forth over the childhood and adolescence until the person is largely self-regulating.

However, at stressful times, it is necessary and appropriate to seek interactive regulation from stable others, temporarily. The loss of the ability to regulate the expression of emotions is the most far-reaching effect of early trauma and neglect; it is through the attachment bond that emotions are regulated (van der Kolk, 1987; van der Kolk, McFarlane, & Weisaeth (1998); Schore, 2003b, pp. 58–107). Again, see Table 6.1 for an overview of the functions of the prefrontal cortex (specifically, the upper right cortex) that are developing in adolescence; the prefrontal system, the hierarchical apex of the limbic system, acts as the senior executive of the emotional brain (Schore, 2003a, 2003b).

To those who may think that adolescence is simply an artifact of some Western cultures, particularly American culture, Luna's (2009) research indicates otherwise. She described her experiments (which controlled for cultural effects) as finding *differences in brain function that distinguish adolescents from children and adults*. In cultures where adolescents are more involved with adults, these differences may not show up behaviorally, but the same growth and pruning still occur (Luna, 2009). A good example of the impact of other mature brains on adolescent functioning is a finding that in predicting behavior problems in adolescence, the support of an adult male presence was more critical than in earlier years (Sroufe et al., 2005, p. 197).

To review, the affect management strategies implicit in attachment styles (as described in detail in Chapter 5) are evident by adolescence. For clinicians (and others, such as parents and teachers) how the adolescent manages emotions (i.e., the attachment style) is not only obvious in his or her characteristic behavior patterns, but also in ways others respond to the adolescent. The differences among the secure and insecure styles will evoke behaviors in current relationships that are similar to the behaviors that initially created the attachment style in early childhood (Karen, 1990).

With the uneven yet plastic brain development of adolescence, there may be a second chance to modulate the affect management strategy from childhood before it becomes inscribed in the rapidly changing neurocircuitry. As stated elsewhere, the immature brain uses mature brains to perform certain functions, such as mood regulation, impulse control, judgment, and moral reasoning (Siegel, 1999). If adolescents are recruiting other brains to reenact the original template of self in interaction with other, there may be opportunities to confound, change, and rework the affect management strategies of the insecurely attached, particularly the avoidant and ambivalent ones. As Sroufe et al. states, "Early experience is not destiny" (2005, p. 240). However, Type "D" generally have need for more structure, hospitalization, medication, etc., before they are able to take advantage of the rewiring opportunities afforded by relationships.

Differences Between Adolescent and Adult Brains

This section addresses the period of rapid growth in the adolescent brain that occurs simultaneously with the reorganizing of connections among many structures of the brain. Part of this reorganization process includes the pruning of disused neural connections. This growth and pruning are affected by environmental experiences and reshape the adolescent brain. A brief review of childhood attachment categories and their characteristic management of affects via the branches of the autonomic nervous system is also provided. The malleability during adolescence affords opportunities to improve on the insecure attachments and perhaps begin to rewire the adolescent brain toward a more secure attachment style of managing affects. With enough environmental pressure, the reverse can also occur: A secure attachment from childhood can be compromised.

The examination of the session between Cori and her therapist that follows this section is an illustration of subtle interactions between two people that have the capacity to alter neural functions, and with enough repetitions, may rewire the brain of the client. Table 6.2 contains a comparison of the ways in which the adolescent and adult differ, many of which are also quite subtle in their expression, as can be seen from the case material.

TABLE 6.2. Comparison of Selected Functions of Adolescent and Adult Brain Functions	
Adults	**Adolescents**
1. Amygdala registers facial expression, and frontal lobe identifies meaning of expression	Amygdala also registers facial expression, but frontal lobe often cannot focus enough to identify correctly the meaning of the facial expression
	(Baird, as cited in Phillips, 2004)
2. Amygdala plays central role in discerning human social signals, especially fear, rage, "gut" feelings; adults recruit more of their brain to do so than adolescents (Damasio et al., 1990, 1994)	Amygdala relied upon too much to process emotions by adolescents; instinctual functioning (Luna, 2009)
3. Adults recruit more of their brain to stay on task than adolescents	Operate more from reflexive, instinctive amygdalar part of brain, leading to impulsivity
	(Luna, 2009; Luna & Sweeney, 2001)
4. Frontal lobes make an assessment, check with memory and other parts of the brain, and coordinate a response; almost all the time, adults handle stress better and get the emotions "right"	Stress can break down frontal cortex functioning; prefrontal cortex continues to mature into the 20s (Giedd, 2005); prefrontal cortex works harder in decision-making (Luna, 2009); ability to recognize emotions via facial expressions poorly developed, so make mistakes
(Baird, as cited in Phillips, 2004)	(Baird et al., 1999)

continued on next page

TABLE 6.2 continued

Adults	Adolescents
5. Corpus callosum connects left and right hemispheres for coordinating sensory and perceptions; over time, the nerves coordinate more and more efficiently (Cozolino, 2006)	Corpus callosum still maturing well into the 20s, as it connects and coordinate the two hemispheres (Harvard Mental Health Letter, 2005a)
6. Spatial working memory matured, meaning brain system integrated and collaborative; uses less neuronal effort to perform certain tasks; spatial working memory efficiently distributed across brain regions	Adolescents (especially younger ones) involve fewer neurons for spatial working memory, increasing the effort to perform same tasks as adults or older adolescents
(Luna, 2009; Schweinsburg, Nagel, & Tapert, 2005)	
7. Adults less influenced by the group when making decisions	Reasoning ability developing, but easily influenced by peers, leading to risky choices and taking chances when peers observing
(Gardner & Steinberg, 2005; Steinberg, 2004, 2005)	
8. Prefrontal cortex exercising "executive functions" such as, anticipation, planning, prioritizing, thinking clearly, impulse control, affect management	Developing prefrontal cortex heavily influences decision-making, and not as influenced by hormones as is widely believed
(Gur, 2005; Kinney, Stengard, Renshaw, & Yurgelun-Todd, 2000; Schore, 1994; Sowell, Thompson, Tessner, & Toga, 2001)	
9. After mid-20s, extensive pruning and myelinization of neural circuitry decreases (Giedd, 2005)	Pruning excess gray matter (neurons and connections); connections left intact strengthened by myelin (white matter) encasing them (Baird, Gruber, & Yurgelun-Todd, 1999)
10. Dopamine helps regulate up–down regulatory neural systems (Buelow et al., 2000)	Dopamine-rich areas of brain change rapidly in adolescence and may be factor in the sensitivity to effects of drugs, alcohol, and sexuality, as dopamine has role in motivation, social motivation, and behavioral reinforcement (Cozolino, 2006; Dougherty et al., 2003; Wallis, Dell, & Park, 2004)

continued on next page

TABLE 6.2 continued

Adults	Adolescents
11. Nucleus accumbens, a region of frontal cortex that directs motivation to seek rewards, is more active in adults	Less activity in nucleus accumbens leads to motivational deficit; this means that adolescents are drawn to high-excitement or low-effort experiences, or both; long-term planning suffers and risk-taking or "laziness" likely
	(Dougherty et al., 2003; Wallis et al., 2004)
12. In adults and preadolescents the pineal gland begins to produce melatonin mid-afternoon to produce sleep around 10 p.m.	Adolescents' melatonin levels rise more slowly so that their nighttime starts later
	(Wolfson & Carskadon, 1998)
13. Basal ganglia prioritizes information in coordination with prefrontal cortex; plays role in movement and coordination (Ratey, 2001)	Active in small and large motor movements, so exposure to music, art, athletics, etc., especially important while this area is developing Ruder (http://harvardmagazine.com/2008/09/the--teen-brain.htm)
14. Cerebellum has role in physical coordination and regulates certain thought processes and activities of higher learning (e.g., math, music, advanced social skills)	Dramatic changes in adolescence, increasing the number of neurons and complexity of their connections; important to utilize those neural circuits as they are developing
	(Cozolino, 2006; Solms & Turnbull, 2002; Wallis et al., 2004)
15. Hormones: Upon orders from the nervous system, released by endocrine glands into the bloodstream and may activate every cell in the body	Although abstract reasoning, memory, and the capacity for planning are fully developed by 15 or 16, the hormonally driven emotional state can affect the execution of those skills, such as interrupting an action underway to think before acting and choose between safer and riskier alternatives
(Johnson, 2003; Passorotti, Sweeney, & Pavuluri, 2009)	(Giedd et al., 1999; Wallis et al., 2004)

Period of Rapid Growth

The neonatal period of development produces the most rapid growth of the biological, psychological, and social aspects of the brain, with the adolescent brain coming in second in rapid growth and development. As with any structure in the body, a time of intense growth is both a blessing and a curse: a blessing for the possibility of enhanced functions and a curse if unforeseen events occur—medical issues, accidents, family strife, falling into an impulsive peer group, and other environmental pressures. These events may begin to mold the plastic and malleable brain during a critical window for the growth of neural circuitries and also, especially in adolescence, the constant pruning of underutilized neural circuitries as well.

Reorganizing of Connections among Structures and Reshaping of the Adolescent Brain

Prior to adolescence, neurons (gray matter) and synapses (intersections between neurons) are numerous, particularly in the cerebral cortex (eventually the site mostly responsible for the management of emotions and behavior). However, during adolescence, more than 15% of the gray matter in the frontal lobes is pruned (Teicher, Andersen, & Hostetter, 1995). Many of the neuronal connections that remain and are used will develop an insulating coat of myelin on the axons, which becomes white matter (myelin makes the signals between neurons travel faster; Ratey, 2001, p. 24). The myelin sheath protects the axons, which carry signals between neurons.

Continued usage improves the communication properties of the resulting neural networks (Hebb, 1949). Synapses form as a result of learning (vs. a nonlearning situation) and can form within 10–15 minutes following such an experience, according to Greenough (2011). The stimulus (internal or external) of the neural networks, if it continues to have an excitatory response (termed *long-term potentiation*; LTP), will allow neurons to "become synchronized in their firing patterns and organized into neural networks" (Hebb, as cited in Cozolino, 2006, p. 42). According to Urion and Jensen (in Ruder, 2011), this cellular excitement (LTP) enhances learning and occurs particularly during adolescence, making exposure to learning to play a musical instrument or to speak a language, for example, easier than in later years. Additionally, new neurons "continue to appear in regions involved with ongoing learning, contributing to the continual growth and shaping of neural networks" (Cozolino, 2006, p. 42).

Spear suggested that "the reorganization of amygdala and prefrontal limbic areas that innervate the hypothalamus and modulate emotional reactivity drive the reorganization of the adolescent brain" (as cited in Schore, 2003a, p. 297). Entering the adolescent stage of development with, for example, either the ambivalent or avoidant styles of insecure attachment categories (i.e., affective regulation strategies) may mean that overpruning of excitatory or inhibitory circuits, respectively, has occurred (Berntson, Cacioppo, & Quigley, 1991; Cozolino, 2006, p. 147). The personality may be characterized by the underutilization of the pruned circuitry. For example, with the avoidant attachment category, low arousal (inhibitory parasympathetic branch) is the result of pruned sympathetic circuitry with the consequence of decreased ability to bear arousing affects. The opposite occurs with the ambivalent attachment category: The excitatory circuitry is retained and the inhibitory circuitry is not as able to tolerate low affects.

Avoidant Attachment Category and Affect Management Issues

Intolerance of more arousing affects can be a consequence of inexperiences with others. For example Pollak, Cicchetti, Hornung, and Reed (2002) and Pollack and Sinha (2002), in comparing neglected, abused, and nonmaltreated children, found that neglected children required more pronounced emotional expressions of the face to identify most emotions. For detailed information about the retrieval of socially relevant information from facial expressions, see Adolphs (2002), Adolphs et al. (2000), and Cole (1987).

Schore correlated the low arousal condition of the avoidant attachment strategy with neglect (2003a, pp. 115–121). The neglected child may consciously give up hope for interactions. Yet, he or she may feel anger about the neglect that is not directly expressed and perhaps not consciously experienced either. Being able to tolerate difficult, arousing emotions would utilize the sympathetic excitatory branch of the autonomic nervous system. For the neglected child who develops an avoidant affect management strategy, the sympathetic branch either has compromised growth or was pruned due to cytotoxic (i.e., cell death) experiences or some combination, leaving the parasympathetic branch as the primary structure managing emotions (Schore, 2003a, pp. 112–115).

A child may dissociate from the emotional pain (excitatory sympathetic nervous system activated) of desiring something that will not happen. The level of arousal is decreased via a system-wide slowing down (parasympathetic nervous system) or shutting down (parasympathetic nervous system-mediated polyvagal system). According to Cozolino such children may be withdrawn, unmotivated, and/or depressed (2006, p. 147). Of course, with neglect there would be no interactive management of pain, the absence of which would have led to chronic low arousal in the first place. If the avoidant strategy persists into adolescence, there may not be the capacity to actively pursue growth opportunities. Given a history of noninvolvement with mature brains, the guidance, mentoring, and learning that adolescent emotional circuitry needs for appropriate development will not occur properly.

Special Case of Low Arousal: Violence

Though somewhat counterintuitive, findings suggest that chronic low arousal (from overutilization of dissociative defenses adopted to cope with abuse) can lead to aggressive outbursts that can be an early marker to antisocial behavior (Raine, Reynold, Venables, Mednick, & Farrington, 1998). The low arousal, in part resulting from the humiliating experience of being rejected, constitutes a self and other template with the linking affect being anger. If this core relationship configuration (Luborsky & Crits-Cristophe, 1998) is evoked via a humiliating or shaming interaction, a sudden outburst of rage may surprisingly occur. Likewise, the abused child, who likely develops an ambivalent/resistant attachment style, will manage affect using the excitatory (sympathetic nervous system) branch. This child may be more actively shamed and humiliated and will also have a self and other template involving an angry self and shaming other. If this template is evoked, there may also be a rage reaction (Schore, 1994, pp. 240–248). As speculated in Chapter 3, it may be that there is a continuum of rage reactions/behaviors that may eventually manifest as antisocial: on one end of the continuum is the more predatory, cooler low arousal, and on the other end is the impulsive ("hot") behavior that erupts without deliberation (Schore, 2003a, p. 292).

Developmentally acquired sociopathy or psychopathy (terms often used interchangeably) may be related to a developmentally hypofunctioning ventro-medial cortex (Bechara et al., 2001), which means that the upper cortex is less involved in threat assessment (safety–danger) and less involved in behavior management, particularly if there is frontal damage (Damasio et al., 1990). The amygdala is therefore heavily influential in threat assessment and in determining behavior in a more rapid and impulsive manner than the upper cortex. The frontal brain regions of children who have been physically abused show electroencephalograph (EEG) abnormalities, leading Teicher et al. (1995) to conclude that stress alters the development of the prefrontal cortex.

On the other hand, others have indicated that those abused individuals who do not perpetuate violence have good right-hemisphere functioning, which is likely a protective factor against becoming violent (Raine et al., as cited in Schore, 2003a, pp. 303–304). Surely, then, these individuals have had some routine access to people in the environment whose modulated personality functioning was available to counteract the effects of abuse. These children were likely to have experienced adequate interactive regulation of affect in order for their right hemisphere, especially the upper right cortex, to be functional and not at the mercy of impulsive, aggressive amygdalar functioning.

Ambivalent/Resistant Category and Affect Management Issues

A child who experiences primary caregivers as inconsistent at best or abusive at worst may need to rely on his or her own efforts to elicit legitimate attention to ordinary needs. Children with this attachment style may be clingy and impulsive (Schore, 1994) and may invite infantilization from others (Karen, 1990). Pollack and Sinha (2002) found that abused children need more information to recognize sad facial expressions, and they need less information to recognize angry facial expressions. The unpredictable possibility of maltreatment leads abused children to utilize partial information about danger, for which they are always on alert (Pollack & Sinha, 2002, p. 790; Schore, 2003a, pp. 291–298). The child who is not abused but subject to extremely inconsistent care will also scan the environment for signs of getting his or her needs met by others.

Being unable to relax a vigilant posture toward others maintains the sympathetic branch activation. The inhibiting of arousal by the parasympathetic branch is not a good survival strategy for those who must actively ensure that their own needs get met or be ready when caretakers do sporadically attend to their needs. The ambivalent/resistant affect management strategy has resulted from the compromised state of the parasympathetic branch due to disuse or pruning—either of which can lead to, or be due to, cell death. As with the avoidant strategy, dissociation is utilized, but in this case the dissociation manages the unregulated, overstimulating, and intense affects that may be directed toward these children. If the ambivalent/resistant strategy continues into adolescence, it is likely that the child will display dyscontrol issues that could include manic, impulsive, or attention-getting behaviors (Cozolino, 2006, p. 148).

Secure and Disorganized/Disoriented Attachment Categories and Affect Management Issues

The secure and the disorganized/disoriented categories of affect management involve both branches of the autonomic nervous system, but in opposite ways. Secure attachment is characterized by appropriate levels of affect for most situations. The sympathetic nervous system and parasympathetic nervous system work together with neither automatically managing affect, regardless of the experience. In contrast, the autonomic nervous system of the disorganized/disoriented attachment category responds unpredictably to situations, such that even the person cannot reliably know how he or she may react. This is the result of extremely unpredictable care, often involving both abuse and neglect. The child was left to manage neglect via dissociation (parasympathetic branch) and to manage intense arousal beyond what could be tolerated by the sympathetic branch—also possibly becoming dissociated to counterregulate the unbearable arousal.

The securely attached child entering adolescence will still undergo the growth and pruning experiences (see Table 6.2) inherent in expectable brain development, so secure attachment does not override those normative growth processes. However, the adolescent's ability to respond to the environment is enhanced by secure attachment and the balanced way that his or her brain has learned to manage emotions and behaviors, particularly via good experiences with the interactively regulated affect of stable others. Unfortunately, the disorganized/disoriented attachment style is likely made worse by the hormonal shifts and other forces acting on an already dysregulated brain (detailed elsewhere in the chapter). See Table 6.3 for summary of suggested relationships between the attachment categories and the autonomic nervous system.

TABLE 6.3
Attachment Categories of Childhood as Managed by Autonomic Nervous System

Secure Attachment
- Homeostatic balance of emotions (autonomic nervous system branches work together; neither sympathetic nor parasympathetic branch is dominant)
- Likely to have had mature brains influencing development of affect regulation strategies

Avoidant Attachment
- Down-regulated/inhibited (inhibitory parasympathetic nervous system or parasympathetic nervous system managing the polyvagal system)
- More extensive pruning of sympathetic branch leading to compromised ability to tolerate arousing affects
- Likely to have been neglected

Ambivalent/Resistant Attachment
- Up-regulated/excitatory (sympathetic nervous system)
- More extensive pruning of parasympathetic branch leading to compromised ability to tolerate low arousal affects;
- Likely to have been subjected to inconsistent intense arousal or abused

Disorganized Attachment
- Unpredictably regulated (parasympathetic nervous system and sympathetic nervous system activating behavior unpredictably)
- Likely to be abused and neglected

Note. Based on Cozolino (2006), Porges (2007), Schore (2003a, pp. 115–121), Siegel (1999, 2007), and Wallin (2007).

Case Illustration: Cori

The following case material comes from the same session as used in Chapter 2, only the focus here is on examining ways in which the interactions reflect the differences between adult and adolescent brain functioning. It would be helpful to use Tables 6.1, 6.2, and 6.3 as reminders of the neurobiological functions that might be illustrated by the exchanges between Cori and the clinician.

> When the clinician first met with Cori, the meeting was tense. The minute Cori walked in the room, the clinician was uncomfortable, guarded, and uncharacteristically found that she could not easily relate to Cori. Cori was unsure about what exactly she was doing talking to a counselor.

> *Cori may be relying more on the amygdala for her reactive sensor of safety–danger, unlike adults whose more mature brain utilizes the prefrontal cortex; self-reflective awareness (right-hemisphere function) is still developing in Cori, as well, so it may be compromised.*

CORI: I don't know why I was sent here (*slightly belligerent, challenging*).

> *The prefrontal cortex is not suppressing the impulse to be belligerent and challenging (excitatory sympathetic branch of autonomic nervous system), as it would in a mature adult brain. Adolescents rely more on reflexive, instinctive amygdalar parts of the brain, leading to impulsivity (Luna, 2009); hence the belligerent pose.*

THERAPIST: (*trying for calm, matter-of-fact demeanor*) Well, your teachers are concerned about your sudden drop in grades, and that sometimes means that a student might be worried about something.

> *In trying for a calm manner, the clinician is relying on the prefrontal cortex for impulse control (inhibitory parasympathetic branch of autonomic nervous system). The nucleus accumbens directs motivation, which in adolescence is also developing, so disciplined activities like studying may suffer naturally; the lack of support in a brain already somewhat unstable may in part account for Cori's drop in grades. Additionally, as adolescent brains engage fewer neurons for spatial working memory, it takes more effort to perform the same tasks as an adult, perhaps contributing to less capacity for efficient task completion (Luna, 2009; Schweinsburg, Nagel, & Tapert, 2005).*

CORI: People in my family don't worry too much about things these days.

> *Based on the family history of Cori in Chapter 1, it seems that the family was functional, with available and effective stress management strategies (work,*

socializing, hobbies, church, friends). If Cori's family is not currently avail-
able to her to emotionally support her in the wake of their losses, her school
performance and rude manner may be compromised. Adolescents' reasoning
ability is more influenced by peer groups than by adults (Steinberg, 2004),
which may account for Cori's susceptibility to being influenced by the family's
current use of down-regulating defense mechanisms, such as denial, suppres-
sion, repression, and blocking/isolation of affect.

THERAPIST: Did they worry about things in the past, but don't right now?

CORI: Naw, not really. We're strong. Like, do you know where I got my name? (*Turns slightly in chair, sideways to clinician; has a matter-of-fact, declarative tone with first comment and slightly aroused tone of voice with the change of subject.*)

> *Cori's dismissive tone of voice and physically turning away may indicate a fear*
> *reaction through which she attempts to distance herself from the clinician*
> *and her own emotions as well (the amygdala may be a playing central role in*
> *detecting danger; Damasio, et al., 1990; Damasio, 1994).*

THERAPIST: Where?

> *The clinician is trying to follow the abrupt change in subject, to the origin of*
> *Cori's name. The clinician feels a sense of disquiet, uncertainty, confusion, as*
> *her last effort was to clarify the affective management style of Cori's family*
> *in the past. Not only did she not get an answer, but also Cori seemed to*
> *completely change the focus.*

CORI: Coretta Scott King. (*Lifts her chin with a little jerk. Slightly proud, though, again, matter-of-fact, as she gives the origin of her name.*)

> *The abrupt change of subject may be a reaction to the clinician, who is*
> *earnestly attempting to connect. Cori's prefrontal cortex may be slow in*
> *processing feedback information (a maturing skill) as Cori's safety–danger*
> *detector, the amygdala, may err on the side of caution, signaling flee or freeze*
> *(a bit) to avoid the clinician; in adolescence, the amygdala is relied upon to*
> *discern social signals and process emotions (Damasio, 1994; Damasio et*
> *al., 1990; Luna, 2009); Cori's smoother social skills from the past may have*
> *deserted her.*

THERAPIST: Oh, really? (*Does not know what to do at that moment and feels slightly anxious.*)

CORI: (*Goes on hurriedly, not really noticing clinician*) Yeah, and my sister Jakki, that's with two k's. You know, she is named after President Kennedy's wife, J-a-k-q-u-a-l-i-n-e (*spelling it out*).

Modulating emotional experiences through interpreting and labeling emotional expressions, a mature brain function, is not occurring; instead, Cori is chattering, perhaps to avoid the clinician's effort to understand her. The *pruning of neurons that are unused*, which occurs throughout adolescence, may compromise previous good development; Cori may be *avoiding processing affect-related meaning, a prefrontal cortex* function.

THERAPIST: Oh, that's a pretty name (*again, does not feel connected*).

CORI: Yeah, and you know what else? My grandmother's dog was named Mary, after the mother of Jesus. (*Gazes away for a few seconds after her words come out in a rush.*)

The ability to read facial expressions, a right-hemisphere function, may be compromised in the *prefrontal cortex*. Cori may be using the *amygdala* to read and perhaps misinterpret, and thereby become overstimulated by the misreading of the clinician's facial expressions; Cori's *gaze aversion* is directing attention away from the clinician (to allow the *parasympathetic* branch to lower arousal); the ability to control the allocation of attention to the possible contents of her own consciousness, a *prefrontal function*, is hampered. *Gaze aversion* may be an automatic response to spike in *sympathetically-driven arousal* (Schore, 2003b, pp. 7–8). Averting the gaze can help *calm* (*inhibitory parasympathetic branch*).

THERAPIST: (*Quiet, but has urge to ask what kind of dog Mary was.*)

CORI: (*Looks at the file cabinet where some student's drawings of a dog and cat are taped on the side.*) You know, I can't remember what Mary even looked like. (*Looks slightly down and her voice is soft and a bit puzzled; seems to be on edge, emotionally.*)

The lowering of arousal may be the beginning of a more homeostatically balanced experience, as Cori may be affected by the lowered affect of the clinician. This dyadic regulation of emotion may be a welcome contrast to Cori's family's recent distancing and isolating ways of managing their own affects.

THERAPIST: (*Still quiet, and feels better about being quiet.*)

The clinician's adult brain is better at handling stress and getting emotions "right" (Baird, Gruber, & Yurglun-Todd, as cited in Phillips, 2004); Cori is beginning to approach the traumatic experiences and needs another stable brain available to help steady her to even begin to tolerate the recent losses.

CORI: I wonder if she is still alive, maybe, you know—somebody found her when, well, after . . . (*looks suddenly withdrawn and her eyes close, as if she is sleeping*).

Cori seems to have been securely attached, meaning that she could manage her emotional life by herself. Or, if she needed others to help her emotionally, she would seek them out and they had a history of generally following through—which would create a <u>homeostatically balanced autonomic nervous system in Cori</u>. However, in the wake of the recent traumas, Cori may be <u>developing an avoidant, dismissing style (inhibitory dominated parasympathetic nervous system)</u>, which could lead to a counterdependent style of apparent self-dependency, if no intervention occurs. She would create a more self-reliant stance and employ the parasympathetic nervous system or even polyvagal system to maintain a "cool" low affect manner; in turn, smooth affective shifts would decrease, as the rigid preference for low affect becomes the norm.

THERAPIST: (*Begins to imagine Mary, the dog, lost in the storm; associates to her own dog's big eyes looking at her beseechingly, and feels a catch in her throat; thinks she should do something, does not know what to do; says nothing.*)

CORI: (*Turns her face back to therapist and says quietly, without making eye contact*) I'm sorry. Have I upset you?

Cori's past history of interactive interpersonal sensitivity may be revived by the clinician's efforts to engage her, however awkward the clinician may feel. Cori may have improved functioning in several areas of her <u>prefrontal cortex</u>, as a result of the connection with the clinician (these include <u>control of mood; processing of emotion-evoking stimuli without conscious awareness; showing more empathy and more adaptive behavior, as she may more accurately assess the danger in the situation</u>). <u>Cori may have engaged cautiously enough that her previous positive expectation of caretaking adults may be surfacing.</u>

THERAPIST: Well, I am upset, thinking about your dog lost like that. I have a dog, and I started to think about him. (*Stops talking and she and Cori look at each other for a few seconds. The clinician has an experience as if a slight "electric current" has passed between them, which had not happened before this interaction.*)

Cori needs the influence of a mature brain to connect (perhaps via mirror neurons; Cozolino, 2006, pp. 186–201; Gallese, 2009, 2010; Siegel, 2007) with her brain to prevent the development of self-regulation strategies (e.g., defenses that begin to habitually dampen or increase emotions) that begin to be employed reflexively, regardless of the situation. Having available another brain that can resonate emotionally with the less tolerable affects will permit more flexibility in Cori's emotion regulation and develop and strengthen her <u>frontal cortex</u>.

CORI: (*Looking slightly away*) You know, Mimi cries about Mary a lot. My mother gets mad at her, though, and . . . (*trails off and looks away*).

Recognition of facial expression occurs via the <u>amygdala</u>, but in adolescents the <u>frontal lobe</u> often cannot focus enough to identify correctly the meaning of the facial expression (Baird, Gruber, & Yurglun-Todd, as cited in Phillips, 2004). Looking away, thereby decreasing the stimulation of mutual gaze, does not help in correctly identifying the meaning of the other's facial expression.

THERAPIST: (*Has urge to ask if Mimi is Cori's grandmother when therapist knows quite well that Mimi is the grandmother; has urge to ask how long the family had the dog. What kind of dog was Mary? Starts to tell herself to stay with Cori in the moment, though emotional flight seems like a good idea. She sees Cori looking at her again, somewhat expectantly.*) Do you miss Mary a lot?

CORI: (*Looks away and starts refastening some clips in her hair, then takes out and reinserts her earrings, then says matter-of-factly:*) Mary lived a good life and was really old. She had arthritis in her back legs. Probably what happened to her out there in the pasture, when Barney (*stepfather*) let her out to pee (*starts to chatter, not so matter-or-fact*) . . . she . . . well . . . maybeeee . . . well . . . whatever. (*Stands up, sits down again abruptly, reworks her barrette in her hair.*) Jakki and I played with Mary a lot when we were little. Before the, well, you know, the storm, not so much. We moved away, you see.

The <u>corpus collosum</u>, responsible for connecting the <u>left and right hemispheres</u> (cognitive–emotional interactions; associates emotions with thoughts), is developing until age 25, so Cori would have erratic abilities anyway. Her matter-of-fact recital of the "facts" of losing the dog were not consonant with the emotional experience of the loss of the dog. As Cori is 10 years away from having a <u>fully mature "switchboard"</u> (the corpus collosum), she is not going to easily <u>connect emotions with thought and conscious perception</u>. The discussion seemed to be making her more deliberate than angry; the <u>basal ganglia</u> (developing in adolescents, larger in girls than boys) <u>coordinate with the prefrontal cortex regarding empathy, suppression of impulses, and management of emotion</u>.

THERAPIST: (*As Cori looks at the therapist, therapist makes a declarative statement, but in low-key voice*) Cori, you must miss Mary. (*Therapist finds an emotional space to be sad with Cori in that moment and feels a "click" with her.*)

Again, the clinician is working to <u>track right brain to right brain</u> and attempts to attune (meet and match; Beebe, 2005) to Cori, in another effort to offer an <u>external source of prefrontal cortex function</u> to Cori's brain.

CORI: Yeah, well, you know Mimi, sometimes she is a Baptist and sometimes she is a Catholic. (*Makes this statement calmly; it is not the flat statements of early in session.*)

THERAPIST: (*Has no idea where this is going, feels incompetent, at a loss for words. Says, in puzzled tone:*) What? (*Worries that she has once again lost a fragile connection.*)

CORI: Mimi bought us a statue of St. Francis (*casts a glance to therapist a bit challengingly*). Are you Catholic?

> The challenging (up-regulated, <u>sympathetic activation</u>) behavior may be Cori's way to autonomously manage the stress of making emotional contact with clinician.

THERAPIST: (*really off balance now*) What?

CORI: Well, you look like you don't know who St. Francis is. You know (*almost sarcastic*), the patron saint of animals?

> The increasingly aysynchronous emotional contact may be the result of Cori's <u>amygdala</u> registering a <u>"gut" feeling</u> that the clinician is coming too close (Damasio, 1994; Damasio et al., 1990); the consequent stress of emotional contact may result in distancing behaviors. Cori's <u>amygdala</u> may be warning her away from making contact with others, as recent disappointments with her family members' self-imposed insulation, making them unavailable for affective management, may make Cori automatically wary of reconnecting with another adult.

THERAPIST: (*happy to know* something; *stammering*) Oh, oh, yes, I did, or . . . do know about St. Francis.

CORI: (*Tucks her chin down and looks at her shoes, reaches down and straightens her skirt which did not need straightening. Starts to cry.*) Mary used to sleep with me and Jakki. No one knows but Mimi, but I have a little dog charm under my pillow that she bought for me at the Dollar Store. (*Suddenly irritation in her voice*) I hate that Dollar Store. Back home, Mama would never let us shop there. (*Starts to imitate her mother*) Only poor people shop there. We can go to Finegold's, just like everybody else. (*Looks up at therapist*) Do *you* shop at the Dollar Store?

> Again, the <u>basal ganglia prioritizes information, and under the press of emotions, it helps with decision making regarding reactions appropriate to the situation; it also helps the prefrontal cortex choose between impulsivity and more deliberate reactions.</u>

THERAPIST: (*Beginning to think that "off-balance" is her middle name, again asks:*) What?

The clinician is <u>mirroring</u> Cori's affective dysregulation.

CORI: (*impatient now*) I said, do you shop at the Dollar Store?

THERAPIST: (*Associating to having to tell her supervisor about her one-syllable interventions, tries to get her mind to work*) Oh, well, actually, I have shopped there before.

Something about Cori's directness, without aggression, drew an ordinary response from the clinician. This may have been the clinician's way of <u>meeting and matching</u> (Beebe & Lachmann, 1994) Cori's question-and-answer approach.

CORI: (irritated) No, I mean, do *you* shop there on a regular basis?

THERAPIST: (*Decides that she must not try to over-think this and be natural*) No, I don't. I don't like it there.

Maybe clinician is <u>matching the more balanced autonomic nervous system of Cori</u> with her response in kind?

CORI: (*somewhat triumphant*) There, you see! That's what I mean! That's what I told Mama but that only made her mad; later, I saw her washing dishes and she was actually crying. She doesn't do that too much. It's usually Mimi and Jakki who are the criers in the family. I try not to show Mama that I don't like the Dollar Store. She doesn't need any more upset. You know what I mean?

The <u>reasoning capacity is weaker in adolescents</u>; without the help of the family talking to her about their situation, Cori is drawing conclusions and making meaning about her mother and how the Dollar Store upsets her mother; actually, the Dollar Store is likely the scapegoat for intense feelings of being devalued, loss of self-esteem, and other complicated emotions. Cori needs the adults to help her cope, but she may be left to her own ways to manage herself, emotionally.

THERAPIST: (*Not knowing which part of Cori's statement to respond to*) Cori, I wonder if sometimes you just don't know what to do? (*Suppresses the urge to elaborate and lets the comment hang in the air between them.*)

The clinician is modeling the use her <u>left-hemisphere abilities to perceive that her right hemisphere was dysregulated</u> and confused emotionally. By serving as an <u>external prefrontal cortex</u> for Cori, the clinician is resonating with the *confusion Cori has induced in her (the clinician), then speculates (left-hemi-sphere reasoning) that Cori may feel unsure.*

CORI: (*Big sigh that makes her shoulders go up and down*) Yeah. (*Long silence; another sigh*) Yeah, you got it.

Cori may have allowed herself to become dyadically/interactively regulated by the clinician, meaning that Cori temporarily "borrowed" the function of the other person to re-regulate herself, which she was unable to do without resorting to defenses that were compromising her functioning. In other words, Cori's attempt to not worry her mother and be a "crier" like her sister and grandmother had cut her off from anyone who would/could interactively regulate her affect. By not having anyone who could be in synchrony, in attunement with her, to be a reliable selfobject, and/or to stay in relationship with her, Cori was unable to employ an internal working model of affect management that would keep her functional. The more she tried to manage her emotions on her own by being soldier-like, with a tough, sarcastic, challenging, and matter-of-fact posturing, the lonelier and more prone to dysregulation she had become.

THERAPIST: (*Now trying not to think, but allows herself to be with Cori somehow*) I know how that feels sometimes.

The clinician provides a simple, plain, not overthought statement, which had to emerge from a more balanced autonomic nervous system.

CORI: (*Walks over to the table with art supplies on it, generally used by the younger kids; she starts drawing for a few minutes.*)

THERAPIST: (*Sits quietly looking out the window; the silence is companionable.*)

Perhaps there are now two people in attunement, much like Cori's experiences with her grandmother in the house smelling of coffee, etc. Cori has dropped her defended posture toward emotionally connecting with the clinician and is now able to use the abilities of the clinician's prefrontal cortex and upper limbic system to coordinate a response and handle stress more interactively.

CORI: (*Walks back to her chair and in a young and shy way hands the drawing of the dog, Mary, to the therapist. Her statement is rather matter-of-fact, however:*) Here, you can put that up by that other dog drawing (*gesturing to the side of the file cabinet with a jerk of her head*). If we are going to talk about that old dog of Mimi's, you ought to know what she looks like.

The hippocampal memory system (more mature than amygdala) may be "reviving" with the interactive regulation of emotion. Cori may be able to engage her left brain as her right brain is more emotionally regulated. She may be more able to think rather than react, as adolescents are more influenced by others than are adults. This phenomenon could be occurring in Cori's brain. Hopefully, adults or her family members (the original group for most people) are available so that Cori can "borrow" their emotional strategies. If so, by properly using stable brains, Cori may be more able to organize her thoughts and weigh the consequences of her behavior.

Discussion of Case

The clinical experience of the adolescent and his or her therapist is different than working with children and adults. Children benefit from play therapy because they manage their emotional lives in fantasy to a large extent. Children displace their emotions into a play situation, and the talented clinician tries to understand the meaning of the play. Bringing to the attention of the child his or her possible emotions is difficult because the capacity for abstract and symbolic thinking does not begin to be developed until adolescence. Children are more concrete in their thinking ability.

With adults, depending on the emotional management strategies, the therapist' use of his or her self will vary. With adolescents, the clinician must be somewhat self-revealing, a difficult technique to employ and not overstep professional boundaries. Adolescents do not generally do well with the "blank slate" often recommended in some therapeutic modalities. It is now known that the ability to arrange one's face to disguise one's inner state is not possible and not really recommended (Dimberg & Olham; Lehkey; 1996; Stenberg, Wiking, & Dahl—all cited in Schore, 2003b, pp. 141–142).

Cori's was suffering from the loss of the constant stream of information that had been exchanged in her family before Hurricanes Katrina and Rita destroyed their lives. Her stressed family members seemed to have become productive and functional in their new home in Texas, but they had not resumed their former warm and emotionally involved attachment style. Their affect management strategies had changed, leaving the mother and grandmother isolated, either crying by themselves or being irritated at the Dollar Store or perhaps other scapegoats. Cori was adopting the family's dismissive emotional management style, which was stressing the development of her adolescent brain (and perhaps of her sister Jakki's brain, as well). As can be seen from the list of mature prefrontal cortex functions in Table 6.1, Cori was not able to exhibit some of these functions unless supported by another brain. Looking at the many differences between the adult and adolescent brain will help the clinician stay aware of some of the functions that adolescents' brains may need to "borrow" temporarily to re-regulate themselves. As the prefrontal cortex's connections to the limbic system, especially the amygdala (affect regulation), are forming during adolescence, experiences with other brains that are able to provide emotional learning and appropriate self-regulation are vital.

CHAPTER 7

Working with Groups
How Selected Principles of Regulation Theory Can Be Applied to Group Work

This chapter explores the recognition of brain functions (with an emphasis on right-hemispheric functions) within the treatment modality of group psychotherapy. For the sake of simplicity, a relatively current textbook on group psychotherapy from a psychodynamic perspective (Rutan, Stone, & Shay, 2007) was chosen for examining certain concepts, but almost any literature on group work could easily be utilized. (*Note*: Assume that technical material on group work is from Rutan et al., 2007, unless otherwise referenced.) Integrating knowledge of current neurobiological research within a practical application helps familiarize the clinician with the process of identifying the psychophysiology that undergirds behaviors in a group.

Many neurobiologically informed clinical treatment principles of regulation theory (Schore, 2003b, pp. 270–281) could be useful in understanding interactions in group work, although regulation theory was originally intended for use in dyadic psychotherapy. The basic premise is that the development of the brain's primary self-regulatory system is the attachment relationship, which will eventually devote neural circuitry to either resiliency or vulnerability when dealing with stress.

Resiliency can be described as the capacity to manage increasingly difficult intensities of affect without resorting to pathological defense mechanisms and behaviors. Vulnerability can be described as automatically employing a patterned and fixed way of coping, regardless of the stressor. According to Schore, ideally, "Coping can occur either by autoregulation or by means of going to others for interactive regulation" (2003b, p. xvii).

Many clients who could benefit from group psychotherapy and/or group counseling have characteristic styles of interpersonally relating that have created relationship problems for them. Often personality traits (see Chapter 5) seem extreme: autoregulating via difficult behaviors involving some combination of over- or understimulating actions: demanding and insistent behaviors or withdrawn and avoidant behaviors. These strategies tend to fall into the insecure attachment categories.

These strategies are not really satisfying, as they tend to repetitively restage the original experiences that created the unsuccessful autoregulation strategy initially (in childhood). Although not necessarily diagnosed with a personality disorder, these clients, nevertheless, may have difficulty with engaging others in a way that is mutually satisfying. It is often the main reason for choosing a group treatment approach—that is, to improve relationship skills.

The group modality can be an excellent practice field for learning the interactive regulation of affect. Hopefully, the emotional regulatory function provided by others in the group or the group itself will eventually increase resiliency at the level of neural circuits in the members. What does this mean? Changing the way that a group member interacts may alter the corticolimbic circuits that are responsible for affect (and therefore, behavioral) regulation (Hariri et al., 2000; Schore, 1994; Siegel, 1999). In a group therapy setting, the nonverbal is as privileged as the verbal, and according to Wallin (2007, p. 262), both forms of communication vary according to the attachment style (Wallin explores the dismissing, preoccupied, and unresolved attachment styles of adulthood).

In a group setting particularly, the smallest of events may elicit a big response, and sometimes, a lasting response, when the group and the leader have to work to understand "what happened?". These abrupt and ragged state changes have great power to disrupt and also to heal. What are they, exactly? They are affective shifts that are associated with orbitofrontal activity and the alteration of behavior in reaction to alterations in the emotional significance of various stimuli (either internal or external) (Dias, Robbins, & Roberts, 1996). These events will activate either the excitatory or the inhibitory messages to neuronal networks (Schore, 2003b, pp. 106–107).

Often group members' personal goals are to enter into "cooperative, loving, interdependent relationships," certainly signs of psychological health (Rutan et al., 2007, p. 6). These goals are difficult to achieve when affective shifts, precipitated by the slightest of signals, often generate difficulties in making smooth emotional connections and heighten the likelihood of conflict. In Western culture where so much is disposable, conflict (i.e., the disruption) can be a reason to dispose of a relationship. What may be missing is an emotional capacity to work within a relationship to address conflict and the skill set to do so (i.e., the healing potential). (Of course, this perspective does not apply to situations of emotional or physical danger.)

The microenvironment of the group therapy modality allows for multiple repetitions of "synchronized energy exchanges" (Schore, 2003b, p. 121). What is the importance of the energy exchange? When new experiences occur, energy is created. This energy begins the process of creating actual structures (dendrites, among them) to connect or strengthen neural circuitry. This neural circuitry could then compete with preexisting circuitry that may have archived dysfunctional patterns. This new circuitry creates the possibility for the development of both self-regulation and the self-and-other emotional regulation that promotes relationship satisfaction, perhaps even reworking less-than-optimal affective management strategies.

Ideally, affect management that is not in itself problematic is described by the phrase from Schore (1994, 1998) that captures the interactive representation in the right hemisphere as the result of a secure attachment (and therefore, sturdy affect management): "regulated-self-in-interaction-with-an-attuning-other." The internalized model of any insecure attachment styles is described as "a dysregulated-self-in-interaction-with-a-misattuning-other" (Schore, 1997c, p. 38).

Schore suggested 20 principles of psychotherapeutic treatment to address those right-hemisphere-activated personality organizations that have their origins in growth-inhibiting early developmental experiences (2003a, pp. 279–281). Those principles that are particularly useful for addressing group development, group dynamics, and the mechanisms and process of change (Rutan et al., 2007) are discussed in this chapter. A typical group psychotherapy session is examined for illustrations of the neurobiology that may underlie the group phenomena implicit in the interactions between and among the group members and the leader.

Stages of Group Development

The ultimate goals of any form of group therapy include (1) greater intrapsychic calm (primarily right hemisphere), (2) improved interpersonal functioning (primarily right brain), and (3) deepened self-knowledge (right and left hemispheres). There are differences of opinion regarding stages of development or whether the concept of stages should even be applied to group therapy. However, Rutan et al. (2007) have a sensible hierarchical concept of group development that identifies four stages of group therapy: formative, reactive, mature, and termination.

Formative Stage

In the first or formative stage members join and form the group by gathering information and thereby orienting themselves to the group. In the formative stage, the group is reflexively assessing safety–danger (managed by the amygdala and other limbic structures). A sense of safety is necessary for trust. A principle of regulation theory (Schore, 2003b, p. 279, #3) is that the clinician should focus on nonconscious (right-hemisphere) states of mind and body. Monitoring body language, tone of voice, prosody, and other cues to internal state will likely occur automatically by the leader(s) and the members of the group, as the most basic of needs is assessed—that is, safety.

Reactive and Termination Stages

The second stage (reactive; belonging) and the fourth stage (termination; separating) are opposite, in that they are, respectively, about making connections and disconnections gracefully. In the reactive stage, both negative and positive emotions and behaviors are tested to determine the degree of authenticity that the group climate might tolerate. A principle of regulation theory (Schore, 2003b, p. 279, #4) especially appropriate to these two stages is that empathy does not only involve matching left brain to left brain using verbal and cognitive skills, but is heavily invested in emotional transactions that invite positive affect and attachment because the reward circuitry of the brain is thereby stimulated (e.g., oxytocin and other calming neuromodulators are elevated with positive encounters). A different principle of regulation theory (Schore, 2003b, p. 279, #6) suggests that the clinician be experienced and attuned to the autonomic states (up- and down-regulated affects) as the clients' and clinicians' right hemispheres stay in synchrony, even if the intensity of the affect rises and falls. In a group, emotional contagion may illustrate this experience. It is the role of the members and the leader to serve as an auxillary cortex (Diamond et al., 1963), sometimes, to manage and contain and ratchet up or down the intensity of affect.

Mature Stage

In the third or mature stage the group works on goals, which in psychodynamic and counseling groups generally involves practicing implementing flexible, sensitive ways members have learned to manage strong emotions and conflict so that they do not cut off emotions or give vent to uncontrollable eruptions. A group that achieves this stage (some do not, but this is not necessarily a problem with the treatment) is increasingly resilient, able to metabolize what regulation theory terms "primitive affects such as shame, disgust, elation, excitement, terror, rage, and hopeless despair" (Schore, 2003b, p. 280, #7). Regulation theory holds that such primitive affects may have been dissociated from consciousness and therefore are not interactively regulated. Such interactive regulation of affect could possibly occur in a group that has reached the mature stage of work. The interactive regulation of affect is a right-brain to right-brain experience, and more particularly, sometimes a limbic-system to limbic-system experience.

A different principle of regulation theory describes the "cocreation of an interpersonal context within the therapeutic alliance that can be nonconsciously sensed by the patient as safe enough to allow deeper self-revelation" (Schore, 2003b, p. 280, #10). Certainly, in a group setting the tolerance, containment, and ability to bear intolerable affects are possible. That is the work of a functional family, also, by which group experiences are deeply influenced, nonconsciously.

Group Dynamics

At each developmental stage of a group, the following group dynamics (forces that influence group functioning) may be expressed differently: leadership, group culture, norms, and roles. For example, leadership may be more active in the beginning formative stage of the group, and as the group gets to the mature, "working though" stage, the leadership will become less active as the group members themselves actively work on issues, with a new set of skills.

Leadership

For most groups the leadership role defines the tasks, roles, and boundaries of the group, especially initially. In regulation theory, the clinician's affective tolerance is described as setting the example for the "range, types, and intensities of emotions that are explored or disavowed" in the clinical relationship (Schore, 2003b, p. 281, #15). As stated elsewhere in this book, the exchange of emotional information happens in less than half a second between two brains. It will be immediately obvious to the nonconscious right brains of the group members which behaviors are tolerable (regarding limits and boundaries) to the clinician's brain. From this nonverbal, nonconscious experience, a dynamic can form in which only certain emotions or intensities of emotions are expressed by the members, as they have assessed the tolerance of the leader (i.e., boundaries). The tasks and roles are more a left-hemisphere experience, although the roles into which the leader might be drawn may be more a nonconscious limbic-system (right-hemisphere) experience.

Group Culture and Norms

Group culture and norms are similar; *group culture* reflects particular ways in which conflicts and affects are expressed and handled, whereas *norms* reference appropriate behavior. Both dynamics are influenced by the leader, the individual members, and the group as a whole. The group may either cohere (group cohesion) or disperse (dissolve), as a function of the attractiveness and sense of belonging. Principle #14 from regulation theory addresses the importance of repairing emotional misunderstandings and ruptures in order for the client(s) to have a new ending to the same old story (Weiss, Sampson, et al., 1986); should their dire expectations be disconfirmed, then the group will be attractive, which is the basis of group cohesion (Schore, 2003b, p. 280). The interactive repair can have a calming effect in that the parasympathetic branch of the autonomic nervous system can be activated, if there is trust. The trust in the group will increase attraction to the group and a sense of belonging—and it may also increase social engagement and calm, parasympathetic nervous system-driven (responsible for physiological state regulation) experiences (Porges, 2007).

Roles

Roles in the group can be generated from two broad sources: (1) the members' characteristic roles taken in social settings (perhaps originating from early family dymanics) or (2) pressure from the group (*role suction* [Redl, 1963], *role responsiveness* [Sandler, 1976], or *role complementarity*), which draws a member to serve a function for the group (nonconscious) and can become an underlying press for the scapegoating dynamic. Rutan et al. (2007) describe MacKenzie's (1997) list of four categories of roles, one of them more activated by the left hemisphere (logical, planning, organized) and the other three activated primarily by the right hemisphere (emotional). The left-brain role is the structural role that is involved in task management. The right brain roles are the following: the sociable (the more attuned personalities), the divergent (the oppositional personalities who may express rebelliousness or differentness for the group via projective identification), and the cautionary (the silent individuals, who often hold shame or humiliation for the group).

Often a person may take on a role whose origins are quite unclear from the history or even from the group process. There is an opportunity in such a case to shed light on nonconscious experiences or conflicts from the past that may be enacted within the group experience. Uncovering and identifying internal working models of self in interaction with other, if problematic yet subtle, is the work of dyadic clinical work, as stated in Principle #12 of regulation theory (Schore, 2003b, p. 280), as well. As noted previously, early internal working models are essentially the attachment history "imprinted in implicit-procedural memory and stored as right hemispheric . . . strategies of affect regulation [that] guide the individual's behavior in interpersonal interactions" (Schore, 2003a, p. 280).

Therapeutic Factors

The influential group therapist Yalom (1975) proposed 11 therapeutic factors. This list has been condensed to four dimensions by Mackenzie (as cited in Rutan et al., 2007, p. 70)—supportiveness, self-revelation, learning, and psychological work—because several of Yalom's factors seemed so similar. We consider each in turn.

Supportive Factors

Group cohesion, altruism, hope, belonging and being accepted into the group are experiences that may attach the members to one another and to the group and the leader via positive affect within the reward circuitry of the brain (particularly in the right hemisphere). Principle #4 of regulation theory reminds clinicians that attachment results from "nonverbal right-brain psychobiological attunement and the use of affect synchronizing transactions for interactively generating and amplifying positive affect" (Schore, 2003a, p. 279). This experience of attachment may activate the reward/pleasure circuitry, which can promote bonding.

Self-Revelation

Self-revelation is both a right- and left-hemisphere experience involving self-disclosure (cognitive) and catharsis (emotionally charged revelations). If experienced in a safe emotional climate (right limbic structures, particularly the amygdala, responsible for safety–danger perceptions,), then difficult or shameful experiences can be revealed without fear of rejection and the resulting aloneness. According to Principle #19, it is the flexible regulation of affect brought about by either the interactive regulation of affect or by appropriate self-regulation that is a primary objective of clinical work (Schore, 2003b, p. 281). A therapeutic factor such as self-revelation, under the right circumstances, can restore or expand appropriate self-regulation of emotions. This shift would involve expansion of the functions of the prefrontal cortex instead of relying on the lower right-brain structures (lower limbic, especially the amygdala).

Learning and Psychological Work

Several types of learning may occur in groups: the explicit learning involved in psychoeducation (left brain); learning via suggestions and advice (left brain); vicarious learning via mirror neurons (Gallese, 2009; Siegel, 2007); and the learning involved in trying out new behaviors (likely a combination of right [less conscious] and left [conscious] hemispheres of the brain). Likewise, psychological work utilizes insight (making the unconscious conscious) and linking the here-and-now group experiences (sometimes reenactments of past interactions that have been out of awareness) to the there-and-then experiences (both a right- and left-brain experience).

Tracking both content and arousal shifts moment to moment can assist in identifying "nonconscious 'hot cognitions' that trigger" a state change (limbic structures, particularly the amygdala), which can both dysregulate the emotional and cognitive functioning of the person in the moment and also be an opportunity for exploring subtle but critical past early experiences imprinted in the neural circuitry (Principles # 9 and #20 of regulation theory; Schore, 2003b, pp. 280–281).

Mechanisms of Change

Mechanisms of change, as described by Rutan et al. (2007, p. 81), are the ways a person uses the therapeutic factors to promote change, either consciously or unconsciously. These mechanisms include imitation, identification, and internalization. These factors are both conscious (left hemisphere) and non/unconscious (right hemisphere) and seem to follow a continuum from more conscious (imitation) to less conscious (identification) to non/unconscious (internalization), as describes by Rutan et al. (2007). The more consciousness is brought to bear, the more the left hemisphere is engaged, and vice versa. The higher right-hemisphere structures can be consciously accessed from the right hippocampal memory structure. However, with many repetitions of imitative learning, including vicarious learning, the self-experience may become represented in the implicit (nonconscious) memory system of the lower limbic system. This "synaptic self" can become inscribed in the neural circuitry by coordinating internal bodily information with external experiences (Schore, 2003a, p. 111).

Imitation

Imitation is a form of learning that includes vicarious learning and modeling. Mirror neurons (Gallese, 2009; Siegel, 2007), which are not consciously used, are automatic, and therefore are more in the realm of nonconscious, may be in part responsible for imitative behaviors. The cerebellum, which manages movement, can be consciously activated. To the degree that nonverbal behaviors (e.g., leaning forward with interest and curiosity) may precede verbal involvement, physical imitation via mirroring may have both conscious and nonconscious influences. Principle #17 of regulation theory suggests that clinicians be alert for opportunities to elevate "emotions from a primitive presymbolic sensorimotor level of experience to a mature symbolic representational level" (Schore, 2003b, p. 281), which would mean becoming verbal about one's experiences, both internally and externally. This step in attempting to verbalize difficult experiences may create fragile new neural circuitry.

Identification

Affective synchrony is one avenue of learning the rhythmic structure of the other and modifying behavior to fit that structure (Lester et al., 1985, p. 24). There can be awareness that one is changing to become like someone else (conscious/left hemisphere), for example, in a mentoring experience. However, nonconscious identifications are likely to have strong emotional elements, such as a feeling of well-being. This element can come about from recreating an inner psychophysiological state similar to others that may involve a limbic-system to limbic-system bond. Additionally, the rapid processing of facial expressions by the right somatosensory cortices generates the same internal somatic sensations that simulate how one would feel while having that same expression on one's own face (Adolphs et al., 2000).

Internalization

Internalization involves a reflexive and nonconscious shift in ways the personality functions. Personality functioning can ideally be scrutinized and verbalized, a conscious process. Both identification (discussed above) and internalization are necessary for changing an insecure internal working model of affect regulation into what Schore described as an "earned secure model" of affect regulation (2003b, p. 281; Principle #20 of regulation theory). A secure attachment has a balanced autonomic nervous system, meaning that emotions and behaviors are not expressed in a rigid way, regardless of the situation. The earned secure internal working model is flexible and therefore adaptive in that it can adjust to changing contexts, both internal and external.

Another Mechanism of Change: Transference

Transference, simply put, is the current experiencing of self-and-other representations that have their origins in past experiences. An experience in the here and now can evoke a response that was first experienced in the there and then of past interactions. An experience that is memorialized in the neuro-circuitry is likely initially to hold deep significance and is often experienced repetitively. The transferences that are most likely to be addressed in a group setting are those involving self-and-other representations (right hemisphere/nonconscious) that were originally stressful, developmentally compromising, and/or traumatic. Additionally, intense affects with somatic components may be a part of the transference and countertransference experience. The clinician's right hemisphere is required to be aware of "countertransferential visceral-somatic responses to the patient's transferential, automatic, facially, prosodicallly, and somatically expressed affects, as well as an attention to the intensity, duration, frequency, and lability of the patient's internal state" (Schore, 2003b, p. 280; regulation theory Principle #8).

Therapeutic Processes of Change

According to Rutan et al. (2007, p. 81), the phrase *processes of change* describes "how the treatment context facilitates the mechanisms of change." Working through the significance of nonconscious internal working models of self in interaction with others is captured by Principle #13 of regulation theory (Schore, 2003b, p. 280): The work of treatment is one of identifying "early-forming, rapid-acting, and, thereby, nonconscious right brain perceptual biases for covertly detecting threatening social stimuli (transferential biases): these stress coping strategies that program motivational expectations of misat-tunement-induced self dysregulation are overtly expressed during stressful transference–countertransference ruptures that occur in 'enactments.'" In other words, the instantaneous perception of subtle cues that remind a person of past and stressful misattunements may skew a group member's perceptions of the present moment. This misperception may encourage acting as if the past experience were occurring in the present. It is the work of the group to challenge (kindly) the misperception via the therapeutic processes of change: confrontation (discovering a problem), clarification (focus on the problem), interpretation (speculate on how the past may be symbolized in current patterns of problematic behavior), and working through (repeated examination of recurring themes implicit in behaviors to promote self-awareness and distinguish past from present).

Confrontation

Rutan et al. state that within the group therapy modality, "confrontation is an attempt to indicate to a patient that a problem exists; it is not an effort to gain or impart understanding per se" (2007, p. 88). Confrontation is a therapeutic process aimed at the right hemisphere in that the feedback is aimed at the underlying reasons for a behavior; the behavior is seen as carrying or symbolizing the meaning. Some types of treatment modalities (e.g., Alcoholics Anonymous or "boot camp" experiences for adolescents or prisoners) focus on the behavior (left-brain observations and admonitions to stop the behavior).

Though not meant to be harsh or shaming in the group therapy modality, bringing something to someone's attention about which he or she was unaware is potentially destabilizing emotionally. Therefore, for the confrontation to serve a therapeutic purpose, the group should be trustworthy (involve multiple alliances) and the speculation(s) about the motivation behind a certain troublesome behavior, for example, must be done with empathy (Rutan et al., 2007, p. 89). Based on Principles #17 and #18 of regulation theory, the therapeutic technique should create "a self-reflective position that can appraise the significance and meaning of affects" (Schore, 2003b, p. 281). Furthermore, the implicit self system (nonconscious; the lack of self-awareness is the target of a confrontation) may be made more able to modulate a wider range of emotions, and the implicit self system will have the opportunity to integrate "these discrete emotions into a variety of adaptive motivational states, utilizing affects as signals, and linking coherent behavioral states to appropriate social contexts" (Schore, 2003b, p. 281).

Clarification

Clarification brings a psychological phenomenon into sharp focus and permits repeating patterns to be examined. Often following a gentle confrontation, group members retrieve memories of similar events or occurrences, and those memories, which were disconnected and nonconscious, can now be organized and highlighted. The group can become one mind, trying for self-awareness and clarity, even if the focus is on one member. As the past templates for certain automatic behaviors or attributions, for example, begin to be pieced together, the opportunity for addressing transference distortions presents itself. Again, transference is the intrusion of a previous way of experiencing the self in relation to others that is evoked by a present-day experience, which, though similar, is not the same but seems vividly the same. Differentiation between past and present is the work of the clarification process.

Interpretation

Interpretations broaden clarification by focusing not only on repeating patterns of behavior, but also by speculating on the non/unconscious motivations and conflicts that underlie the behavior under examination. The focus can be on a group member or on the group's reaction to the leader, to one another, or to the group itself. Rutan et al. (2007) caution that timing is critical; a premature speculation about what is outside one's awareness can be as problematic as one that is offered in the emotional heat of the moment. Additionally, the clinician is cautioned to be aware of his or her (countertransferential) motivation for offering an interpretation—for example, to shut down affect prematurely for the comfort of the therapist.

Working Through

The multiple relationships in the group setting offer multiple opportunities to examine the same themes again and again, each time perhaps with a greater grasp of the meaning of the past as enacted within the group. With so many brains to register what happens in the group, a shared reality-attuned perception may be quite likely to emerge, even more so than in some other treatment modalities. There is always the caveat that the group perception could become skewed, however, as a group dynamic (e.g., consensual validation) of selective perception may occur. The training and experience of the leader are critical in those instances.

For lasting change to occur, a period of time is required. The processes of change (confrontation, clarification, and interpretation) are necessary but not sufficient for such lasting change. Why not? Because it is quite difficult for an individual by him- or herself to become aware of the self-protective measures that were put into place in the past (as probably the best possible solution to the situation) but which may be obsolete in the present.

Case Example

The following is a transcript of the 4th of 12 group sessions with adults between the ages of 25 and 35. The purpose of the group was to improve relationship skills. There were five men and five women. One woman dropped out at the third session because of babysitter problems. The group meets from 5:45 to 7:15 every Tuesday evening at a Family and Children Services Center, a United Way Agency serving a neighborhood of mixed ethnicity, race, and class that borders a large university. Many college students live in the area and take advantage of the services, which are set up on a sliding fee scale. There are programs for at-risk youth, an adult day care located in the building, child-care services for clients who are receiving mental health services, and an anger management program.

The group had begun with male and female co-therapy leaders. One of the leaders was a social work intern who had contracted mononucleosis and had to drop out of the internship for 6 weeks. The student would have returned for the last two or three sessions, if at all. The student left the agency at session two of this group.

(*Note*: This chapter's commentaries are presented in short phrases, similar to notations one might make as session notes are studied to understand the underlying neurobiology of the exchanges.)

Members: Franklin, Ron, Evie, Hallie, Anna, Brian, Mario, Cici, Karl, Ava

THERAPIST: Welcome, everyone. I am sorry to announce that Mina will not be back to our group. Her message said that she could not work out the baby-sitting arrangements and wished she could tell you goodbye herself (*silence of minute or so*).

> *Defenses: blocking of affect (inhibition of thinking and impulses); repression (moving from conscious awareness of an idea or affect to avoid anxiety); denial (minimizing experience by lack of awareness). Each member likely utilizing different mechanisms, and some may not be silent as a defensive process; defenses likely managed by the parasympathetic branch of the autonomic nervous system (brain trying for low affect, perhaps to counterregulate the possible upset of the announcement).*
> *Other comments: Group is in the formative stage of group development, assessing safety and danger to determine if trust is possible (right-hemisphere reacting, particularly the amygdala, which may be overly sensitive, should the member have trauma background).*

FRANKLIN: Mina? I can't believe it! She was goin' on so about how much she had her eyes opened and all that. What was she goin' on like that for (*disbelievingly; louder with each word he spoke*)?

> *Defenses: acting out (direct expression of impulses to remain unaware of wishes or affects that accompany them); managed by the sympathetic branch of the autonomic nervous system (brain trying for high affect, perhaps to counterregulate the possible sadness of the announcement).*

RON: (*equally loud*) Ah, man, don't give her a hard time. You know how she is about that little boy of hers. Besides, I saw you looking at her all the time with that look.

FRANKLIN: What? Hey, I never said anything about you looking at the ladies here. Besides, we are supposed to be thinking about how we get along with our so-called "significant others . . . " (*Loud exchange of accusations flies between Ron and Franklin.*)

Defenses: acting out (direct expression of impulses to remain unaware of wishes or affects that accompany them); maybe each is using self-assertion (actively taking care of oneself, verbally or through action); though each defense mechanism is sympathetically activated, the behaviors seem closer to acting out than self assertion, because self-assertion is a more adaptive defense that acting out.

Other comments: There was an abrupt affective shift, activated by the excitatory message to neuronal networks; nonverbal (right brain) as important as the verbal communication (left brain, linguistic): "I saw you lookin' at her all the time"); disruptions in relating are often the result of conflict and lack of a skill set to constructively address conflict.

EVIE: (*talking over Franklin in conciliatory way*) Guys, guys, what's with the attitude? I mean, we *are* here because we are worried about how we get along with other people. Franklin, why are you being sarcastic about our "significant others"?

Challenging to Ron and Franklin. Defenses: self-assertion (actively taking care of oneself, verbally or through action); maybe acting out via the sarcastic tone of voice; self-assertion is a homeostatically balanced reaction (the parasympathetic and sympathetic branch of the autonomic nervous system work in concert, with neither the excitatory sympathetic nervous system nor the inhibitory parasympathetic nervous system preferred over the other, regardless of the situation); may be using parasympathetic nervous system to stay calm and permit social engagement.

Other comments: Evie may be taking the sociable role of attuned personalities (right brain).

HALLIE: (*in a sing-song voice, chiming in with Evie*) Yeah, what are you worked up about? Seems like that just came out of the blue.

Chiming in with Evie. Defenses: identification (recreating an inner psychophysiological state similar to others); can be either parasympathetic nervous system or sympathetic nervous system activated, depending on the state being matched.

Other comments: This could be a limbic-system to limbic-system bond. Additionally, the rapid processing of facial expressions by the right somatosensory cortices generates the same internal somatic sensations that simulate how one would feel while having that same expression on one's own face.

RON: (*starts talking, as if no one else had said anything since his last remark*) And anyway, I saw her over at the HEB, and she didn't say anything about leaving us (*puzzled*).

> *Lack of awareness and puzzlement. Defenses: blocking of affect; inhibition (renouncing certain functions to avoid anxiety from various sources of conflict); parasympathetic nervous system (inhibitory branch of autonomic nervous system) managing the low affect.*

BRIAN: (*quietly, but looking right at Ron*) Us? Leaving us? You're actin' like she did something to us . . . like on *purpose*. And you two talked at the HEB? We signed that paper that said that we would not socialize till the group was over. (*He gets louder with each word.*)

> *Defenses: Challenging and loud. Defenses: Acting out or self-assertion or perhaps a combination of both (excitatory sympathetic branch)*

RON: (*starts stuttering*) Wh-wh-wh-ell, hell, you know how it is at the store? People just ttttttttalk in the checkout line.

> *Off-balance and stuttering. Defense: regression; sympathetic nervous system (excitatory) branch of autonomic nervous system.*

KARL: (*who had hardly spoken up during the previous session, asks in matter-of-fact way*) Were you in the checkout line?

RON: (*really flustered and reddening in the face*) Actually, no, if you must be exact, fer Christ's sake. We were standin' over by the cold cuts section. What difference does that make?

> *Ron's being flustered and red in the face in response to an apparently nonaggressive question. Defense: regression (excitatory sympathetic nervous system branch of autonomic nervous system); the nonverbal (loudness) can vary according to attachment style; the clinician may want to note that this member may exhibit a variation of the childhood ambivalent style, which is activated by the excitatory (sympathetic nervous system) branch of autonomic nervous system; this may indicate that the member may have particular difficulty bearing low affect, such as sadness or loss.*

ANNA: (*turning her whole body to face the therapist; appears upset/angry*) Why are you letting him go on? I paid my good hard-earned money to come here to figure out my mistakes with my boyfriend, and this sounds just like all the endless, stupid bickering that we do at the supper table. (*Stops herself from talking further by abruptly snapping her mouth shut.*)

Angry in confronting therapist. Defense: self-assertion and/or acting out; both regulated by the <u>excitatory sympathetic branch of autonomic nervous system.</u>

Other comments: A <u>confrontation</u> (sympathetic nervous system-activated) of the aggressive type; in group work, <u>confrontation</u> should occur in a safe environment, bringing something to a member's attention about which he or she had been unaware; safety–danger is registered quickly by the right brain, particularly the <u>amygdala.</u>

THERAPIST: (*Interrupted by Evie before she can speak*)

EVIE: (*definite and accusing tone of voice, ignoring Anna's complaint*) What difference it makes is that you acted like you *just happened* to be in the checkout line, but I'll bet that you talked to her as long as she would talk to you over the cold cuts.

Tone of voice. Defense: acting out (<u>excitatory sympathetic nervous system activated</u>).

THERAPIST: (*tries to speak again*) Excuse me for interr—

ANNA: (*somewhat pleadingly to the therapist*) I can't stand how mad you guys are. Can't you put a stop to all this?

THERAPIST: (*a little apologetically*) I *would* like to get a word in, or actually I have a question. I wonder what is fueling all this high emotion all of a sudden. It started with talking about Mina's absence and has seemed to snowball. Why don't we all stop for a minute and ask ourselves how we are feeling or what we are thinking right now.

Anna asking for help and therapist trying to manage the emotionality in the group. Defense: self-assertion (activated by <u>excitatory sympathetic nervous system branch of autonomic nervous system</u>).

Other comments: Leader models both <u>verbal</u> (left brain) <u>and nonverbal</u> (right brain) affect management; <u>nonconscious right brains</u> of group members will quickly resonate with limits tolerated by leader.

MARIO: (*speaking more quickly than usual*) AAAHHH, you know people like me and mebbe some uh the rest of you can't be quiet for a minute. I can tell you right now that I know that I am mad at you for letting everyone get so hot and crazy actin' in here. It seemed like we were havin' decent conversations for a few weeks and now this.

Defenses: self-assertion and maybe acting out (regulated by the <u>sympathetic branch of autonomic nervous system</u>).

Other comments: Mario's speaking quickly but revealing his emotion ("mad") by verbally labeling therapeutic factor of self-revelation is interesting *in light of the emotionality in the group; usually, self-disclosure is more likely to occur when there is more trust and safety than seems to be in the group at this point; the <u>amygdala registers safety–danger; however, perhaps Mario was experiencing safety from the clinician's attempt to contain the emotionality.</u>*

THERAPIST: Mario, I know that you are more a man of action, but just for a minute, if you could let the action be focused inward, then whoever wants to can report on how they are feeling or what they have been thinking. OK? In fact, I will time 60 seconds on my watch. OK?

Trying to manage the emotionality. Defenses: anticipation (planning); sublimination (allow impulses to be channeled rather than dammed up or diverted); affect acknowledged leading to modest satisfaction results; <u>clinician trying to model homeostatically regulated defense mechanisms; parasympathetic nervous system–sympathetic nervous system working together.</u>

MARIO: (*grudgingly*) OK.

THERAPIST: (*waits for exactly 60 seconds*) OK, would someone like to tell us what you reflected on about how the beginning of our group affected you?

Defenses: self-assertion; anticipation; sublimation.

(*Long pause. Two try to talk at the same time, look down, and then to the surprise of the group, Karl speaks up first.*)

KARL: I was just thinking that I had made myself a promise to be quiet during these meetings. My girlfriend made me come here, and I was gonna be damned if I was doing any talkin' (*becoming belligerent*).

Self-revealing, though in somewhat hostile manner; girlfriend made him join group. Defenses: acting out via hostility; displacement (solving conflict by assigning impulse to different person/situation than original one); did not take responsibility for coming to group.
    Other comments: Self-revelation, a therapeutic factor, may be in response to clinician trying to contain the emotional contagion (<u>right-brain to right-brain communication among several group members</u>).

THERAPIST: (*curious*) So, did you have a secret agenda from the group, about the not talking, I mean?

KARL: (*looks down and then directly at group members, one at a time*) I really did. She made me mad, actin' like everything is all my fault, like men are too dumb to "relate" and all kinda crap like that. So I thought "I'll show her."

Seems deliberate and self-disclosing, maybe even vulnerable. Defense: self-assertion (actively taking care of oneself, verbally or through action; excitatory branch/sympathetic nervous system).

ANNA: (*carefully*) Did that make you mad, that Ron wasn't really in the checkout line? That he maybe really talked to her in secret, sort of. (*turning to Ron*) I'm not saying that you two did something wrong, Ron (*looks directly at Ron*). But what I was thinking during our 60 seconds of forced quiet was that was just like my Dad; he was always acting all innocent, saying, "Well, I just ran into her at the store" and sh--- like that. My mom was always on him for that.

> *Trying to understand Ron by asking direct questions; vulnerable about similarity between Ron and her father's behavior. Defense: self-assertion (actively taking care of oneself, verbally or through action; excitatory sympathetic nervous system branch).*

KARL: Yeah, well, maybe I understand your dad; I keep little and sometimes big secrets all the time. I can't stand to be bossed around, so when I do something nobody knows about, well, I don't know, it's just better for awhile.

> *Self-revealing and vulnerable. Defense: self-assertion (actively taking care of oneself, verbally or through action; excitatory sympathetic nervous system branch.*

RON: (*muscles his way into the conversation between Anna and Karl*) Anna, you can cuss in here; you don't have to act so proper. And what I was thinking about during our 60 seconds was that I was always being accused of doing something wrong when I was a kid. My mother acted like she had eyes everywhere and would accuse me of the weirdest sh-- (*looking at Anna*) Yeah! I said, a cuss word!

> *Becomes aggressive verbally toward Anna, who had been self-disclosing and vulnerable. Defenses: verbally acting out (direct expression of impulses to remain unaware of wishes or affects that accompany them) activated by excitatory sympathetic nervous system branch of autonomic nervous system.*

BRIAN: (*a little louder than the last time he spoke up*) What is it with you and the rules, Ron?

> *Maybe emotional contagion with Brian, like Ron, also being verbally aggressive. Defense: verbally acting out (direct expression of impulses to remain unaware of wishes or affects that accompany them).*
>
> *Other comments: Emotional contagion is activated by the excitatory sympathetic nervous system system; the norm may be forming in the face certain kinds of emotions, and it could dissolve/disperse attractiveness and sense of belongingness. Social engagement is not being encouraged in a calm manner at this point (Porges's polyvagal system; see Chapter 4 for details).*

THERAPIST: (*intervening between Ron and Brian and refocusing on the effort to reflect on their personal reactions*) Brian, would you mind telling us what you were thinking about and maybe feeling during the minute we were quiet?

BRIAN: (*startled a little*) Well, it seemed a little forced, and my mind was blank.

Surprised by focus on him; became self-revealing. Defenses: self-assertion (actively taking care of oneself, verbally or through action); "blank" may reflect isolation of affect (splitting affect from content, resulting in not being consciously aware of either idea or affect) or blocking (inhibition of thinking and impulses).

Other comments: Clinician may be clarifying (bringing psychological phenomenon into sharp focus) by asking Ron about what was on his mind.

THERAPIST: (*turning toward Brian*) Going back to your comment on the "socializing outside the group" agreement. You have said before that it irritates you when your boyfriend doesn't do what he promises. Do *you* ever want to go back on your word or not have to be so reliable? To not have to follow the rules?

FRANKLIN: (*cuts off Brian before Brian can answer*) You know what, Brian. My mind was a blank, too. I hate it when someone tells me what to do; I wonder if Mina did not come back because I was looking at her. My girlfriend is always on my case for looking at other women. I know that she could have the little boy here at the agency while we do group. None of this I'm saying probably makes any sense. But I think maybe I should have been more, well, polite to her, especially when she was sayin' all that personal stuff last time. I dunno (*trails off*).

Franklin is emotionally overstimulated (interrupting the therapist) with fears of own guilt; Franklin, like Brian, is "blank." Defenses: self-assertion (actively taking care of oneself, verbally or through action); "blank" may reflect isolation of affect (splitting affect from content, resulting in not being consciously aware of either idea or affect) or blocking (inhibition of thinking and impulses); identification (with Brian); or even dissociation (<u>mediated by parasympathetic nervous system/polyvagal system</u>; see Chapter 4).

(*The group is quiet for a minute or so.*)

Defenses: blocking of affect (inhibition of thinking and impulses); repression (moving from conscious awareness of an idea or affect to avoid anxiety); denial (minimizing experience by lack of awareness); even dissociation (<u>mediated by parasympathetic nervous system/polyvagal system</u>).

CICI: (*speaking for the first time*) You know, I realized that when you asked us to be quiet, I had been so quiet inside after all the arguing started, that I did not want to be quiet. In fact, I wanted to yell at all of you to SHUT UP! (*Everyone laughed, but not at her.*)

> *Cici had opposite reactions: When things were externally noisy, she was quiet inside and when externally quiet, she was internally noisy. Defenses: in reaction to external noise, blocking of affect (inhibition of thinking and impulses); in reaction to external quiet, thoughts or emotions for which the stimulation (sympathetic nervous system) may be intolerable.*

THERAPIST: Brian, looking back on the first part of the session, what would you speculate that your reaction was?

BRIAN: You don't give up, do you?

THERAPIST: I don't mean to be pushy, but maybe Franklin saw himself in you, you know, about being blank, and he sort of commented over you, or so I thought. And you did not get a chance to say anything about yourself, so I thought I *would* give it another try.

BRIAN: OK, OK, I was thinking, "Wouldn't you just know it. First the other leader ups and gets sick and then Mina just leaves. No warning, nothing. Seems like that happens to me a lot."

> *Brian forthcoming about his experience; more vulnerable, though somewhat challenging to therapist about effort to invite him to respond. Defenses: "Blank" may reflect blocking of affect (inhibition of thinking and impulses); repression (moving from conscious awareness of an idea or affect to avoid anxiety); denial (minimizing experience by lack of awareness; challenging may be a form of self-assertion (actively taking care of oneself, verbally or through action).*

HALLIE and CICI: (*speaking almost at the same time*) What happens to you a lot? (*Both giggle.*)

BRIAN: (*thoughtfully, wistfully*) Well, you know, you know. Well, people leaving, not doing what they are supposed to, you, ummm, I mean, if someone is committed to you, they should do what they say and keep their word.

> *Putting into words his wishes in vulnerable manner. Defenses: self-assertion (actively taking care of oneself, verbally or through action).*
>
> *Other comments: From other group members, an attempt at clarification (bringing something into sharp focus); even, perhaps, an interpretation (which broadens clarification, permitting the recognition of a repeating pattern (i.e., "What happens to you a lot?"). Recognizing and becoming self-aware are excitatory, active behaviors (sympathetic nervous system) and verbal interventions generated by left hemisphere.*

(*Hallie starts crying.*)

EVIE: Hallie, what's the matter?

HALLIE: (*crying more loudly*)

> *Upset, vulnerable, does not seem to employ defense; difficult to tell as her demeanor is not described.*

EVIE: (*looking at the whole group accusingly*) See, you made her cry with all this.

> *Accusing—maybe worried that she was somehow at fault. Defenses: maybe projection (assigning quality of oneself to another) and/or injustice collecting.*
> *Other comments: Evie accusingly looks at the group: this may be quite an aroused reaction on Evie's part; perhaps the conflict has evoked a past self-and-other template (right hemisphere) wherein she had to take on adult responsibilities for conflict management?*

RON: (*irritated*) Wait just a damn minute, *who* did something to her?

> *Demanding. Defenses: difficult to determine if verbally acting out (direct expression of impulses to remain unaware of wishes or affects that accompany them) or self-assertion (actively taking care of oneself, verbally or through action). The arousal of these defenses is from the excitatory sympathetic nervous system branch of the autonomic nervous system.*

THERAPIST: (*ignoring Ron*) Hallie, when you are a little more composed, could you tell us why you are crying?

(*The group waits, with less tension than during the whole session.*)

HALLIE: I feel like an idiot—I can't believe that I started bawling like that. (*Stops and starts, trying to find words to express herself.*) I wish I could have told Mina that I liked having her here. She could talk about herself so perfectly, and I wish I could do that. Last time, talking to us about all that private stuff, made me want to tell her things about myself. And now she isn't here.

> *Vulnerable and willing to self-disclose painful experience of missing group member. Defenses: self-observation (homeostatically balanced between the excitatory and inhibitory branches); an adaptive behavior.*
> *Other comments: The clinician may have made the group a little safer by asking Hallie why she was crying and, for the moment, ignoring Ron's outburst; members may be nonconsciously (right-hemisphere) resonating with the limits set by both the leader and the group.*

THERAPIST: Is it possible that others are missing Mina, too? Or maybe put in mind of missing someone else from another time in your life?

Therapist perhaps hoping for self-assertion, self-observation.

(*Big silence, then Cici starts talking about the air show, in detail, that her boyfriend took her to last weekend.*)

FRANKLIN: Cici, you know I like planes as much as the next guy, but I swear I can't figure out why you are talking about this now.

> *Defenses: self-assertion, self-observation (homeostatically balanced between the excitatory and inhibitory branches); an adaptive behavior.*

CICI: (*startled into being quiet for a second*) You know, when Hallie was crying, all I could think of was the last part of the air show when the military jets flew the missing man formation. You know, for our boys in Iraq?

ANNA: (*a little frustrated in tone of voice*) You guys, I don't understand any of this. First you're mad, then people are crying, and now the time is almost out. What good did this do, anyway?

> *Defenses: Anna and Cici both trying for self-observation (adaptive, homeostatically balanced defense mechanism).*

THERAPIST: You have asked a really good question. What *does* this group session have to do with getting along better with some people in our lives? (*No one responds.*) It might be that there were strong reactions to Mina and the meaning of her suddenly quitting. Maybe we should start to ask ourselves what happens in our relationships when something suddenly happens to us? (*no response*) For example, the group started to become agitated and irritable with each other right after I said that Mina wasn't coming back. Does anyone have an idea about why that happened? (*No response, but group's body language made it seem more like members were considering this question.*)

> *Defenses: initially, perhaps blocking of affect, isolation of affect, dissociation— all inhibitory processes (parasympathetic nervous system) employed in reaction to an upsurge in arousal (sympathetic nervous system).*
>
> *Other comments: Initially, the defenses may be indication of the vulnerability of an automatic coping strategy (a fixed and patterned way of coping, regardless of the stressor); as individuals, the members may have trouble managing much excitatory arousal; clinician attempting clarification and perhaps interpretation (bringing into sharp focus what may be a pattern of coping) may be trying to move the group from reactivity (belonging, even with the differences; excitatory); the lessening of tension, noticed via body language, may hint that group members may be able to have more mature (i.e., interactive regulation of affect) ways to respond, which would reflect a balance between the inhibitory and excitatory arousal systems.*

MARIO: Look, I am suspicious of all that "touchy-feely" psychobabble, but, for real, it made me mad that Mina wasn't here. Maybe it's just women, or just Mina, but I can't ever just come right out and say what I really mean, like she did. Don't get me wrong, it's not like I want to run off at the mouth about my *feeeelings* (*a little sarcastically*).

> *Defenses: At end of comment the sarcasm is verbal acting out (direct expression of impulses to remain unaware of wishes or affects that accompany them); at the beginning of the comment, Mario seemed to be trying to be more self-aware and employ self-observation (higher-level adaptive defense, meaning homeostatically balanced between the sympathetic and parasympathetic branches).*

THERAPIST: Sometimes feeling mad about something can cover up kinda down or sad feelings. Sometimes it's easier to be mad about missing someone . . .

ANNA: I know what you are going to say, that women feel sad and men feel mad! (*Therapist looks a bit surprised because that remark or criticism was directed at her and was not at all what she, the therapist, was thinking.*) That's more psychobabble—*my* first thought about Mina, was "Good, she's gone, now somebody else can have a turn."

> *Defenses: projection (diminishes anxiety by disowning own feelings/wishes and fears and "putting them" into others).*
> *Other comments: An experience in the here and now can evoke a response that was first experienced in the there and then of past interactions; for an experience to be memorialized in the neurocircuitry, it was likely initially of deep significance and repeatedly experienced. The transferences that are most likely to be addressed in the group are self-and-other representations (right hemisphere and nonconscious) that were originally stressful, developmentally compromising, and/or traumatic.*

THERAPIST: Anna, it seems that somehow it's better for you that Mina is gone. Why is that?

ANNA: (*surprised*) I did not mean that; it just sorta flew out of my mouth. In fact, I actually sort of liked her.

> *"it just sorta flew out of my mouth": Defenses: acting out (direct expression of impulses to remain unaware of wishes or affects that accompany them).*
> *Other comments: Confrontation by clinician—"it seems that somehow it's better for you"—which is bringing something to Anna's attention that was out of her awareness.*

THERAPIST: Well, maybe it's both: Maybe you liked her and had some other reaction to her, too.

ANNA: Yeah, yeah, she made me upset, talking about that little boy of hers so much. My mother gave me to my oldest sister when I was about 3 and had herself a high old time with that stupid boyfriend of hers. She never gave up anything for me, like Mina gave up the group.

CICI: Now that I think about it, I remember thinking at that air show, "What about flying the *missing mom* formation?" Anna, I know what you mean. Our dad always had two or three jobs, so we never saw him. The kids used to make fun of me that I did not even have a dad, 'cause he never showed up for anything at school; Mom, not so much either. My older brother was always there, though, watching out for me, and he came to everything. Everyone knew that they had to deal with him if they messed with us little kids.

> *Defenses: Both Anna and Cici seem to be more self-revealing, which may be self-observation (moving toward trying to use words to express experiences, rather than behavior)*

HALLIE: I did want to say something about my dream before this is over (*members groan, though not unkindly*). Well, I know I always talk about my dreams (*determined*), but my therapist always asks me about my dreams, and I always find out something important. Like, I had a dream that somebody at work left on a trip and never said anything to anyone about leaving.

> *Defense: self-assertion.*

RON: Hallie, you had a dream just like that last week about the girl in Aruba going missing. Your dreams seem just alike to me.

> *Defenses: seems to be devaluing Hallie's dream; maybe denial (minimizing experience by lack of awareness).*

THERAPIST: Though we only have a couple of minutes, if we are going to talk a little bit about Hallie's dream, it might be a good idea to talk about what her dream might have meant to you.

> *Invites higher-level behavior, such as self-disclosure (conscious awareness of own inner experience). Defenses: Clinician suggesting use of adaptive, higher-level defenses such as self-observation (homeostatically balanced, using both excitatory and inhibitory branches of autonomic nervous system to work together for less polarized reactions (too high/too low affect).*
>
> *Other comments: Clinician modeling use of intellectual/cognitive processes (left brain) to try to understand emotional meaning (right hemisphere) of Hallie's dream to group members; also an educational therapeutic factor of*

suggestions and advice (left brain) plus therapeutic factor of vicarious learning, as some members reveal the meaning of Hallie's dream to them (mirror neurons); and even trying out new behaviors (both left [imitative, somewhat] and right hemispheres); clinician trying for a posture of psychological work, as opposed to reactivity, which would utilize insight (making the non/unconscious, conscious). The group modality is an excellent practice field for learning the interactive regulation of affect that may improve resiliency by altering corticolimbic circuits responsible for affective and behavioral management and regulation.

RON: I know, I know, you said that last time. OK (*takes a breath*), I don't like her dreams because they make me think of my girlfriend always saying, "Oh, go ahead, when the going gets tough, the tough get going."

Tries for self-revelation, self-awareness. Defenses: self-observation leading to self-revelation.

Other comments: Perhaps imitation (using vicarious learning and modeling) may lead to a moment of identification with clinician (recreating an inner psychophysiological state similar to others), in that Ron takes a breath, as if to prepare himself to do something hard—that is, to be reflective rather than reactive.

FRANKLIN: What the hell does that mean?

Defenses: Aggressive verbally; acting out? (direct expression of impulses to remain unaware of wishes or affects that accompany them); these defenses are arousing and managed by the sympathetic branch of the autonomic nervous system.

RON: She means that when we fight, that I grab my truck keys and leave. There she is standing at the door of the apartment, yelling at me to come back and be a man and finish our "talk." *Some talk.* All she does is yell at me about everything I do wrong.

(*The group is quiet for a few seconds.*)

Defenses: Maybe group is reacting to the openness of Ron's self-revealing remarks; perhaps the silence is a higher level of defense (anticipation: planning) or more heavily defended, using isolation of affect (splitting affect from content, resulting in not being consciously aware of either idea or affect); or blocking (inhibition of thinking and impulses); or suppression (conscious decision to postpone focus on conflict or situation).

THERAPIST: (*trying to wrap up the session*) We seem to be talking about both the reality of Mina's leaving as well as some of the meanings to us that someone leaving or someone lost to the group might have . . .

Defenses: Therapist trying to link current experience with losses from the past, perhaps being a bit intellectual, or using intellectualization (thinking rather than feeling affect to defend against anxiety from unacceptable impulses); or clinician may be trying to link right and left hemispheres (nonconscious = emotional; conscious = cognitive); as an insight for Ron and as modeling for the group the psychological work of linking the here-and-now group experiences (sometimes reenactments of past interactions that have been out of awareness) to the there-and-then experiences (both right- and left-brain experiences). Tracking both emotions and cognitions as they affect each other.

FRANKLIN: Well, hold on there therapist, don't act like you didn't tear up when Cici was crying over there. You can't act like it was just us.

Defense: self-assertion. Other comments: Confrontation of clinician by Franklin, bringing to attention something ("tearing up") about which the clinician may have been in denial or may have suppressed.

THERAPIST: You're right, Franklin. I was trying to hide my tears there for a while. Sorry if I acted like I wasn't affected. I guess I wondered if I could have done something to help her stay in the group and felt guilty when we were quiet for 60 seconds.

Self-revealing, self-disclosing expression. Defense: self-observation (a balanced defense with the excitatory and inhibitory branches working well together).
Other comment: Main reason for choosing group treatment—improve relationship skills; the brain's primary self-regulatory system is the attachment relationship.

BRIAN: (*imitating the therapist*) Well, it's almost time to end this session. Would anyone like to make a remark before we close? Or maybe we should have another 60 seconds of silence to really screw us up until next week!

(*Everyone laughs in a way that seemed comfortable and starts to leave.*)

Defenses: acting out (direct expression of impulses to remain unaware of wishes or affects that accompany them); or perhaps humor (tender; adaptive as does not contain aggression) or wit (more aggressive than humor, therefore, less adaptive); perhaps affiliation (bonding).

THERAPIST: Well, Brian, you actually did take the words right out of my mouth. It is time to close. See you all next week.

EVIE: (*with her hand literally on the doorknob*) Well, I wish I had a little of the group's time.

Defenses: help-rejecting complainer, masochism. Evie will not be able to really ask for or receive in this group meeting, at least, not at this meeting; help-

rejecting complaining is a way to manage dependency needs; a person asks for help and then immediately ensures that he or she will not receive the help; the person both wants and fears dependency.

Concluding Comments

As noted previously, the ultimate goals of group therapy are greater intrapsychic calm, improved interpersonal functioning (both primarily right-hemisphere processes), and deepened self-knowledge (both right and left hemispheres). Insecure attachment strategies tend to repetitively restage the original experiences that created the unsuccessful autoregulation affect management strategy initially. The clinical goal is to provide some experience with secure attachment (regulated self in interaction with an attuning other) and to compete with the insecure attachment style (a dysregulated self in interaction with a misattuning other) that is imprinted into the neural circuitry. The synchronized energy exchanges make possible multiple repetitions that may create change via growth of new dendrites that connect with or strengthen existing neural circuits. In turn, these fortified neural circuits may improve affective and behavioral self-management, thereby also improving the possibility of relationship satisfaction. The group modality is an appropriate setting for such growth opportunities.

CHAPTER 8

Integrating Selected Neurobiological Concepts into the Supervisory Process

In preceding chapters, selected foundational concepts were described and illustrated with case material. These concepts include the functions of certain parts of the brain that affect physiological arousal (bodily and affective); the significance of understanding adaptive and maladaptive ways a person's brain manages arousal or the lack thereof, using the concept of defense mechanisms; and ways the interactions between the brains of two or more persons are biologically programmed to perceive threat and how that capacity might develop into adaptive or maladaptive coping responses.

This final chapter has a focus on two defense mechanisms—projective identification and dissociation—as a way to explore how the transfer of affect and other experiences may occur, both in the clinical encounter (in this case, between the supervisee intern and the client) as well as in the supervision process (between the supervisee and the supervisor). In current clinical supervision, the demands of short-term treatment and financial constraints (to name a few pressures) contribute to an emphasis on goal setting and measuring of same, often at the expense of examining the clinical contributions of the reactions the people are having to each other in the therapeutic alliance. In earlier times in the clinical world this process was discussed in terms of the *transference* and *countertransference* (Freud, 1958b). More recently, the neurobiological substrata of defensive processes (particularly, projective identification and dissociation) have been understood as the mechanisms of transference–countransference. These processes are so complex and intertwined that a complete discussion was beyond the scope of earlier chapters to give them the attention they deserve. Though a similar, if not identical or parallel, process may occur between a supervisor and supervisee, often short-shrift is paid to that fact. It is worth highlighting the parallel process between the supervisee and client as replicated within the supervisee and supervisor experience.

Selected Supervision Issues

The academic aspects of teaching clinical theories and technique, though critical to the acquisition of skills to address the treatment of mental health issues, is beyond the scope of this chapter. Of interest to us here are those neurobiological phenomena that may have a profound effect upon the ongoing development of the professional use of self. Of course, these phenomena may heavily impact academic teaching as well, but the illustration is confined to the supervision process for clinical work with persons who have mental health issues.

Clinical supervisors (and teachers) in the mental health field should help their supervisees (and students) bear difficult emotions, wishes, thoughts, and other reactions (McWilliams, 2004, p. 299). Many contemporary therapeutic modalities that favor a cognitive–behavioral approach do not emphasize the clinician's reaction to the therapeutic situation as a source of information, but rather as, perhaps, the student's or therapist's personal problem, if it is addressed at all. Other modalities maintain the idea that clinicians should strive for a nonresponsive facial and body language reaction to their clients—something that is almost impossible, as recent findings in child development and related fields have clearly addressed (Aron, 1991, 1992; Greenberg, 1991; Hoffman, 1983; Lachmann & Beebe, as cited in Moskowitz, Monk, Kaye, & Ellman, 1997; Siegel, 2003).

Issues that are generally common to many therapeutic approaches have been chosen to illustrate both the interactions between the supervisee and the client and also between the supervisor and the supervisee. These issues include the following:

- Emotional safety and comfort
- Degree of self-disclosure between supervisor and supervisee
- Supervisor possibly overwhelming the supervisee unwittingly
- Balance between the supervisor helping the supervisee become aware of his or her contribution to the therapeutic dyad, yet not cross the boundary into personal therapy with the supervisee.

In addition, the neurobiological underpinnings of adaptive and defensive projective identification (object constancy perhaps being a special case of projective identification), transference, and countertransference are briefly described, and material from a session between the supervisee and the client is examined for illustrations of these clinical constructs. To illustrate the parallel process in supervision, a sample of the supervision discussion also is examined.

As most supervisors find, a parallel process can occur between the supervisee and supervisor that mirrors some of the dynamics or experiences in the clinician–client relationship (Feldman, as cited in Parad & Miller, 1963, pp. 299–306; Hamilton, as cited in Parad, 1958, p. 34–35; Kottler & Blau, 1989, pp. 72–72, 99–103; Weissman, Epstein, & Savage, 1983, pp. 242–243). In the case illustration that follows, the social work intern was excited and interested in learning about the practical application of the neurobiological underpinnings of the therapeutic relationship.

The intern is a serious, bright, talented young woman whose undergraduate major had been Spanish literature and education. I have found myself favorably biased toward those who come to the mental health professions with such a background. Their disciplined deconstruction of the narrative line of a story, speculating on the motivations(s) of the characters, and generally drenching themselves in the experiences literature offers can often put them far ahead of others. There is a close similarity between the way literature is studied today and the clinical skill necessary to understand the themes and templates addressed in psychotherapeutic work.

However, teaching a right-brain approach to those accomplished in the left-brain academic world can become a challenge. The current mental health treatment climate has a heavy emphasis on "doing" something or reaching a preset "goal," both of which are clearly more left-brain endeavors. With the limited time that managed care currently allows for mental health care, the structure implicit in goal setting is inevitable—and not necessarily negative. However, learning about and appreciating the clinical intricacies of the brain-to-brain connections are often lost in the interest of the time pressure imposed by third-party payors' severe limits on number of sessions (e.g., 4–10 sessions for serious psychiatric diagnoses). However, preserving the value of the treatment alliance does not have to be abandoned with fewer sessions. There need not be a choice between "doing" something versus creating a connection with the client, which in itself has the potential to become therapeutic. Certainly there is ample evidence that the treatment alliance is a most important curative factor, regardless of the treatment modality (O'Neill, 2002), so anything that promotes such an alliance is valuable.

Always trying to privilege the therapeutic alliance in my own practice, I have struggled *not* to prematurely interpret, *not* to hunt for the affect management strategies of clients but to let them emerge, yet to *find* ways to apply the research findings (a left-brain endeavor) about the ways that two right brains synchronize. I have been trying to teach a subtle point: that the ambient atmosphere that can occur when two right brains are in synchrony can set the stage for an encounter that can be therapeutic. Conversely, when the two right brains are asynchronous (e.g., not in "sync" or not "clicking"), barriers to therapeutic progress may occur. The approach described in this chapter is about "being with" or "not being with" and the neurobiological consequences of those moments between clinical dyads—the client–therapist dyad as well as the therapist–supervisor dyad.

One way that I sometimes work with a supervisee is to go over almost verbatim material. We try to both think and feel our way through the exchanges, both the verbal and nonverbal. I sometimes find myself talking too much when I should just let the two of us let our left and right brains have some space to unhurriedly work out the kinks in our considerations. Sometimes, supervisees avoid my eye contact, or vice versa, when the encounter becomes too intense, or at times, too sad. Sometimes there is some kind of asynchrony between us and I worry that a supervisee is indulging my excited, maybe long-winded, teaching. Sometimes I think to stop us and ask how this is going for him or her. Sometimes I only think of that in the car going home, chagrined! Sometimes I feel incompetent, especially when at my most "brilliant." Other times, there is a delicate moment that just happens, and we seem to know that the climate for the teachable moment has occurred. Like a soap bubble, it pops and we go on. We do, somewhat awkwardly, try to talk about those times, though probably not often enough. It is very hard. And always I feel like I learned a lot, always hoping that the supervisee did, as well.

To move to the details of the process for deconstructing the clinical issues and highlighting the neurobiology of case material, it is helpful to refer to copies of the defense mechanisms and their brief definitions. The definition of terms (e.g., attunement),and the schematic of the human nervous system noting the functions under study are useful, too. For the case of Mary considered in this chapter, the functions of the autonomic nervous system and related constructs are then examined. However, projective identification and dissociation are the focus, particularly because these defensive maneuvers affect transference and countertransference and the parallel processes in supervision. Finding examples of behaviors that seem to illustrate neurobiological constructs can be tedious and daunting, at times. Though the following exercise in speculating about some of the neurobiological actions that may undergird the therapeutic encounter can be done alone, it is recommended to work with others, especially when first attempting to apply neurobiology to interpersonal encounters. However, before addressing the case material, the following sections define and briefly discuss adaptive and defensive projective identification, transference, and countertransference.

Projective Identification

Projective identification is an awkward term that currently invites instant rejection in the larger mental health treatment community. To recent graduates of clinical programs, the term is often associated with an old-fashioned psychoanalytic world of a century ago. To compound the problem, seminal contributors to the clinical literature have never agreed on one definition. Bearing these issues in mind, I have tried to make the following discussion of this vital concept as friendly as I am able. A brief review of affect regulation experiences is necessary before discussing adaptive and defensive projective identification, dissociation, and object constancy (concepts that capture shared psychological processes from infancy, which may become compromised by certain experiences).

Humans are born unable to regulate their emotions, their bodily functions, and their behavior. However, the baby brain is preprogrammed to immediately seek out another brain and body that can regulate those vital functions. Though this chapter focuses more directly on emotional regulation, bodily regulation is clearly part of emotional management via the selected neurobiological constructs discussed.

What are regulatory processes? What do those processes have to do with projective identification and the supervision process? Virtually the same unconscious dyadic communication process learned in infancy persists throughout life and occurs in the dyadic experience between people, including the therapist–client dyad and the supervisor–supervisee dyad.

A brief discussion on the origins of certain affect regulatory processes is in order before the case illustration. The baby must signal somehow that he or she is in need, and an other must be able not only to receive the signal, but also to properly address the signaled need—that is, to regulate the baby's functions.

Early theorists who observed children coined the term *projective identification* (Klein, 1946) to describe the signaling–receiver experience. How that signal–receiver phenomenon actually works and what is actually signaled are two different constructs in the literature. The "how" can be thought of as the process of signaling–receiving, and the "what" can be thought of as the content. The *process* of signaling–receiving is projective identification, and the *content* that is signaled is captured by the transference–countertransference process, described in the next section of this chapter. When an old familiar template for interacting with another person is restaged in a current relationship, this "enactment" is the transference–countertransference experience (and the process through which it unfolds is projective identification).

Adaptive Projective Identification

In a perfect world the attuned caregiver (or therapist or supervisor) responds in a timely fashion to the baby's (client's or supervisee's) signals, eventually microregulating the physiology (Schore, 2003a, pp. 71–88; Sroufe, 1996) as well as the emotional apparatus of the baby. The process of properly attending to the infant's needs will structure the neural circuitry, so that the infant's internal state (barring constitutional factors, trauma, medical or other stressful factors) will be able to regulate itself over time. Process builds structure, which leads to *expecting* the process, building more structure, and on and on. For example, the baby signals distress by uncomfortably wriggling; the caregiver has a somewhat synchronous somatic reaction, then responds by fixing the problem; the baby learns that signaling distress brings comfort. Additionally, over time, the baby learns to approximate some of the comforting strategies and creates some self-comforting strategies appropriate to the developmental stage (e.g., stroking a blanket or thumb-sucking). These repeated experiences are eventually inscribed within the upper right brain, hippocampal, and other memory systems. The memories stored in the hippocampus are easily retrievable because they are "memories of emotions" versus "emotional memories," which are stored in the lower memory systems (e.g., the amygdala) and are not available to deliberate, conscious attempts to access (LeDoux et al., 1989). Memories encoded in consciously inaccessible ways are subject to being enacted within the therapeutic or supervisory dyad (and in other relationships, too).

The therapeutic process (and the parallel process in supervision) will most likely be negatively affected by the difficult amygdalar "memories of emotions" (vs. the hippocampal "emotional memories"), as those unconscious experiences may be revived via state-dependent recall—that is, cues or triggers that are sensory experiences in the present and are similar to those in the past. The client may not be able to distinguish between past and present, unconsciously, which invites the "model scene" (Lichtenberg, 1989), essentially a past stressful or traumatic way of experiencing others currently.

The therapist may have an unconscious synchronous somatic reaction to the quality of the somatic state of the client, particularly the state of arousal. This physiological reaction is a somatic marker (Damasio, 1994, as cited in Schore, 2003b, p. 29) that may lead to somatic countertransference (Lewis, as cited in Schore, 2003b, p. 29), meaning that the therapist's right-hemispheric state is resonating with the client's right-hemispheric state.

To return to the origins of the regulation of emotions, eventually neural pathways become stronger and stronger as they are dedicated to various self-regulating tasks. It is the sensitive dosing of the properly synchronized care that eventuates in self-regulatory behaviors. Or, when under stress and temporarily unable to self-regulate, the person (or child) will seek out others who can re-regulate the stressed coping system. The microprocess of signaling needs is the beginning of adaptive projective identification.

The repetitive microregulations over time will lead to states becoming traits—that is, imprinted in the neural circuitry (Hebb, 1949). For example, "the detection and complex processing of the smallest change within a human face occurs within 100 milliseconds" (Lehky, as cited in Schore, 2003b, p. 98), and that such facially expressed state changes are mirrored (Dimberg & Ohman, as cited in Schore, 2003b, p. 98) and synchronously matched by an observer's right hemisphere within 300–400 milliseconds, at levels beneath awareness (Stenberg et al., as cited in Schore, 2003b, p. 98). This process occurs whether the projective identification is adaptive or maladaptive and there is no awareness (consciousness) of the process.

So, what happens? Projection begins as a signal; identification begins as the signal is received. Hopefully, acting appropriately on the baby's signaled need will then occur. Should the caregiver not respond appropriately to the signal, the misread cue can be followed by a repair. Perfect attunement is not the goal, and not even desirable. The infant brain will use less-than-optimal care to begin to incrementally take over some of the functions, provided that, on average, attunement and synchrony occur enough to transform external nurturing into internal self-regulation. In the clinical experience, an opportunity to rewire the neural circuitry is possible, as the clinician may provide some of the missing or compromised functions (particularly arousal management) in much the same way as should have occurred when the person was younger.

This attachment bond formation (i.e., the arousal management function) occurs within the physiology of the brain. The caregiver's face (and later possibly the clinician's face) triggers the anterior pituitary gland to produce endorphins that stimulate the production of dopamine (an arousing neurotransmitter) in the subcortical reward center, leading to pleasure, bonding, and attachment (Schore, 2003b). With multiple repetitions, this physiological process can lead to the secure attachment bond, in which the person has a homeostatically balanced autonomic nervous system. In the case of an older adolescent or an adult, there is the hope that an insecure attachment strategy may eventually become an earned secure attachment, with the concomitant adaptive capacity to manage the emotions more constructively, using the same neural pathways and processes that should have occurred in childhood.

To reiterate from previous chapters: Homeostatically balanced means that the brain prefers neither the excitatory branch (sympathetic) nor the inhibitory branch (parasympathetic) to manage affect and behavior. The flexibility and adaptability inherent in a balanced arousal system indicate that adaptive signaling–receiving has occurred and will likely continue to occur, as the person will likely choose relationships in which there is no need for defensive projective identification. In sum, the interactive regulation of affect can lead to the type of attunement that, in turn, creates an attachment strategy involving appropriate and nonproblematic self-regulation. This type of regulation has its beginnings in adaptive projective identification strategies (Schore, 2003b, pp. 98–107).

An attuned caregiver will struggle to contain his or her own reactions—an effort that is important for the child to sense (Schore, 2003b). The attuned interaction is therefore not simply mirrored but *metabolized* by the caregiver. It is important for each person in a dyad to know, on some level, that a reciprocal impact has been made (Winnicott, 1958). Likewise, the attuned clinician/supervisor will be somatically and emotionally affected by the interaction and hopes to be able to contain his or her own reactions to the client/supervisee, or failing in that, have an awareness of the reactions to the client, and be able to address such verbally.

Maladaptive or Defensive Projective Identification

The signals in maladaptive (defensive) projective identification are activated by the same process as in adaptive projective identification. At this point, however, there is a difference in the content of what is projected. Ridding the brain of, to give some examples, a difficult affect, wish, behavior, or intensity of affect is one of the goals of defensive projective identification. With adaptive projective identification, the process benignly tries to signal a need and recruit another to meet that need—which is usually a good thing, depending on the context and developmental stage, of course.

Why would a brain have to "rid" itself of anything? The primary reason is that stressful and traumatic experiences are often memorialized in subcortical neural circuitry, out of conscious awareness. Traumatic memories and affects have been preserved in the implicit (low right brain, subcortical) memory system. The hippocampal and other memory systems in the brain are available to consciousness, have more of a narrative line, and are more in summary form. In contrast, disturbing memories and affects in the subcortical systems are disorganized, chaotic, and not "online"—not able to be deliberately remembered in an organized way by ordinary means (Greatrex, 2002; Panksepp, 1999; see Bliss, 2010 for examples of indirect retrieval of emotional memories).

It is these disturbing experiences that are likely to be projected or ejected out of a person's own brain. Ideally, the upper frontal cortex would have had attachment experiences that promoted development of upper brain structures critically involved in detecting changes of emotional state and breaches of expectation (Nobre, Coull, Frith, & Mesulam, 1999). In part, tolerating and managing such experiences play a critical role in mediating internal and external worlds (Schore, 1994, p. 465), making projecting such difficult states unnecessary. The capacity of the upper cortical structures to tolerate difficult affects is key in metabolizing one's own affective experiences and precluding undue subcortical influence.

How does the ejected material actually "move" from one brain to another? It is through the actions of the person who is nonconsciously miserable about experiencing such memories and/or affects, the origins of which are often unknown to the person. What actions? Pressure (acting out) is brought to bear on the intended receiver of an experience that needs ejecting, often in the form of repeated attributions—for example, "You are arrogant because you have whiter skin than I do." The receiver generally identifies with the projection (although introjection likely occurs initially, which means taking into the self an identical experience). The receiver is carefully, though nonconsciously, choosing to be a good receptacle of the attribution, in this case a Hispanic woman with light skin. The light-skinned receiver is sensitive about her fair complexion, as she has been the butt of many aggressive comments and accused of thinking she is better than darker-skinned Hispanics. Once the receiver has emotionally resonated with the attribution and all its implications, the sender can dissociate from whatever his or her discomfort is with the experience because it has been "downloaded" into the mind of another person. When "download complete" occurs, the sender may truly not have any awareness of the psychological ejection of a part of him- or herself. This "ejection" is merely the sender's attribution of a trait, emotion, wish, fear, and so on, with which the "receiver" begins to resonate.

In a clinical encounter, this dissociative moment is critical, because it is a sign that the client has just "off-loaded" a fragment of an extremely stressful or traumatic experience. Suddenly, the clinician may feel alien to him- or herself, perhaps experiencing excitement, rage, elation, terror, disgust, shame, or hopeless despair (Heiman, 1950; Schore, 2003b, p. 280), which are particularly distressing because the clinician may have no idea of the origin (nor would the client). Meanwhile, the client can appear a bit blank, parasympathetically dominated in affect, perhaps as in a trance, if only for a moment. If the clinician's intuition (right brain) is working hard, he or she might ask, "What does it mean to you that I am light-skinned?", or something similar.

The client often is bewildered, not at that moment experiencing the difficult affect or memory, and wondering why the clinician is even pursuing the topic, typically assigning any interest in the topic to the clinician, even though the client initiated the discussion or the affective encounter. A clinician who does not resonate with the ejected (projected) material may show signs of boredom, irritation, anger, hostility, not understanding, behaving in a way that he or she does not approve of, or in a foreign or terribly familiar way (Strupp, as cited in Schore, 2003a, p. 88). Because the projected and then dissociated material is ever in danger of being re-experienced (via reintrojection) by the projector, often there is considerable acting out. The purpose of the acting out is to keep the ejected material "alive" in the receiver. For example, the light-skinned clinician's sensitivity to being accused of arrogance can be easily evoked by a mere comment, which may keep the emotions associated with those past experiences actively experienced in the present moment (Foster, Moskowitz, & Javier, 1996).

The client will sense this deflection of the attributed (i.e., projected or ejected) material and then may ramp up his or her efforts to signal that the clinician should receive the ejected/projected experience. "Prolonged blindness" on the part of the clinician may occur (Spezzano, as cited in Schore, 2003b, p. 88), wherein the clinician is no longer scanning for implicit external signals of internal disorganization, and the client continues to send out signals of intensifying stress.

The distress/bid for interactive attention is mediated by corticotrophin releasing factor (CRF), a stress hormone, increasing heart rate, blood pressure, respiration, muscle tone, and hypervigilance, followed by dissociation (high levels of parasympathetic nervous system dorsal motor vagal activity; Schore, 2003a, p. 67). Clients who respond at sensorimotor levels do so because that is where their earliest attempts at mutual regulation went awry (Bach, 1998, p. 188). Extreme projective identifications are associated with insecure attachments (Murray, 1991, p. 76).

Object Constancy: An Example of Defensive Projective Identification

Object constancy is another older term, like projective identification and transference–countertransference. It refers to the ability of the mind to retain a mental image of the function of another person who has provided positive experiences such as approval, soothingness, comfort, encouragement, or admiration (Mahler et al., 1975, pp. 109–112; Kramer & Akhtar, 1994, p. 27). With enough repetitions, the brain will take on those functions for itself and, when under stress, can generate self-approval, self-comfort, self-admiration, and so forth. When under enough stress, the brain of a person will also seek another person's brain to temporarily provide that function until it is restored and can resume its autonomous functioning.

A continuum likely exists regarding the degree of object constancy a brain has developed over time. Those with a less sturdy ability to retain an image of soothingness, etc., may be more likely to utilize defensive self-protective behaviors (i.e., maladaptive defense mechanisms), which become increasingly problematic for them and for others around them. Winnicott's (1958) concept of the capacity to be alone as a developmental achievement implies that an internalization of an at least benign, if not comforting, representation of an other, makes for adaptive defenses. A compromised ability for object constancy is the likely result of an insecure attachment, in which the child does not experience the caretaker as reliable and appropriately responsive—and therefore does not experience sufficient repetitions to stimulate the neurocircuitry to self-regulate affect.

In my clinical experience I have often observed behavior that I have come to think of as "reverse object constancy." It is likely a variant of projective identification in which a person creates extremely difficult emotional states in others *in order to be remembered* because he or she is fearful of being entirely forgotten without some action on his or her part. It may be a lingering pre-state of mentalization (Fonagy, 1998), wherein the person is unable to keep in his or her own mind the internal world of another person. This is in contrast to the psychological goal of ridding the mind of certain experiences, rather than a way to ensure that the other keeps the projector in his or her mind. It may be a way to avoid the terrifying experience of being entirely forgotten. In the case illustration to follow, the client may have had so many caretakers that she makes herself memorable by her acting-out behaviors. Object constancy, at its most functional, may serve as a protective factor against the development of problematic defensive behaviors and inner experiences. However, the content of this example of defensive projective identification is something noxious that is unconsciously chosen to be unforgettable to the receiver of the projection. This is the reverse of the function of object constancy, in which the brain of the developing child is remembering the other's benign or helpful functions. For example, the light-skinned clinician may not be able to easily forget the accusation from her client that she is arrogant because of her skin color. And the client may have resorted to a familiar way to be remembered by her clinician. The client may not have the confidence that she will be remembered unless she takes charge and controls the clinician's memory of her in an emotionally assaultive manner.

Transference—Countertransference

The supervision process, even with new clinicians, will almost always have elements of the intersubjective experience of the clinician and client that are experienced by the clinician as problematic. In other words, the supervisor–supervisee experience may mirror certain aspects of the supervisee–client experience, particularly those elements or dynamics that should be the focus of clinical scrutiny, eventually. There are certainly multiple opportunities to teach about treatment theories, techniques, and strategies, which is largely a left-hemisphere endeavor. However, more often than not, concerns arise about the felt experience of the supervisee with the client and the often-resulting confusion and consternation, a right-hemisphere experience. Regardless of the level of clinical experience, there can be a bit of a crisis of confidence if the right brain of the clinician is somewhat dysregulated within the treatment alliance, or worries about the lack thereof. A discussion of the historical clinical thinking about this right-brain to right-brain experience follows.

Transference–countertransference is also an awkward term that seems dated today, reminiscent of the work of early psychoanalysts, no longer mentioned in many clinical programs that are not psychodynamic in orientation. That is unfortunate because the concepts and phenomena are critical to clinical work. The brain is associational, needing few cues to rapidly compare past experiences with elements of current perceptions. The brain is also economical in its energy output; it does not need to see the whole dog to conclude that it is a dog. It is the stressed and traumatized brain that uses a normal process (i.e., needing few details to compare past with present) to its disadvantage. For example, a person who endured sexual molestation when the perpetrator was drinking may, at the smell of that type of alcohol or the tinkle of ice in the glass, have a massive reaction, blurring past and present. This is an involuntary occurrence, using a select sensory experience imprinted in the lower, subcortical regions of the brain, which are either–or in their associations involving safety and danger. If something is a little bit dangerous, the lower limbic system will experience *huge* danger.

Transference

When transference occurs, the client "relocates" an experience that happened in the past into the present, with the clinician. Traumatic memories are often the content of such transferences. The content may be a negatively valenced emotion, a wish, a level of arousal (high or low), a quality of the client or of someone else, a fear, an attitude, and so on, endlessly (Horowitz, 1983). This material is transferred to the mind of an other via projective identification. Many contributors to the literature have focused in minute detail on what the content of the transferred experience might be, often as a function of their theoretical orientation. Examples of the content are in the next section on countertransference.

Countertransference

What is countertransference? It is the clinician's nonconscious reaction to the transferred experience of being with the client. There is a bodily experience in the clinician to the imagery, affects, or thoughts that have been induced nonconsciously by the client. According to Zagon (2001), the key structures involved in the "heightened therapeutic moment" include the right amygdala (involved in unseen fear) and the right insula (which generates a cortical image of the internal condition of stomach, lung, bowels, pancreas, liver). Recognition of the physical responses and wondering about their meaning is an important skill to learn for any clinician—and not easy to accomplish, rivaled only by doing something clinically useful with the information.

Staying in the implicit, subcortical, right hemisphere (the target of the transferred experience) with clients can be taxing; likewise with supervisees. Some supervision styles may be quick to criticize new clinicians for being "overidentified" with the client, "taking empathy too far," or needing their own therapy to address the emotions and other experiences that get stirred up. There are certain times when all that and more may be true. However, the first response, in my opinion, should be to consider the clinician's reactions as a source of data and develop ways to appreciate the information inherent in the interactions, particularly the possibility of helping the client improve in the management and regulation of his or her affect (not to mention helping the new clinician bear intolerable affects, etc., which belong to another). Recognition of the clinician's unusual reaction (detailed above in the section on defensive projective identification), such as boredom, irritation, and so on, is a tip-off about the countertransference that may have occurred in response to the client's attempt to transfer an experience to the right brain of the clinician.

Various clinicians have addressed the content of transference and, consequently, the countertransferential responses. Some examples include Bion's "me/not-me" concept (1962), which seems similar to Racker's (1968) concordant–complementary identification. The concordant identification is one in which the clinician identifies with the "me" (or the self of the client), whereas in the complementary identification the clinician identifies with the "not-me" (or the internalized representation of the other) internal world of the client.

Kernberg's (1975) work with borderline pathology and (in his opinion) the ubiquitous use of projective identification addresses the object relationship (i.e., internalized self, internalized object [i.e., the other], and linking affect) to determine which elements or parts of the elements of the object relationship might be projected. In Kernberg's theory of object relations, what is projected is the same as what is transferred by the client and identified with by the clinician; Kernberg's approach is a more finely grained perspective than others with respect to projecting (transferring) the sense of the self, the sense of the other, and/or the affect. Many discussions of countertransference address ramifications of the clinician being treated as if he or she were similar to, or identical with, a figure from the past, which may be true. However, the ideas of Kernberg and like-minded others who more minutely examine the subtle experiences that are created in the brain of another person are more easily explained by recent findings in neuroscience, which address how affect is transferred from brain to brain.

Other clinicians exploring the transference of affective states include Miehls (1997), Dicks (1993), and Middelberg (2001), whose work with couples has led them to identify the reciprocal feedback loop between partners and some common, often polarized, mental contents that may be split between the partners (e.g., the pursued–pursurer of Middleberg's discussion). The "identification" aspect of the reciprocal interactions in the couple are likely the same phenomenon as countertransference, that is, a response to the transferred material, whatever it is. Silverman and Lieberman (1999) illustrated the mechanism for the intergenerational transmission of violent relational patterns between a young child and her mother as resulting from projective identification and the dissociated effect on the child of the frightening content projected by the mother. Again, the reciprocal interaction could be restated to say that the mother "transferred" her own fears to the child. The child's nonconscious identification is very much like countertransference.

Kohut's theory (1971) is that the "selfobject" function of the brain of the caretaking other (either in the past or the clinician) is eventually inscribed in the brain function of the client. That process could easily be a product of projective identification learned early on. Later, in the therapeutic encounter, the early relationship templates become the content of the narcissistic transferences as described in his theory. A useful selfobject function memorialized in the neural circuits seems similar to the experience of object constancy (Mahler et al., 1975).

For L. Horowitz, L. (1983), projective identification brings about certain past transferential templates leading to role suction, group spokesman, and scapegoating. In group work, the revival of such powerful roles creates countertransference issues in almost any group therapist. Waska states that projective identification is often at the core of the transference, so certainly the clinician will be induced to participate in a countertransferential manner (2007, p. 45). In Schamess's 1984 paper he describes the transference–countertransference process as a primitive form of communication, which for some people is the best they can do. It is the job of the clinician to properly read the clues to the client's inner state, which will be projected toward, or attributed to, the clinician.

The more deliberate and emotionally thoughtful structures of the right brain, in particular, are *not* involved in projective identification nor in transference–countertransference, as all these processes are nonconsicous (Smith, 1990). In those whose brains have stored distressing and potentially debilitating affects and memories outside of awareness, it is the lower subcortical structures, such as the amygdala and some neural pathways not mediated by self-reflective states (Greatrex, 2002, p. 191; van der Hart, Nieuwenhuis, & Steele, 2006, p. 190), which contain those experiences. LeDoux (1996) and Panksepp (1999) describe how fear-conditioned memories (in the low right brain) are stored in such a way as to not be communicable to upper brain structures for processing and working on. Eradicating a fear-conditioned memory, connected as it was to danger, is quite difficult. Ideally, the right ventral medial prefrontal (orbitofrontal) cortex plays a primary role in optimizing cautious and adaptive behavior in potentially threatening situations (Sullivan & Gratton, 2002).

According to Ogden (1982), projective identification may serve the following functions for traumatized individuals: as a psychological process that is simultaneously a type of defense, a means of communication, a primitive form of object relationship, and a pathway for psychological change. Change may be thwarted by clinicians themselves using defensive projective identification and acting out in the countertransference. According to Schore, toxic affects (e.g., shame, envy, vulnerability, impotence) can be moved back to the client and expressed defensively via sarcasm, teasing, ridicule, and efforts to control the client in some way (2003b, p. 91).

Whether or not the clinician recognizes countertransference bodily signals, and whether or not he or she can regulate those bodily signals, determines whether or not the countertransference is destructive or constructive, desymbolizing or symbolizing, reactive or reflective, defensive or adaptive (Schore, 2003b, p. 91). Though some (Klein, 1946, 1975; Steiner, 1979; Waska, 2007) have described the projective process as a *fantasy* of translocating one's own conflicted material to another brain, albeit nonconsciously, in fact, in light of the somatic experiences that occur in the targeted brain of the projections (transference), there is an undeniable *reality* to the identification (countertransference). Smith (1990) makes the clear distinction between countertransference and countertransference *acting out*. The countertransference is unconscious (i.e., the identification with the projected material and attendant somatic reactions), whereas the ways in which a clinician behaves, though driven by unconscious influences, are a primary means of bringing the unconscious experience to the attention of the clinician.

Illustrations of Concepts: Mary as an Adult Client

The case illustration that follows examines a session with the client, Mary, who was discussed in Chapter 5 (pp. 136–138) as the case of "Little Mary." Fifteen years have passed and Mary and her family have received social and other services from multiple agencies. An intern, Graciella, is assigned to Mary and has seen her three times. The session interchange and the process of the intern being supervised are examined in relation to the concepts discussed in this chapter, including the interactions and behaviors that illustrate projective identification and transference and countertransference.

To recap, Mary's hospitalization occurred at age 8, following her removal from an abusive home situation. In the hospital her behavior was described as chaotic and unpredictable, with no obvious pattern for managing her emotions behaviorally. Mary's autonomic nervous system was described as "uncoupled," which we now know means that she unexpectedly swung between the excitatory sympathetic branch of the autonomic nervous system and the inhibitory parasympathetic branch of the autonomic nervous system. Her behaviors and defense mechanisms were described as "wild," and she used few adaptive defense mechanisms. Reactive attachment disorder of childhood was a preliminary diagnosis in the first few days of Mary's hospitalization.

Moving to the present, the 20-year-old client is presented in a staff meeting of social work, psychology, psychiatry, and marriage and family student interns at a nonprofit mental health agency that serves as a training program and internship site for licensed professional counselors. Because Mary has been a client at the nonprofit mental health clinic on and off for several years, she has worked with several clinicians-in-training and is well known to permanent agency staff and administrative staff as well. The agency is located on the edge of a college in which Mary has been an on-and-off student since she graduated from high school. The college is one of the main industries in the medium-sized city. The agency is within walking distance and on bus lines to the most disadvantaged areas of the city. Mary still lives with a foster family (the eighth one) that adopted her when she was 16.

One of the senior clinicians on the agency staff was the caseworker when Mary and her siblings were placed in foster care as children; a supervisor himself of the first of Mary's interns, he had encouraged clinicians currently treating Mary to get the records from her foster care and hospitalizations. He made an appointment with Mary to reveal that he was the current intern's supervisor and to discuss her reactions to that fact, offering to resign as that intern's supervisor, if she wished.

Mary declined the offer and records were secured with her permission. Obviously an issue in Mary's care at the agency is that her family had come to the attention of many agencies over the years (e.g., police, child protective services, attendance officers from the schools). Confidentiality issues were unusually complicated as the city was small. The social service and social control agencies observed varying levels of confidentiality regarding Mary's extended family and their legal and social problems.

The following is a supervision meeting concerning the third session of the intern's work with Mary. The intern, in her late 20s, is a graduate student in the local college that Mary also attends. Graciella taught high school Spanish and Spanish Literature for a few years, but is now studying social work. Her ambition is to become able to address mental health needs of adolescents who were similar to the disadvantaged students she had taught.

SUPERVISOR: What questions do you have about the session?

GRACIELLA: (*quiet*) I am questioning my suitability for the counseling profession, after this session with Mary.

SUPERVISOR: What is worrying you?

GRACIELLA: A lot (*looking down and worrying whether she can be genuine with this supervisor, whom she hardly knows*).

SUPERVISOR: (*finding herself careful*) Are the worries vague or do you have some specific concerns?

GRACIELLA: (*grasping for something to say*) You probably heard that Mary stormed out of my office in the middle of our session.

SUPERVISOR: Yes, the office staff said something about it.

GRACIELLA: (*looking up for the first time*) Yes, I heard them say, "Oh, poor Graciella, she got stuck with Mary."

SUPERVISOR: Where were they when they said that?

GRACIELLA: In the coffee room.

SUPERVISOR: That is completely unacceptable—we cannot have that kind of talk where clients can hear, at least. (*Musing to herself, we should not have that kind of talk, period, but people are people.*)

GRACIELLA: (*Now worrying that she will have contributed to shaming other staff, and being the new staff member, that's no way to get along with coworkers— and she tried so hard to get this internship, everyone wants to work here, and other self-critical and obsessive thoughts.*) Will they know I told on them? (*Regrets her choice of words immediately, as she knows she sounds like a second-grader.*)

SUPERVISOR: (*ignoring her question*) What happened in the session? Give me a synopsis before we go over the transcript you have.

GRACIELLA: (*Feeling like she has to be professional and give a report, but still wondering if the supervisor will answer the question about her "telling on" the staff*) Mary was upset that I had not read her file. She wants me to write her a letter or some documentation for a medical withdrawal from school. I tried to stay focused on the letter, but when I asked her for details about why she had missed so many classes, she got mad that I had not read the file and that I would have known the answer to the questions, even though at the beginning of the session, she was mad at me for seeming to assume that her word wasn't a good substitute for reading others' words about her, or something like that. When I tried to ask her, she was upset and attacked me for being a light-skinned Mexican.

SUPERVISOR: Wait a minute—that is confusing. Why don't we go over the transcript, line by line, and figure out what happened? (*Gives Graciella a handout.*) We can use this list of the steps of a defense mechanism, projective identification, which is related to transference and countertransference, to try to track what may have occurred between you and Mary. OK?

GRACIELLA: (*Now completely sure that she is making a fool of herself and feeling helpless to stop the process*) OK.

Figure 8.0 presents the chronological steps that occur in the process of projective identification, with the attendant dissociation. Projective identification is the process that drives the reciprocal influences within the therapeutic moment (which can be labeled transference–countertransference, i.e., the actual content embedded in the exchange; Freud, 1958a, 1959a; Schore, 2003b, pp. 28–31). The process begins with an experience between two people (in these cases, between the intern supervisee and client as well as between supervisor and supervisee):

> ### FIGURE 8.0.
> ### Steps Involved in Projective Identification During a Therapeutic Encounter.
>
> - Sudden rupture of therapeutic alliance occurs
> - Right brain nonconsciously compares current misalliance (cue–trigger) and earlier empathic failures, instantly activating "hot cognitions" (Greenberg & Saffran, 1984)
> - Early interactive representations encode expectations of imminent dysregulation
> - Brain suddenly shifts dominance from left-hemispheric linear mode of processing to right-hemispheric nonlinear processing
> - Dysregulating transaction occurs
> - Reconstructs "model scene" (Lichtenberg, 1989)
> - Introduces into consciousness a chaotic state that had been defended against
> - Dreaded state of mind ensues (M. J. Horowitz, 1987)
> - Bodily state evoked via state-dependent recall
> - Splitting triggered (the instant evaporation of the positive and sudden intensification of the negative transference)
> - Leads to malignant transference reaction = hyperarousal or hypoarousal
> - Self disorganizes (explosively or implosively; increased right-hemispheric activation)
> - Somatic countertransference (therapist resonates with the client's right-brain state)
> - Resulting in "somatic markers" = physiological responses that receive or block the client's distress-inducing projective identifications
> - Depending on therapist's reaction, may have enactment
> - Leading to negative therapeutic reaction
> - Hopefully, interactive repair will occur, with attempts to reattune (therapist must be able to manage emotional therapeutic withdrawal)
> - Can lead to "working through" process of interactive repair (Tronick, 1989) = therapist recognizing and regulating the negative affect within own self
> - If therapist autoregulates successfully, can resonate with client's internal state of arousal dysregulation, modulate it, communicate it back prosodically in a more regulated form, and then verbally label own state experiences and client's as well
> - Moving from desymbolizing to symbolizing with "words during states of high emotional arousal is an important achievement in self-regulation" (Dawson, 1994, p. 358)
> - Can lead to internalization of therapist's regulatory function and reflective awareness
> - Cortical and sensory–limbic connections are reworked in long-term dynamic psychotherapy (McKenna, 1994; PET imaging study by Schwartz, Stoessel, Baxter, Martin, & Phelps, 1996)
>
> See Schore, 2003b, pp. 28–31

The supervisor and supervisee reviewed the transcript of the third session, identifying the defense mechanisms, particularly projective identification and dissociation. They speculated on clues to transference and counter-transference, as well. The supervisor used the format in Figure 8.1 to deconstruct the projective identification and resulting transference–countertransference dynamics as they unfolded in the session.

As the session is examined, a parallel process between supervisor and supervisee emerges and mirrors some of the dynamics between Gabriella and Mary. The supervision dyad deconstructs, step by step, the interactions between Graciella, the intern, and Mary, the client, using this template. The template is also useful in deconstructing the parallel process occurring between the supervisor and the intern.

Review of Case Illustration

The following material is the result of the supervisor and supervisee's work on the session in minute detail, identifying defense mechanisms and their underlying neurobiological mechanisms in the commentaries. Also the work is to identify the structure of the interview, using the concepts in the template (underlined in the session notes) in Figure 8.1 for reference, which tracks the projective identification process as it drives the content of transference and countertransference.

MARY: (*as she is sitting down*) I was wondering if you read that big file of mine yet?

THERAPIST: No, I haven't yet. Do you want me to?

MARY: I thought you had to do that?

THERAPIST: (*Now unsure of herself: Does she have to read it? Is it a technique issue or agency policy? She wants to do the right thing, whatever that is.*) I'm not actually sure if I have to; could you let me check with my supervisor on that?

> Here Mary may be beginning to create in the intern's mind Mary's own experience of uncertainty via projection (attributing qualities of the self to another; often this dynamic becomes active when we treat the other in ways that could create those qualities that we are seeking to disown). Projection is an active defense, utilizing the sympathetic (excitatory) branch of the autonomic nervous system.

MARY: Aw right, I guess so. Anyway, to change the subject, what about that medical withdrawal I need to drop this semester?

THERAPIST: We may be back to the subject of the file; do you think that I need to read your file so I can understand why you need a medical withdrawal?

MARY: (*irritated*) You could just ask me, don't you think?

THERAPIST: (*Thinking about staff meeting in which one of the senior clinicians declared that she never read the previous file, citing "contaminating my thinking" as the reason; intern realizing that that viewpoint had influenced her own attitude.*) Yes, why don't you fill me in on your situation at school (*relieved that there is some direction to go with the topic; had felt stuck, not knowing what to do, maybe guilty, as there really was implicit agreement to read the file*).

> The clinician is feeling unsure, somewhat dysregulated, and doubting herself— which is not entirely a negative, as being overconfident invites errors as well. Graciella's inner experience may be matching Mary's, and, if so, it seems uncomfortable and aroused (excitatory sympathetic nervous system branch of autonomic nervous system). Graciella is experiencing several difficult emotions in quick succession: relief, stuckness, and guilt.

MARY: (*resigned, a bit*) It's pretty simple, really. Here it is the end of September, and I had to miss three classes already. I won't be able to keep up now.

THERAPIST: Why did you miss classes?

MARY: (*Looks away, folds arms over her chest, shakes her head slowly back and forth, and says in aggrieved way*) If you had talked to my other counselor, I wouldn't have to go through all this again.

> Though posture and head shaking seem to reflect low affect (inhibitory parasympathetic branch of autonomic nervous system), in fact, the accusatory comment is more highly aroused (excitatory sympathetic nervous system) and more like verbal acting out (direct expression of impulses to remain unaware of wishes or affects that accompany them).

THERAPIST: (*sudden rush of feeling bad, maybe shamed (?) and a little irritated, too*) I apologize, I think I did nod my head last week when you asked if I was going to read your file. (*Knows the apology is not heart-felt.*) But I think we could talk about it today, right? And I could at least know what has been going on (*feels like that is a weak response, a bit too distant and intellectual, maybe?*).

> The defense of intellectualization (left hemisphere) may be employed. Intellectualization is thinking about, rather than feeling, affect to defend against anxiety from unacceptable impulses. If so, what were the unacceptable impulses? Maybe some negative and uncomfortable reaction to the aggression (accusatory tone by Mary, i.e., "If you had talked to my other counselor . . . ").

MARY: (*silent for a long minute or so*) Sooo, OK, here it is. My little half-brother got put in jail down on the coast, so I had to leave for a while to get him out of jail. (*Stops talking and sits very still, different from the aroused* [excitatory sympathetic nervous system] *state of only moments ago; seems a bit paralyzed.*)

> Mary may be employing dissociation (still and a bit paralyzed) to cope with the current and perhaps past emotions being evoked by her little brother being in jail. Dissociation is a drastic modification toward a numbing affective state (inhibitory parasympathetic nervous system driven); can be so "shut down" (Porges's [2007] polyvagal theory) that much physical action is impossible.

THERAPIST: (*Has a bad feeling about herself; doesn't know what to do; asks a concrete question.*) How old is he?

> The question reflects a left-hemisphere data collection action, not a right-hemisphere connected and empathic effort (synchrony). Graciella is trying to collect herself (so may have disconnected; asynchrony) with a seemingly innocent question, but she is totally off the mark. This instantaneous yet subtle move to a disconnected state is the beginning of the sudden rupture of the therapeutic alliance.

MARY: (*dully*) 17.

THERAPIST: How can you legally do that—he is a minor?

MARY: Not really, he has been an emancipated minor for a while.

THERAPIST: Oh. (*Thinking, "Now what do I do here?"; uncertain, feeling like a school teacher in problem-solving mode.*) OK, Mary, I can see that this is making you feel bad, so let's try to think about this rationally—

MARY: (*whips up head, body getting tense*) Rationally? Rationally? (*loud*) Here's rational! You know what he was in jail for? Well, do you?! (*fully angry now*).

> Graciella was pushed to self-protective behaviors (e.g., concrete question, "rational" comment), giving up "lending" her more vulnerable right brain to Mary for the moment, which may have been instantaneously experienced by Mary as another rejection in a long line of rejections.
> Mary may have nonconsciously restaged a toxic and well-worn self-and-other configuration (an enactment) with Graciella, whose nonconscious cooperation was seamless. Graciella may have become another person who is supposed to be a helper, but really backs away under pressure (parents, multiple foster home parents). Weiss and Sampson (1986) would speculate that Mary was trying to test Graciella to determine if an old template of danger would recur or if a "new story with a different ending" would happen within the therapeutic dyad.

This would be an example of Mary's right brain <u>nonconsciously comparing</u> <u>current misalliance</u> (cue–trigger likely provoking retreat to the left brain by Graciella) and earlier empathic failures, instantly activating "hot cognitions" which, for Mary, may be ones of rejection.

THERAPIST: (*off-balance emotionally, uncertain*) No, I . . .

Graciella's brain suddenly shifts dominance from left-hemispheric linear processing to right-hemispheric nonlinear processing, as did Mary's brain, but earlier in the session, beginning with, "Rationally? Rationally? (loud) Here's rational!"

MARY: (*aggressive and angry*) I'll tell you. It was "driving while Mexican." Do you know what that's like? I bet you do—you are Mexican, for sure, but oh, so light, aren't you?

The hot cognitions (rejections) invite <u>early interactive representations that</u> <u>encoded expectations of imminent dysregulation.</u>

THERAPIST: (*stunned by what feels like an attack; trying to compose herself*) Mary, I am not sure exactly . . .

MARY: (*getting in a rage, but has lowered her voice to cold and angry tone*) Yeah, I know, we have to be quiet with these thin walls here—I've heard *that* before.

THERAPIST: (*self-protectively*) I was not going to say anything about the noise, but I wondered if we can stay on the track of your medical withdrawal.

MARY: You are just like all the rest, aren't you?! You do *not* want to hear about "driving while Mexican" or anything else; let's just fill out this form, blah, blah.

The <u>dysregulating transaction reconstructs the "model scene" that recreates</u> <u>earlier transactions:</u> either a single traumatic one; multiple traumatic scenes; or scenes that happened repetitively and were not necessarily traumatic in themselves, but the accumulation of stressful experiences imprinting into the neural circuitry is every bit as toxic as trauma.

THERAPIST: (*Thinking about the students she had taught on the Texas–Mexico border that inspired her to become a therapist and how Mary reminded her of them.*) Look, Mary, I do *not* know what your life has been like, and I *am* a light-skinned Mexican, as you can plainly see, but I will try to understand it the best I can. Could we just both take a few deep breaths and try to calm down a little. I really would like to help you with your school paperwork.

MARY: I'm going to the ladies room. (*Jumps up and leaves the office.*)

THERAPIST: (*In tears the minute Mary leaves the room and upset with herself, feeling helpless, stupid, inept, and like she is maybe in the wrong profession and should go back to teaching. Takes her own advice in the form of a few deep breaths, drinks from her water bottle, and blows her nose, which is what she is doing when Mary returns.*)

> *The model scene introduces into consciousness a chaotic state, which had been defended against (paradoxically, Graciella's trying to calm them both, and trying to reconnect may have sent Mary out of the room in a state of extreme avoidance (inhibitory branch of autonomic nervous system) to counterregulate the abrupt oscillations in arousal. Mary may have wished for, but rarely experienced, someone trying to stay connected to her during painful arousal (remembering her history of many broken foster home placements, for which Mary may blame herself, however nonconsciously). Mary may assume that she can push people away effectively; perhaps this is generally true.*

MARY: Oh, great, now I've really done it. Now I have made the counselor cry. Didn't you wonder why I have so many counselors at the therapy store here? You aren't the first one to cry, for sure.

> *Mary may be experiencing the dreaded state of mind, a bodily state evoked due to state-dependent recall. Mary has successfully driven away another "helper." This may trigger splitting, which is the instant evaporation of the positive transference and a sudden intensification of the negative transference.*

THERAPIST: I'm trying to get a hold of myself, Mary, so we can try to do something important for you, and I don't just mean the letter to the school, you know.

MARY: (*not as angry as when she left the room a few minutes previously*) Yeah.

THERAPIST: (*Feels like she is taking a chance, lowers her voice*) Mary, you know, if you have a big file like you say, then you have probably been through a lot.

MARY: (*looks up, not defiant any more*) Graciella, I can be a perfect bitch; ask anyone around here—ask anyone in town, actually. Everybody knows our black sheep of a family. Every time I get a new counselor or teacher, I live in fear that they will read that !@#%*@! file. It reads like a made-for-TV movie or for *Intervention*—you know, that cable thing about drug addicts—that's us, all over and worse.

> *This interaction could have led to a malignant transference reaction, either with a hyperaroused (sympathetic nervous system) or a hypoaroused (parasympathetic nervous system) client with a disorganizing attachment style:*

either explosive (sympathetic nervous system) or implosive (parasympathetic nervous system low or polyvagally numbing). Either reaction would be a right-hemispheric activation.

THERAPIST: Are you saying that you did *not* want me to read the file?

MARY: That's exactly what I am saying.

THERAPIST: (*back to uncertainty*) Oh.

Graciella is trying to stay in synchrony (attuned via right hemisphere) because the left-hemispheric behaviors evoked a dysregulated transaction in the therapeutic dyad (asking concrete question motivated by Graciella's attempt to protect herself emotionally from Mary's aggressive behaviors; e.g., "Rationally? Rationally? Here's rational! . . . but oh, so light, aren't you?").

Graciella had been resonating with the client's right-brain state (somatic countertransference), particularly when Graciella started crying when Mary left the room. This bodily reaction resulted in somatic markers that are physiological responses that receive or block the client's distress-inducing projective identifications. Depending on the clinician's reactions, an enactment can occur. Fortunately, Graciella did not block Mary's inept but genuine attempts to reconnect ("I can be a perfect bitch") by staying in the intellectual problem-solving mode that drove Mary away initially. Graciella actually tried to receive Mary's distress-inducing projections, which may have been the battered self-esteem and negative self-criticisms.

If Graciella had resorted to the more protective left-hemispheric way of relating (intellectual, action-oriented, problem-solving, question-asking), she may have distanced herself emotionally from Mary, who nonconsciously, at least, if not consciously, has been acutely aware of the therapist's withdrawal, however slight it may have been. Mary may have experienced familiar rejection in the face of her effort to actually seek help. At that point, there could have been another edition of the familiar experience of the rejecting other in relation to the self, who wishes to be helped with the linking affect of anger (likely the basic self, other, and linking affect configuration; Kernberg, 1976). Graciella's blocking of Mary's effort to induce in her Mary's own battered self-esteem and self-criticisms may have led to a negative therapeutic reaction.

MARY: (*despairing*) I know, I am hopeless, aren't I?

THERAPIST: (*earnest, leaning forward*) You know, as long as we can talk about things, we will probably do OK, I think. But, to be honest, you really shook me up. I will just try my best.

This interaction may constitute an interactive repair, with Graciella trying to resynchronize with Mary in an awkward but authentic manner. For the interactive repair to work properly, Graciella's brain must both resonate with Mary's mental experience (e.g., low self-esteem) and, after the right brain registers that difficult moment, Graciella's left brain must also be able to think about what happened and make some intervention. The use of the right and left hemispheres in this way constitutes a therapeutic withdrawal, which is different from the earlier withdrawal when Graciella fled to the left brain for re-regulation of her own affect, leaving Mary stranded in her chaotic emotionality and acting-out behavior.

Therapeutic withdrawal can lead to a working-through process made possible by an interactive repair in which the therapist recognizes and regulates the negative affect within his or her own self.

If Graciella auto-regulated successfully (e.g., "to be honest, you really shook me up"), then the possibility exists that Graciella can resonate with Mary's internal state of aroused dysregulation, modulate it, communicate it back prosodically (tone of voice) in a more regulated form, and then verbally label her own and Mary's emotional state experiences.

MARY: That's my problem—I don't always try my best. Like the school thing. I hate to drop out again for a "medical withdrawal" (*sarcastic tone of voice*).

THERAPIST: What do you mean?

MARY: (*serious now*) Look, I really like school, it saved me many a time. Sometimes it was the only thing that made sense, but I had to go help my brother. He just got obnoxious with a cop down at the beach, and, well, you know what happens.

Mary is more self-revealing and no longer externalizing (actively experiencing in the external world parts of one's own personality; e.g., self-rejecting), projecting, or acting out. As Mary risked being more genuine in response to Graciella's increased genuineness, they moved from desymbolizing to symbolizing with words during the state of high emotional arousal. This shift is an important achievement in self-regulation. Of course, this movement from desymbolizing to symbolizing must happen repeatedly in order to create and strengthen neural circuitry to compete with the automatic negative-state-inducing neural circuitry.

THERAPIST: (*surprised*) You mean that you don't want the medical withdrawal, after all?

MARY: (*thoughtful*) Maybe, maybe not. Those classes aren't that hard . . .

THERAPIST: (*thoughtful*) Why don't you let me talk to my supervisor; maybe the agency could write a note to your faculty so that all the absences won't be unexcused? After all, your psychiatrist is here, maybe we could work something out. I cannot promise, but let me call you tomorrow after I get some advice about all this. It's new to me, OK?

MARY: (*tentatively*) Might work, might not. But OK, if you want to go to all that trouble.

THERAPIST: (*carefully*) OK, if you promise to remember that I am just trying and not sure about all these policies.

MARY: (*still a little tentative, cooperative*) OK.

> Being able to put emotions into words while still experiencing them, at least somewhat, can lead to the client's internalization of the therapist's regulatory functions, especially reflective self-awareness. Cortical and sensory–limbic connections are reworked in long-term dynamic psychotherapy (McKenna, 1994; PET imaging study by Schwartz et al., 1996).

Parallel Process in Supervision

After the supervisor and the intern reviewed the session notes to illustrate the projective identification process, their own interactions were seen to be similar, revealing a parallel process: As the session is examined, a parallel process between supervisor and supervisee emerges and mirrors some of the dynamics between Graciella and Mary.

Graciella took the process recording session notes (this is a transcript of the recorded session with commentary from Gabriella about tone of voice, posture, some of her internal thoughts and emotions, etc.) to her supervisor, noting to herself that she was reluctant to do so. Graciella and the supervisor then listen to the recording, turn it off and discuss it, and then listen some more. Later, the parenthetical comments were added for the transcript.

SUPERVISOR: What questions do you have about the session?

GRACIELLA: (*quiet*) I am questioning my suitability for the counseling profession, after this session with Mary.

SUPERVISOR: What is worrying you?

GRACIELLA: A lot (*looking down and worrying whether she can be genuine with this supervisor, whom she hardly knows*).

> The lack of safety due to the newness of the professional relationship mirrors what Graciella and Mary also were experiencing; each dyad had only met three times.

GRACIELLA: (*after completing the exercise on the therapy session with Mary by tracking the moment-to-moment projective identification process*) You know, I did not know how forthcoming I could be with you, since we've only met a few times. I now see how you are about Mary and me in the session and I realized that I did the same as Mary. I brought up a "safe" topic in the beginning, too?

SUPERVISOR: Explain what you are thinking.

GRACIELLA: Well, I brought up Mary storming out of the office, which was not the most shameful thing on my mind. And Mary brought up the medical withdrawal, but from going over the session, being rejected was the shameful thing that she did not want to talk about.

SUPERVISOR: So what was harder than Mary storming out of your office?

GRACIELLA: Looking back on it, it was my crying that I did not want to bring up. And because the crying was not recorded, I would have never had to tell you about it, really. (*Graciella and the supervisor now replay a portion of their last session to consider their interaction from this more authentic, but vulnerable, perspective. This portion of their session was also noted earlier in this chapter.*)

SUPERVISOR: (*finding herself careful*) Are the worries vague or do you have some specific concerns?

GRACIELLA: (*grasping for something to say*) You probably heard that Mary stormed out of my office in the middle of our session.

SUPERVISOR: Yes, the office staff said something about it.

GRACIELLA: (*looking up for the first time*) Yes, I heard them say, "Oh, poor Gabriella, she got stuck with Mary."

SUPERVISOR: Where were they when they said that?

GRACIELLA: In the coffee room.

SUPERVISOR: That is completely unacceptable, we cannot have that kind of talk where clients can hear, at least. (*Musing to herself, "we should not have that kind of talk, period, but people are people."*)

GRACIELLA: (*Now worrying that she will have contributed to shaming other staff, and being the new staff member, that's no way to get along with new coworkers— and she tried so hard to get this internship, everyone wants to work here, and other self-critical and obsessive thoughts.*) Will they know I told on them? (*Regrets her choice of words immediately, as she knows she sounds like a second-grader.*)

GRACIELLA: (*stopping the recording*) Now I remember being grateful that I could worry about upsetting staff members for telling on them, rather than talk about crying in front of Mary.

SUPERVISOR: I missed that entirely; I got caught up in being disturbed about staff behavior and confidentiality, especially for Mary with her family's infamous behavior in town. I started worrying about my professional responsibility and liability and lost focus on you and Mary.

GRACIELLA: I think that's where I got sidetracked, feeling like a tattletale, like when I was a kid; I was the Goody Two-Shoes in the family.

SUPERVISOR: This is a good segue into discussing the difference between supervision and therapy. Though supervision is not for your own therapy, there are times when your personal reactions are important to understand a therapeutic moment. We have to work together to not cross boundaries, yet appreciate that none of us is unaffected, sometimes deeply, by what happens to our brains. If I think that something is too personal for the supervision, I would recommend that you take the matter to your own therapy. On the other hand, if you feel pressured by me, I hope you will let me know.

GRACIELLA: OK, I hope I can. Being the Goody Two-Shoes makes it hard for me to be direct. But here goes: When we were talking about the model scene leading to the dreaded state of mind and triggering splitting negative and positive states, or whatever that is on the list, that happened when you ignored my question.

SUPERVISOR: What question?

GRACIELLA: I think it is coming up soon on the tape. (*Presses the tape:*)

SUPERVISOR (*on tape*): (*ignores her question*) What happened in the session? Give me a synopsis before we go over the transcript you have. (*Now turns off the tape:*) Oh, that question. Yes, and (*looking at the list of steps for projective identification*) that can lead to a malignant transference, either hyperaroused or hypoaroused.

GRACIELLA: I felt a thump in my chest, which means hyperarousal—

SUPERVISOR: (*interrupting*) Yes, but then you went on to summarize the session in a "teacher voice"!

GRACIELLA: Yes, I remember being hurt and deciding to give a report, kind of like a medical report: no emotion.

SUPERVISOR: Sorry for interrupting you just then. I get excited about examining sessions in this way. You know, I was an English major, so I like following the story line, just like you did in teaching literature. But that has limitations, because the backdrop of the physiology can be missed.

GRACIELLA: Uhmmm. Looking at the steps, I can see that what happened next in giving my report: I was trying to not be so aroused, so I went "professional" [see Kottler, 1993, on pressure for therapists to "perform"].

SUPERVISOR: Let's listen to the tape some more. (*Turns on the tape:*)

GRACIELLA (*on tape*): (*Feeling like she has to be professional and give a report, but still wondering if the supervisor will answer the question about her "telling on" the staff*) Mary was upset that I had not read her file. She wants me to write her a letter or some documentation for a medical withdrawal from school. I tried to stay focused on the letter, but when I asked her for details about why she had missed so many classes, she got mad that I had not read the file and that I would have known the answer to the questions, even though at the beginning of the session, she was mad at me for seeming to assume that her word wasn't a good substitute for reading others' words about her, or something like that. When I tried to ask her, she was upset and attacked me for being a light-skinned Mexican.

SUPERVISOR: Wait a minute—that is confusing. Why don't we go over the transcript, line by line, and figure out what happened?

GRACIELLA: (*Now completely sure that she is making a fool of herself and feeling helpless to stop the process*) OK.
(*Turns off tape and resumes analysis with supervisor:*) I can see, or hear, in this case, that I was <u>dysregulated</u>. I never heard of that word before, but it works for me. I started babbling and wasn't able to track the sequence of the session. Also, I left out the crying, I can see that now. Like Mary, I was upset, then did something to get control of my upset—which, for me, has always been to do something academic or intellectual. Looking back, I feel set up by Mary's accusations, especially the racial comment about being light. That's a bomb where I come from.

SUPERVISOR: Since Mary brought this into the session, we should speculate on the meaning of the racial comment; but, to backtrack, let's not miss the way you counterregulated yourself, going from being upset about tattling and my not being responsive to your upset by ignoring your question, to your recital of the session. I thought that you were not in high arousal at that time, but going toward <u>hypoarousal</u>, by the "just the facts, ma'am" style of police reporting.

GRACIELLA: OK, that seems right. I was trying for composure and low emotionality. I was intimidated, so I tried to be like a news journalist, I guess.

SUPERVISOR: It is good to know how we might react to different emotions from others. Going back to the racial comment. What are your thoughts or reactions about that?

GRACIELLA: I know you said that this is not my therapy, but here is what I think right now. I hope it's OK to tell you a little about my past.

SUPERVISOR: It's fine, just so what we discuss is useful to your work and you do not feel that I have tried to become your therapist.

GRACIELLA: (*laughs*) Maybe I might want you to be my therapist. But seriously, Mary could not know what a hot button the light skin crack was.

SUPERVISOR: Maybe she made a good guess; you never know about how sensitive clients perceive things about us.

GRACIELLA: Yeah, well, anyway. Here is the thing. I am the youngest of 14 children and the lightest. I look like my aunt, who was a teacher. Some of us were born in Mexico and some here in the U.S. There are only four of us who finished high school, much less college, and now for me, grad school. So Mary's story is familiar; in fact, I am trying to help the "Marys" of the world who are like most of my brothers and sisters. We were not mistreated, though, just poor. But we all had experiences with the racists. Even me. But for me, it was my own people who were against me because I am so light.

SUPERVISOR: I appreciate your candor. We all identify with each other, including supervisors with supervisees. Keeping an "open brain" is the goal, but not so easy to do. We have been examining the *process* of interactions between the therapist–client dyad and the therapist–supervisor dyad; let's now turn to the examination of the *content* of the interactions between you and Mary. It is time for some preliminary speculations about the effects of Mary's childhood experiences on ways she learned to manage arousal, which may have become inflexible and maladaptive ways of dealing with stress in adulthood. Disordered personality functioning can be a consequence of such maladaptive strategies. Those maladaptive strategies may manifest in interactions between therapist and client, some of which we have just described. And, of course, sometimes the dynamic in the therapy may find expression within the supervisor–supervisee interactions, as we have just seen.

> *The supervisor and the intern use descriptions of the attachment categories of childhood and adulthood, comparing them to criteria of similar personality disorders. Illustrations in the clinical encounter as well as in the available*

history about Mary lead to a list similar to the one in Table 8.1, which details the similarity between the descriptions of the behaviors of the disorganized/ disoriented/Type "D" attachment strategy and the criteria for borderline personality disorder, as currently listed in the DSM-IV-TR (American Psychiatric Association, 2000, p. 710). From the first clinical encounter, examples of the arousal management strategies implicit in the attachment strategy as well as the diagnostic criteria are enacted between the client and the clinician.

TABLE 8.1.
Comparing Criteria Mary Meets of Disorganized/Disoriented Attachment and Borderline Personality Disorder

Disorganized/Disoriented Attachment Category[a]	Borderline Personality Disorder[b]
Behaves erratically and inconsistently, often sending opposing messages at the same time	Pattern of unstable or intense interpersonal behavior characterized by alternations between extremes of idealization and devaluation or impulsivity in at least two areas that are potentially self-damaging; inappropriate, intense anger or difficulty controlling anger, affective instability due to a marked reactivity of mood or unstable self-image or sense of self
Appears confused and engages in undirected movements or expression (Main & Solomon, 1990)	

[a]Note. Based on Crittendon, 1988; Main & Solomon, 1990.
[b]From *The Diagnostic and Statistical Manual of Mental Disorders, Fourth Edition, Text Revised.* See Appendix B for complete DSM diagnostic criteria for the disorder referenced above.

Concluding Comments

As can be seen in the description of Mary's behavior, she can be unpredictable, an indication of an unbalanced/uncoupled autonomic nervous system. However, it could be speculated that her arousal system may have been positively impacted by her last living situation with a stable family. She does seem to take on the role of a caretaker toward her brother and is attempting to manage college, albeit with difficulty being persistent. Defense mechanisms include highly aroused behaviors and symptoms such as acting out (angry accusation of racism; rescuing her brother in jail, leaving her classes), devaluation (critical of therapist), as well as forms of low affect (for which she was prescribed medication for depression).

As can be seen in the session, Mary became dysregulated easily, as the nonconscious templates of past self–other experiences were inadvertently (yet, inevitably) triggered by the intern (the dysregulated self in interaction with the misattuned other; Schore, 2003b, p. 27). This dysregulated experience is the therapeutic target (Knapp, 1992), regardless of the therapeutic modality. Whether or not a particular theory embraces the concepts of transference–countertransference, there are inevitable mutual influences within the therapeutic moment that can often reveal unconscious processes (Freud, 1959b; Schamess, 2006; Stolorow, Brandchaft, & Atwood, as cited in Schore, 2003b, p. 27). Again, these unconscious processes, containing past problematic transactions, are possible even if no deliberate attention is paid to them. These transactions may be able to decrease the negative effects of childhood abuse if positive attunement, bonding, and (perhaps) an eventual corrective attachment occur (Kaufman & Henrich, 2000; Kaufman, Plotsky, Nemeroff, & Charney, 2000).

The childhood attachment style of disorganization and disorientation might predict that Mary will experience symptoms of the borderline condition (Table 8.1) (van der Kolk, 1987). Though Mary's behavior as an adult is not as severely disturbed as suggested by some of the criteria, the connection between Mary's childhood neglect/abuse and adult problematic behaviors is not hard to see. For clinicians, this connection may yield valuable information, not only for making a good assessment and diagnosis, but also in planning for Mary's treatment and predicting how the therapeutic alliance may be affected—always with the caution that more information is necessary to make a diagnosis about Mary's behavior. Making a diagnosis is not, per se, important, except as an exercise through which to discern and understand the organization of the behaviors. Once the affect management strategies implicit in the attachment category (as well as in the diagnosis) and the defense mechanisms are identified, the corrective emotional experience needed within the therapeutic alliance is clarified. For example, as Mary does not have a predictable set of coping strategies for arousal management, the clinician must be prepared to overcorrect for either too high or too low arousal. If Mary becomes too excitable, the clinician will need to resonate with Mary's distress and then try to help her calm down, and vice versa, with painfully low affect.

Mary's depression is being addressed by the agency psychiatrist. Though there is no medication specifically identified for borderline personality disorder, there are many choices available for common symptoms of this condition: Problems with anxiety, depression, or sleep all respond to various medications. For any clinician, particularly one new to the work, the gathering of information, such as has been done for Mary, may also promote empathy for the client's issues: in Mary's case, apparently wild and erratic behaviors. Mary may eventually work with as many clinicians as she had foster homes, which may be an artifact of the agency policy (e.g., short-term work in a training agency where interns do not typically stay more than one or two semesters). However, it could be speculated that breaking and making new "attachments" over and again may be quite familiar to her. With the continuing possibility of treatment staff, it would be useful to rapidly put together information so as to have the best treatment alliance possible in the shortest amount of time.

The permeability of interpersonal emotional boundaries is illustrated both by the intern's taking on some of Mary's emotions and by the same process as it was mirrored between the intern supervisee and her supervisor. Experiencing and managing difficult affects and their intensity are inevitable requirements between any two people in any kind of relationship. Exploring with the trainee ways to address the ever-likely transfer of emotions was essential in the supervision process. As exemplified, certain subtle shifts occurred between the dyads that created emotional safety, which, when detected, made for a more relaxed and trusting interchange (Charnus & Livingston, as cited in Edward & Sanville, 1996, pp. 386–403). Enhancing the professional use of self will contribute utility to a treatment alliance, the goal of any therapeutic modality.

Epilogue

Of interest to clinicians are those neurobiological phenomena that may have a profound effect upon the ongoing development of the professional use of self, with the goal ever in mind of helping our clients. A common and most difficult clinical experience is the rupture of the alliance with our clients, which may invite a host of negative self-attributions on the part of the clinician about his or her "professional" self. The therapeutic connection is known to be one of the most important factors in treatment, a fact supported not only by common sense and practice wisdom, but also borne out by "two well-cited meta-analyses demonstrating that the therapeutic alliance is the most consistent and strongest predictor of treatment success within the clinician-client experience" (Horvath & Symonds; Martin, Garske, & Davis as cited in Muran & Barber, 2010). That being the case, mental professionals devote effort via consultation and continuing education to honing our skills in order to promote a therapeutic alliance, and are often distressed over a rupture to that alliance. The rupture is the only way that unresolved trauma can be addressed, however, as verbal techniques will not be enough for healing (Schore, 2003a; 2003b).

The neurobiological perspective on the therapeutic alliance is that a positive alliance will either be stored in the hippocampus (memories of emotions) or in the amygdala as implicit procedural memories that are "the way things were," in a neutral or positive sense. However, it is the negative treatment alliance that may be enacted within the clinical relationship. This difficult alliance embodies past traumatic memories which are not accessible via "talk therapy," though some talk may occur about the trauma. These emotional memories will be stored in the amygdalar memory system and may emerge as flashbacks or be relived in the present, or both. The past may merge with the present when a traumatic experience is evoked, inadvertently and almost inevitably, in the treatment relationship. It is somewhat of a paradox that the difficult and sometimes almost unbearable ruptures, impasses, or derailments actually hold out the possibility (at the level of neural circuitry) of repair and healing from the past insults to development.

This book has used clinical cases to focus on certain arousal management structures in the brain, with the main goal of tracking affect and intensity of affect between the client and clinician. The focus of *affect* (right hemisphere) is a departure from the more conventional focus on the *meaning* (left hemisphere) of the content of client–clinician interactions (Schore, 2012, pp. 222–252). For example, somewhat tediously deconstructing the parallel process between a supervisor and a supervisee as it mirrors the supervisee–client interactions illustrates the ubiquity of microregulation of affect between people. It certainly is an example, in the case of Graciella and her supervisor, of how the confidence of both clinicians (supervisor and supervisee) in their professional selves was derailed after several mini-ruptures occurred, with both questioning their own competence.

Each chapter of this book has explored the social synapse (Cozolino, 2006), that is, the interpersonal space between people in which "synaptic shadows" (Siegel, 2012) are created by previous experiences, as well as the way that the past shapes both current and future perceptions, emotions, thinking, anticipation, planning, and behaviors (Siegel, 2012), sometimes consciously but primarily unconsciously. Most important, without embracing any particular theory, this book has sought to emphasize the incredible neurobiological impact of the clinician on the client(s), and the client's own neurobiological effect on the clinician. When the neurobiological exchange in this dyad is fully understood, powerful change can be made in strengthening the therapeutic relationship and improving the lives of clients.

Identifying Defense Mechanisms

Worksheet 2.1.
Identifying Defense Mechanisms

Example of self-protective (defended) behavior that is focus of clinical attention.

Defense and definition of defense

Example of self-protective (defended) behavior which is focus of clinical attention.

Speculation about anxiety or experience which defense seeks to manage

Coping styles of defense (Conte & Plutchick, 1995)

  Avoid (withdraw from)

Minimize (reduce)

Substitute (doing unrelated pleasurable activities to solve a problem)

Help-seeking (by retreating to immature behaviors)

Replacement (improving weaknesses)

Mapping (getting information before acting)

Blaming (attributing cause to someone else)

Reversal (doing opposite of feeling state)

Is defense more active, high arousal or more passive, lower arousal?

Part of the autonomic nervous system which manages the level of stimulation which accounts for the level of arousal in the brain, sympathetic or parasympathetic?

Or is the defense homeostatically regulated with the SNS and PNS coupled together and functioning as a team?

Or are both the PNS and SNS active simultaneously?

Or is the PNS avoiding others and managing affect in a dissociative manner?

Or is PNS managing affect using another defense, though the affect is in low arousal range?

Is defense flexible or rigid? Support your answer.

Is defense problem-solving oriented or a form of self-deception? Support your answer.

Does defense intend to adapt person to environment or is it an attempt to change the external environment (Hartmann, 1958)? Explain.

Which part (SNS or PNS) of the autonomic nervous system is less sturdy and needs to be strengthened?

Which part of the brain of the clinician may help strengthen the above part of autonomic nervous system affect/emotion tolerance? Explain the dyadic experience between the client and clinician that has the potential of improving (stimulating) affective/emotional tolerance.

Is defense adaptive or maladaptive? Explain.

Diagnostic Criteria

Diagnostic criteria for 301.0 Paranoid Personality Disorder

A. A pervasive distrust and suspiciousness of others such that their motives are interpreted as malevolent, beginning by early adulthood and present in a variety of contexts, as indicated by four (or more) of the following:

1. suspects, without sufficient basis, that others are exploiting, harming, or deceiving him or her
2. is preoccupied with unjustified doubts about the loyalty or trustworthiness of friends or associates
3. is reluctant to confide in others because of unwarranted fear that the information will be used maliciously against him or her
4. reads hidden demeaning or threatening meanings into benign remarks or events
5. persistently bears grudges, i.e., is unforgiving of insults, injuries, or slights
6. perceives attacks on his or her character or reputation that are not apparent to others and is quick to react angrily or to counterattack
7. has recurrent suspicions, without justification, regarding fidelity of spouse or sexual partner

B. Does not occur exclusively during the course of Schizophrenia, a Mood Disorder With Psychotic Features, or another Psychotic Disorder and is not due to the direct physiological effects of a general medical condition.

Note: If criteria are met prior to the onset of Schizophrenia, add "Premorbid," e.g., "Paranoid Personality Disorder (Premorbid)."

Diagnostic criteria for 301.20 Schizoid Personality Disorder

A. A pervasive pattern of detachment from social relationships and a restricted range of expression of emotions in interpersonal settings, beginning by early adulthood and present in a variety of contexts, as indicated by four (or more) of the following:

1. neither desires nor enjoys close relationships, including being part of a family
2. almost always chooses solitary activities
3. has little, if any, interest in having sexual experiences with another person
4. takes pleasure in few, if any, activities
5. lacks close friends or confidants other than first-degree relatives
6. appears indifferent to the praise or criticism of others
7. shows emotional coldness, detachment, or flattened affectivity

B. Does not occur exclusively during the course of Schizophrenia, a Mood Disorder With Psychotic Features, another Psychotic Disorder, or a Pervasive Developmental Disorder and is not due to the direct physiological effects of a general medical condition.

Note: If criteria are met prior to the onset of Schizophrenia, add "Premorbid," e.g., "Schizoid Personality Disorder (Premorbid)."

Diagnostic criteria for 301.81 Narcissistic Personality Disorder

A. A pervasive pattern of grandiosity (in fantasy or behavior), need for admiration, and lack of empathy, beginning by early adulthood and present in a variety of contexts, as indicated by five (or more) of the following:

1. has a grandiose sense of self-importance (e.g., exaggerates achievements and talents, expects to be recognized as superior without commensurate achievements)
2. is preoccupied with fantasies of unlimited success, power, brilliance, beauty, or ideal love
3. believes that he or she is "special" and unique and can only be understood by, or should associate with, other special or high-status people (or institutions)
4. requires excessive admiration
5. has a sense of entitlement, i.e., unreasonable expectations of especially favorable treatment or automatic compliance with his or her expectations
6. is interpersonally exploitative, i.e., takes advantage of others to achieve his or her own ends
7. lacks empathy: is unwilling to recognize or identify with the feelings and needs of others
8. is often envious of others or believes that others are envious of him or her
9. shows arrogant, haughty behaviors or attitudes

Diagnostic criteria for 301.82 Avoidant Personality Disorder

A. A pervasive pattern of social inhibition, feelings of inadequacy, and hypersensitivity to negative evaluation, beginning by early adulthood and present in a variety of contexts, as indicated by four (or more) of the following:

1. avoids occupational activities that involve significant interpersonal contact, because of fears of criticism, disapproval, or rejection
2. is unwilling to get involved with people unless certain of being liked
3. shows restraint within intimate relationships because of fear of being shamed or ridiculed
4. is preoccupied with being criticized or rejected in social situations
5. is inhibited in new interpersonal situations because of feelings of inadequacy
6. views self as socially inept, personally unappealing, or inferior to others
7. is unusually reluctant to take personal risks or to engage in any new activities because they may prove embarrassing

Diagnostic criteria for 301.6 Dependent Personality Disorder

A. A pervasive and excessive need to be taken care of that leads to submissive and clinging behavior and fears of separation, beginning by early adulthood and present in a variety of contexts, as indicated by five (or more) of the following:

1. has difficulty making everyday decisions without excessive amount of advice and reassurance from others
2. needs others to assume responsibility for most major areas of his or her life
3. has difficulty expressing disagreement with others because of fear of loss of support or approval. **Note:** Do not include realistic fears of retribution
4. has difficulty initiating projects or doing things on his or her own (because of a lack of self-confidence in judgment or abilities rather than a lack of motivation or energy)
5. goes to excessive lengths to obtain nurturance and support from others, to the point of volunteering to do things that are unpleasant
6. feels uncomfortable or helpless when alone because of exaggerated fears of being unable to care for himself or herself
7. urgently seeks another relationship as a source of care and support when a close relationship ends
8. is unrealistically preoccupied with fears of being left to take care of himself or herself

Diagnostic criteria for 301.4
Obsessive-Compulsive Personality Disorder

A. A pervasive pattern of preoccupation with orderliness, perfectionism, and mental and interpersonal control, at the expense of flexibility, openness, and efficiency, beginning by early adulthood and present in a variety of contexts, as indicated by four (or more) of the following:

1. is preoccupied with details, rules, lists, order, organization, or schedules to the extent that the major point of the activity is lost
2. shows perfectionism that interferes with task completion (e.g., is unable to complete a project because his or her own overly strict standards are not met)
3. is excessively devoted to work and productivity to the exclusion of leisure activities and friendships (not accounted for by obvious economic necessity)
4. is overconscientious, scrupulous, and inflexible about matters of morality, ethics, or values (not accounted for by cultural or religious identification)
5. is unable to discard worn-out or worthless objects even when they have no sentimental value
6. is reluctant to delegate tasks or to work with others unless they submit to exactly his or her way of doing things
7. adopts a miserly spending style toward both self and others; money is viewed as something to be hoarded for future catastrophes
8. shows rigidity and stubbornness

Research criteria for depressive personality disorder

A. A pervasive pattern of depressive cognitions and behaviors beginning by early adulthood and present in a variety of contexts, as indicated by five (or more) of the following:

1. usual mode is dominated by dejection, gloominess, cheerlessness, joylessness, unhappiness
2. self-concept centers around beliefs of inadequacy, worthlessness, and low self-esteem
3. is critical, blaming, and derogatory towards self
4. is brooding and given to worry
5. is negativistic, critical, and judgmental towards others
6. is pessimistic
7. is prone to feeling guilty or remorseful

B. Does not occur exclusively during Major Depressive Episodes and is not better accounted for by Dysthymic Disorder.

References

Abelson, R. P. (1983). Computer simulation of "hot"cognition. In S.S. Tomkins & S. Messick, Eds.), *Computer simulation of personality* (pp. 277–308). New York, NY: Wiley.

Abelsohn, D. (1983). Dealing with the abdication dynamic in the post divorce family: A context for adolescent crisis. *Family Process, 22*, 359–383.

Adolphs, R. (2002). Recognizing emotion from facial expressions: Psychological and neurological mechanisms. *Behavioral and Cognitive Neuroscience, 1*, 21–61.

Adolphs, R., Damasio, H., Tranel, D., Cooper, G., & Damasio, A.R. (2000). A role for somatosensory cortices in the visual recognition of emotion as revealed by three-dimensional lesion mapping. *Journal of Neuroscience, 20*(7), 2683–2690.

Ainsworth, M. D. S., Blehar, N. C. Waters, E., & Wall, S. (1978). *Patterns of attachment: A psychological study of the strange situation.* Hillsdale, NJ: Erlbaum.

Allen, J. G., Fonagy, P., & Bateman, A.N. (2008). *Mentalizing in clinical practice.* Arlington, VA: American Psychiatric Association.

Amaral, D. G., Price, J. L., Pitkanen, A., & Carmichael, S. T. (1992). Anatomical organization of the primate amygdaloid complex. In J.P. Aggleton (Ed.). *The amygdala: Neurobiological aspects of emotion, memory, and mental dysfunction* (pp. 1–66). New York, NY: Wiley Liss.

American Psychiatric Association. (1994). *Diagnostic and statistical manual of mental disorders* (4th ed.). Washington, DC: Author.

American Psychiatric Association. (2000). *Diagnostic and statistical manual of mental disorders* (4th ed., text rev.). Washington, DC: Author.

American Psychiatric Association. (2010). DSM-5 *development*. Retrieved May 29, 2010, from http://www.dsm5.org/Proposed/Revisions/Pages/ Personality and PersonalityDisorders.

Anderson, A. K., & Phelps, E. A. (2001). Lesions of the human amygdala impair enhanced perception of emotionally salient events. *Nature, 411*, 305–309.

Aoki, C., & Stekevitz, P. (1988). Plasticity and brain development. *Scientific American, 259*, 56–68.

Applegate, J. S., & Shapiro, J. R. (2005). *Neurobiology for clinical social work: Theory and practice*. New York, NY: Norton.

Arlow, J. (1977). Affects and the psychoanalytic situation. *International Journal of Psychoanalysis, 58*, 157–170.

Aron, L. (1991). The patient's experience of the analyst's subjectivity. *Psychoanalytic Dialogues, 1*, 29–51.

Aron, L. (1992). Interpretation as expression of the analyst's subjectivity. *Psychoanalytic Dialogues, 2*(4), 475–507.

Bach, S. (1998). On treating the difficult patient. In C.S. Ellman, S. Grand, M. Silvan, & S.J. Ellmans (Eds.), *The modern Freudians: Contemporary psychoanalytic technique* (pp. 185–195). Northvale, NJ: Aronson.

Badenoch, B. (2008). *Being a brain-wise therapist: A practical guide to interpersonal neurobiology*. New York, NY: Norton.

Baird, A. A., Gruber, S. A., Fein, D. A., Maas, L. C., Steingard, R. J., Renshaw, P. F., et al. (1999). Functional magnetic resonance imaging of facial affect recognition in children and adolescents. *Journal of the American Academy of Child and Adolescent Psychiatry, 38*, 195–199.

Baird, A. A., Gruber, S. A., & Yurgelun-Todd, D. A. (1999, November). *Development of frontotemporal networks: Implications for psychopathology*. Poster session presented at Society for Research on Psychopathology, Montreal, Canada.

Barbanell, L. (2006). *Removing the mask of kindness: Diagnosis and treatment of the caretaker personality disorder*. Northvale, NJ: Aronson.

Barbas, H. (1995). Autonomic basis of cognitive–emotional interactions in the primate prefrontal cortex. *Neuroscience and Biobehavioral Reviews, 19*, 499–510.

Baron-Cohen, S., Ring, H. A., Bullmore, E. T., Wheelwright, S., Ashwin, C., & Williams, S.C. (2000). The amygdala theory of autism. *Neuroscience and Biobehavioral Review, 24*(3), 355–364.

Bartholomew, K., & Horowitz, L. M. (1991). Attachment styles among young adults: A test of a four category model. *Journal of Personality and Social Psychology, 61*, 226–244.

Basch, M. (1975). Toward a theory that encompasses depression: A revision of existing causal hypotheses in psychoanalysis. In E. J. Anthony & T. Benedek (Eds.), *Depression and human existence* (pp. 485–534). Boston: Little, Brown.

Beebe, B. (2005). Mother–infant research informs mother–infant treatment. *Psychoanalytic Study of the Child, 60,* 6–46.

Beebe, B., & Lachmann, F. M. (1988). Mother–infant mutual influence and precursors of psychic structure. In A. Goldberg (Ed.), *Progress in self psychology* (Vol. 3, pp. 3–25). Hillsdale, NJ: Analytic Press.

Beebe, B., & Lachmann, F. M. (1994). Representation and internalization in infancy: Three principles of salience. *Psychoanalytic Psychology, 11*(2), 127–164.

Beebe, B., & Lachmann, F. M. (2002). *Infant research and adult treatment.* Hillsdale, NJ: Analytic Press.

Bechara, A., Dolan, S., Denburg, N., Hindes, A., Anderson, S. W., & Nathan, P. E. (2001). Decision-making deficits, linked to a dysfunctional ventromedial prefrontal cortex, revealed in alcohol and stimulant abusers. *Neuropsychologia, 39,* 376–389.

Bellah, R. N., Madsen, R., Sullivan, W. M., Swidler, A., & Tipton, S. M. (1985). *Habits of the heart.* New York, NY: Harper & Row.

Benes, F. M. (1989). Myelination of cortical–hippocampal relays during late adolescence. *Schizophrenia Bulletin, 15*(4), 585–593.

Benjamin, J. 1988. *The bonds of love: Psychoanalysis, feminism, and the problem of domination.* New York, NY: Pantheon Books.

Berntson, G. C., Cacioppo, J., & Quigley, K. S. (1991). Autonomic determinism: The modes of autonomic control, the doctrine of autonomic space, and the laws of autonomic constraint. *Psychological Review, 98,* 459–487.

Berzoff, J., Flanagan, L. M., & Hertz, P. (1996). Inside out and outside in: *Psychodynamic clinical theory and practice in contemporary multicultural contexts.* Northvale, NJ: Aronson.

Bion, W. R. (1962). *Learning from experience.* London: Heinemann.

Bjork, J. (2004). Incentive-elicited brain activation in adolescents: Similarities and differences from young adults. *Journal of Neuroscience, 24*(7), 1793–1802.

Blair, R. J. R. (2004). The roles of orbital frontal cortex in the modulation of antisocial behavior. *Brain Cognition, 55,* 198–208.

Blakeslee, S. (2007, February 6). A small part of the brain, its profound effects. *New York Times.* Available at http://www.sandrablakeslee.com/articles/insula_feb07,php.

Blanck, G., & Blanck, R. (1979). *Ego psychology II: Psychoanalytic psychology*. New York, NY: Columbia University Press.

Blanck, R., & Blanck, G. (1986). *Beyond ego psychology: Developmental object relations theory*. NY: Columbia University Press.

Bleiberg, E. (2001). *Treating personality disorders in children and adolescents: A relational approach*. New York, NY: Guilford Press.

Bliss, S. (2010). The "internal saboteur": Contributions of W. R. D. Fairbairn on understanding and treating self-harming adolescents. *Journal of Social Work Practice, 24*, 227–237.

Bourne, L. E., & Russo, N. F. (1998). *Psychology: Behavior in context*. New York, NY: Norton.

Bowlby, J. (1977). The making and breaking of affectional bonds: I. Aetiology and psychopathology in light of attachment theory. *British Journal of Psychiatry, 130*, 201–210.

Bowlby, J. (1988). *A secure base* (2nd ed.). New York: Basic Books.

Brenner, C. (1974). On the nature and development of affects: A unified theory. *Psychoanalytic Quarterly, 43*, 532–556.

Brody, P. (1992). *The central nervous system: Structure and function*. New York, NY: Oxford University Press.

Brown, L. M., & Gilligan, C. (1992). *Meeting at the crossroads: Women's psychology and girls' development*. Cambridge, MA: Harvard University Press.

Buchanan, T. W., Tranel, D., & Adolphs, R. (2009). The human amygdala in social function. In P.L. Whalen & E. A. Phelps (Eds.), *The human amygdala* (pp. 289–318). New York, NY: Guilford Press.

Buck, R. (1994). The neuropsychology of communication: Spontaneous and symbolic aspects. *Journal of Pragmatics, 22*, 265–278.

Buelow, G., Hebert, S., & Buelow, S. (2000). *Psychotherapist's resource on psychiatric medications: Issues of treatment and referral*. Canada: Brooks/Cole Thomson Learning.

Carter, R. (2009). *The human brain*. New York, NY: DK Publishing.

Cassidy, J. (1994). Emotion regulation: Influences of attachment relationships. *Monographs of the Society for Research in Child Development, 59*, 228–249.

Charmandari, E., Kino, T., Souvatzoglou, E., & Chrousos, G. P. (2003). Pediatric stress: Hormonal mediators and human development. *Hormone research, 59*(4), 161–179.

Charnus, L. A., & Livingston, P. G. (1996). Clinical supervision: Its role in "containing" counter-transference responses to a filicidal patient. In J. Edward & J. Sanville (Eds.), *Fostering healing and growth: A psychoanalytic social work approach* (pp. 386–403). Northvale, NJ: Aronson.

Cicchetti, D. (2004). An odyssey of discovery: Lessons learned through three decades of research on child maltreatment. *American Psychologist, 59*(8), 731–741.

Cicchetti, D., & Toth, S. L. (1991). A developmental perspective on internalizing and externalizing disorders. In D. Cicchetti & S.L. Toth (Eds.), *Internalizing and externalizing expressions of dysfunction: Rocheste r symposium on developmental psychopathology* (Vol. 2, pp. 1–19), Hillsdale, NJ: Erlbaum.

Clark, A. J. (1991). The identification and modification of defense mechanisms in counseling. *Journal of Counseling & Development, 69,* 223.

Cole, J. (1987). *About face.* Cambridge, MA: MIT Press.

Cole, P. M., Michael, M. K., & O'Donnell Teti, L. (1994). The development of emotion regulation and dysregulation: A clinical perspective. *Monographs of the Society for Research in Child Development, 59,* 73–100.

Conte, H. R., & Plutchik, R. (Eds.). (1995). *Ego defenses: Theory and measurement.* New York, NY: Wiley.

Cozolino, L. (2002). *The neuroscience of psychotherapy: Building and rebuilding the human brain.* New York, NY: Norton.

Cozolino, L. (2006). *The neuroscience of human relationships: Attachment and the developing brain.* New York, NY: Norton.

Craig, A. D. (2002). How do you feel?: Interoception—the sense of the physiological condition of the body. *Nature Reviews Neuroscience, 3,* 655–666.

Critchley, H. D., Weins, S., Rotstein, P., Ohman, A., & Dolan, R. J. (2004). Neural systems supporting interoceptive awareness. *Nature Neuroscience, 7,* 189–195.

Crittendon, P. M. (1988). Relationships at risk. In J. Belsky & T. Nezworski (Eds.), *Clinical implications of attachment theory* (pp. 136–174) Hillsdale, NJ: Erlbaum.

Dahl, R. E., & Spear, L. P. (2004). Adolescent brain development: A period of vulnerabilities and opportunities. *Annals of the New York Academy of Sciences, 1021,* 1–22.

Damasio, A. R. (1994). *Descartes' error: Emotion, reason, and the human brain.* New York, NY: Putnam.

Damasio, A. R. (1999). *The feeling of what happens: Body and emotion in the making of consciousness.* New York, NY: Harcourt, Brace.

Damasio, A. R., Tranel, D., & Damasio, H. (1990). Individuals with sociopathic behavior caused by frontal damage fail to respond autonomically to social stimuli. *Behavioural Brain Research, 41,* 81–94.

Darwin, C. (1872). *The expressions of emotions in man and animals.* London: John Murray.

Dawson, G. (1994). Development of emotional expression and emotion regulation in infancy. In G. Dawson & K.W. Fischer (Eds.), *Human behavior and the developing brain* (pp. 346–379). New York, NY: Guilford Press.

Demos, V. (1991). Resiliency in infancy. In T.F. Dugan & R. Coles (Eds.), *The child in our times: Studies in the development of resiliency* (pp. 3–22). New York, NY: Brunner/ Mazel.

Diamond, M. C., Krech, D., & Rosenzweig, M. R. (1963). The effects of an enriched environmenton the histology of the rat cerebral cortex. *Journal of Comparative Neurology, 1223,* 111–120.

Dias, R., Robbins, T.W., & Roberts, A.C. (1996). Dissociation in prefrontal cortex of affective and attentional shifts. *Nature, 380,* 69–72.

Dicks, H. V. (1993). *Marital tensions: Clinical studies towards a psychological theory of interaction.* London: Karnac.

Dimberg, U., & Ohman, A. (1996). Behold the wrath: Psychophysiological responses to facial stimuli. *Motivation and Emotion, 20,* 149–182.

Dince, P. R. (1977). Partial dissociation as encountered in the borderline patient. *Journal of the American Academy of Psychoanalysis, 5,* 327–345

do Amaral, J. R., & de Oliveira, J. M. (2009). *The limbic system, the neocortex, the primitive brain.* Retrieved June 2, 2009, from http://www.healing-arts.org/n-r-limbic.htm.

Dougherty, D. M., Bjork, J. M., Harper, R. A., Marsh, D. M., Moeller, F. G., & Mathias, C. W. (2003). Behavioral impulsivity paradigms: A comparison in hospitalized adolescents with disruptive behavior disorders. *Journal of Child Psychology and Psychiatry and Allied Disciplines, 44,* 1145–1157.

Edelman, G. M. (1989). *The remembered present: A biological theory of consciousness.* New York, NY: Basic Books.

Edward, J., & Sanville, J. (Eds.). (1996). *Fostering healing and growth: A psychoanalytic social work approach.* Northvale, NJ: Aronson.

Eichenbaum, H. (1992). The hippocampal system and declarative memory in animals. *Journal of Cognitive Neuroscience, 4*(3), 217–231.

Epstein, R. (2007). The myth of the teen brain. *Scientific American Mind, 18*(2), 56–63.

Ericyas, A. H., Topalkara, K., Topaktas, S., Akyuz, A., & Dener, S. (1999). Suppression of cardiac parasympathetic functions in patients with right hemispheric stroke. *European Journal of Neurology, 6,* 685–690.

Farmer, R. C. (2009). *Neuroscience and social work practice: The missing link.* Thousand Oaks, CA: SAGE.

Feldman, Y. (1963). Understanding ego involvement in casework training. In H. J. Parad & R. R. Miller (Eds.), *Ego-oriented casework: Problems and perspectives* (pp. 292–306). New York, NY: Family Service Association of America.

Field, T. (1985). Attachment as psychobiological attunement: Being on the same wavelength. In M. Reite & T. Field (Eds.), *The psychobiology of attachment and separation* (pp. 415–454). Orlando, FL: Academic Press.

Fine, C., Lumsden, J., & Blair, R. J. R. (2001) Dissociation between "theory of mind" and executive functions in a patient with early left amygdala damage. *Brain, 124*, 287–298.

Florsheim, P., Henry, W. P., & Benjamin, L. S. (1996). Integrating individual and interpersonal approachs to diagnosis: The structural analysis of social behavior and attachment theory. In F. W. Kaslow (Ed.), *Handbook of relational diagnosis and dysfunctional family patterns* (pp. 81–101). New York: Wiley.

Fonagy, P. (1998). Attachment and borderline personality disorder. *Journal of American Psychoanalytic Association, 48*(4), 1129–1146.

Fonagy, P., Gergely, G., Jurist, E., & Target, M. (2004). *Affect regulation, mentalization, and development of the self*. New York, NY: Other Press.

Fosha, D. (2000). *The transforming power of affect: A model for accelerated change*. New York, NY: Basic Books.

Fosha, D. (2010, March). *Energy, vitality, pleasure, truth, desire, and the emergent phenomenology of transformation: Transformational theory and the healing-based practice of AEDP*. Paper presented at the conference of the UCLA–Lifespan Learning Institute, Los Angeles, CA.

Fosha, D., Siegel, D .J., & Solomon, M. (Eds.). (2009). *The healing power of emotion: Affective neuroscience, development, and clinical practice*. New York, NY: Norton.

Foster, R. P., Moskowitz, M., & Javier, R. A. (1996). (Eds.). *Reaching across boundaries of culture and class: Widening the scope of psychotherapy*. Northvale, NJ: Jason Aronson.

Freed, A. O. (1980). The borderline personality. *Social Casework: Journal of Contemporary Social Work, 61*, 548–558.

Freud, A. (1966). *The ego and the mechanisms of defense. The writings of Anna Freud*. New York, NY: International Universities Press. (Original work published 1936.)

Freud, S. (1957). On the history of the psychoanalytic movement. In J. Strachey (Ed. & Trans.), *The standard edition of the complete psychological works of Sigmund Freud* (Vol. 14, pp. 2–26). London: Hogarth Press. (Original work published 1914.)

Freud, S. (1958a). The dynamics of transference. In J. Strachey (Ed. & Trans.), *The standard edition of the complete psychological works of Sigmund Freud* (Vol. 12, pp. 99–108. London: Hogarth Press. (Original work published 1912.)

Freud, S. (1958b). Recommendations to physicians practicing psycho-analysis. In J. Strachey (Ed. & Trans.), *The standard edition of the complete psychological works of Sigmund Freud* (Vol. 12, pp. 111–120). London: Hogarth Press. (Original work published 1912.)

Freud, S. (1959a). Further Recommendations in the technique of psycho-analysis: Observations on transference-love. In E. Jones (Ed.), *Collected papers* (Vol. II, pp. 312-322). London: Hogarth Press. (Original work published 1915.)

Freud, S. (1959b). Repression. In E. Jones (Ed.), *Collected papers* (Vol. 4, pp. 84–97). London: Hogarth Press. (Original work published 1915.)

Frijda, N. H. (1988). The laws of emotion. *American Psychologist, 43,* 349–358.

Fuchs, T., Sattel, H., & Henningsen, P. (Eds.). (2010). *The embodied self: Dimensions, coherence and disorders.* Stuttgart: Schattauer.

Furness, J. B. (2006). The organization of the autonomic nervous system: Peripheral connection. *Autonomic Neuroscience: Basic & Clinical, 130*(1-2), 1–5. Available at www.elservier.com/locate/autneu.

Fuster, J. M. (1999). *Memory in the cerebral cortex: An empirical approach to neural networks in the human and nonhuman primate.* Cambridge, MA: MIT Press.

Gacano, C. B. (Ed.). (2000). *The forensic assessment of psychopathy: A prac-titioner's guide.* Mahwah, NJ: Erlbaum.

Gainotti, G. (2012). Unconscious processing of emotions and the right hemisphere. *Neuropsychologia.* Retrieved January 11, 2012, from http://jour-nals1.scholarsportal.infol.ezproxy.library. yorku.ca/sh.

Gallese, V. (2009). The two sides of mimesis: Girard's mimetic theory, embodied simulation and social identification. *Journal of Consciousness Studies, 16*(4), 21–44.

Gallese, V. (2010). Embodied simulation and its role in intersubjectivity. In T. Fuchs, H. Sattel, & P. Henningsen (Eds.), *The embodied self: Dimensions, coherence and disorders* (pp. 77–92). Stuttgart, Germany: Schattauer.

Gardner, M., & Steinberg, L. (2005). Peer influence on risk taking, risk preference, and risky decision making in adolescence and adulthood: An experimental study. *Developmental Psychology, 41*(4), 625–635.

Gazaniga, M. S., Ivy, R. B., & Mangum, G. R. (2000). *The new cognitive neurosciences* (2nd ed.). Cambridge, MA: MIT Press.

Gellhorn, E. (1964). Motion and emotion: The role of proprioception in the physiology and pathology the emotions. *Psychological Review, 71,* 457–472.

George, N., Dolan, R. J., Fink, G., Baylis, G. C., Russell, C., & Driver, J. (1999). Human fusiform gyrus extracts shape-from-shading to recognize familiar faces. *Nature Neuroscience, 2,* 574–580.

Giedd, J. N. (2005). Structural magnetic resonance imaging of the adolescent brain. *Annals of the New York Academy of Sciences. 1021*, 77–85.

Giedd, J. N., Blumenthal, J., Jeffries, N. O., Castellanos, F. X., Liu, H., Zijdenbos, A., et al. (1999). Brain development during childhood and adolescence: A longitudinal MRI study. *Nature Neuroscience, 2*(10), 861–863.

Gilligan, C. (1987). Adolescent development reconsidered. In C.E. Irwin (Ed.), *Adolescent social behavior and health* (pp. 63–92). San Francisco: Jossey-Bass.

Giovacchini, P. L. (1982). *A clinician's guide to reading Freud*. Northvale, NJ: Aronson.

Goldberg, A. (Ed.). (1996). *Basic ideas reconsidered. Progress in Self Psychology, 12*, 169–190.

Goldberg, J. R. (1993). What is normal adolescence? *Family Therapy News, 24*(2), 18–20.

Greatrex, T. (2002). Projective identification: How does it work? *Neuropsychoanalysis, 4*(2), 187–197.

Green, A. (1977). Conceptions of affect. *International Journal Psychoanalysis, 58*, 129–156.

Green, R. L., & Ostrander, R. L. (2009). *Neuroanatomy for students of behavioral disorders*. New York, NY: Norton.

Greenberg, J. (1991). Countertransference and reality. *Psychoanalytic Dialogues 1*, 52–73.

Greenberg, L. S., & Saffran, J. D. (1984). Hot cognition: Emotion coming in from the cold. A reply to Rachman and Mahooney. *American Psychologist, 44*, 19.

Greenough, W. T. (1986). What's special about development? Thoughts on the bases of experience-sensitive synaptic plasticity. In W. T. Greenough & J. M. Juraska (Eds.), *Developmental neuropsychology* (pp. 387–407). Orlando, FL: Academic Press.

Greenough, W. T. (2011). *Beckman Inst Greenough*. Retrieved April 24, 2011, from http://s/psych.uiuc.edu/people/showprofile.php?id=61.

Greenspan, S.I. (1981). *Psychopathology and adaptation in infancy and early childhood*. New York, NY: International Universities Press.

Grings, W. W., & Dawson, M. E. (1978). *Emotions and bodily responses*. New York, NY: Academic Press.

Gunnar, M., & Quevedo, K. (2007). The neurobiology of stress and development. *Annual Review of Psychology, 58*, 145–173.

Gur, R. C. (2005). Brain maturation and its relevance to understanding criminal culpability of juveniles. *Current Psychiatry Reports, 7*, 292–296.

Hallowell, E. M. (2006). *CrazyBusy*. New York: Random House.

Hamilton, G. (1958). A theory of personality: Freud's contribution to social work. In H. Parad (Ed.), *Ego psychology and dynamic casework* (pp. 11–37). New York, NY: Family Service Association of America.

Hariri, A. R., Bookheimer, S.Y., & Mazziotta, J.C. (2000). Modulating emotional responses: Effects of neocortical network on the limbic system. *NeuroReport, 11*, 43–48.

Hartmann, H. (1958). *Ego psychology and the problem of adaptation.* New York, NY: International Universities Press. (Original work published 1939.)

Harvard Mental Health Letter. (2005a). The adolescent brain: Beyond raging hormones. *Harvard Medical School, 22*(1), 1–3.

Harvard Mental Health Letter. (2005b). The biology of child maltreatment: How abuse and neglect of children leave their mark on the brain. *Harvard Medical School, 21*(2), 1–3.

Hebb, D. O. (1949). *The organization of behavior: A neuropsychological theory.* New York, NY: Wiley.

Heiman, P. (1950). On countertransference. *International Journal of Psycho-Analysis, 31*, 81–84.

Hellige, J. B. (1993). *Hemispheric asymmetry: What's right and what's left.* Cambridge, MA: Harvard University Press.

Hickok, G. (2008). Eight problems for the mirror neuron theory of action understanding in monkeys and humans. *Journal of Cognitive Neuroscience, 21*(7), 1129–1243.

Hofer, M. A. (1994). Hidden regulators in attachment, separation and loss. *Monographs of the Society for Research in Child Development, 59*, 192–207.

Hoffman, I. (1983). The patient as the interpreter of the analyst's experience. *Contemporary Psychoanalysis, 19*(3), 389–422.

Horowitz, L. (1983). Projective identification in dyads and groups. *International Journal of Group Psychotherapy, 33*(3), 259–279.

Horowitz, M. J. (1983). *Image formation and psychotherapy.* New York, NY: Aronson.

Horowitz, M. J. (1987). *States of mind: Configural analysis of individual psychology.* New York, NY: Plenum Medical.

Horvath, A. O., & Symonds, B. D. (1991). Relation between working alliance and outcome in psychotherapy: A meta-analysis. *Journal of Counseling Psychology, 38*, 139–149.

Howes, C. (1999). Attachment relationships in the context of multiple caregivers. In J. Cassidy & P.R. Shaver (Eds.), *Handbook of attachment: Theory, research, and clinical applications* (pp. 671–687). New York, NY: Guilford Press.

Izard, C. E., Porges, S. W., Simons, R. F., Haynes, O. M., Hyde, C., Parisi, M., et al. (1991). Infant cardiac activity: Developmental changes and relations with attachment. *Developmental Psychology, 27,* 432–439.

Jackson, J. H. (1931). *Selected writings of J. H. Jackson: Vol. 1.* London: Hodder and Stoughton.

Jacobs, W., & Nadal, L. (1985). Stress-induced recovery of fears and phobias. *Psychological Review, 92*(4), 512–531.

Jacobs, B. L., van Praag, H., & Gage, F. H. (2000). Depression and the birth and death of brain cells. *American Scientist, 88,* 340–345.

Johnsen, B. H., & Hugdahl, K. (1991). Hemispheric asymmetry in conditioning to facial emotional expressions. *Psychophysiology, 28,* 154–162.

Johnson, M. D. (2003). *Human biology: Concepts and current issues* (2nd ed.). San Francisco, CA: Benjamin Cummings.

Johnson, M. H. (2005). Subcortical face processing. *Nature Reviews Neuroscience, 6,* 766–774.

Jordan, J. V. (2000). *Toward connection and competence* (Work in progress, No. 83). Wellesley, MA: Stone Center Working Paper Series.

Jordan, J. V. (2004). Personality disorder or relational disconnection? In J.J. Magnavita (Ed.), *Handbook of personality disorders: Theory and practice* (pp. 120–147). New York, NY: Wiley.

Kandel, E. R. (2005). *Psychiatry, psychoanalysis, and the new biology of the mind.* Arlington, VA: American Psychiatric Publishing.

Karen, R. (1990, February). Becoming attached. *The Atlantic Monthly,* 35–70.

Kaslow, F. W. (Ed.). (1996). *Handbook of relational diagnoses and dysfunctional family patterns.* New York, NY: Wiley.

Kaufman, I. (1963). Psychodynamics of protective casework. In H. J. Parad & R.R. Miller (Eds.), *In ego-oriented casework: Problems and perspectives* (pp. 191–205). New York, NY: Family Service Association of America.

Kaufman, J., & Henrich, C. (2000). Exposure to violence and early childhood trauma. In C.H. Zeanah, Jr. (Ed.), *Handbook of infant mental health* (2nd ed., pp. 195–207). New York, NY: Guilford Press.

Kaufman, J., Plotsky, P. M., Nemeroff, C. B., & Charney, D. S. (2000). Effect of early adverse experiences on brain structure and function: Clinical implications. *Biological Psychiatry, 48,* 778–790.

Kawasaki, H., Adolphs, R., Kaufman, O., Damasio, H., Damasio, A. R., Granner, M., et al. (2001). Single-neuron responses to emotional visual stimuli recorded in human ventral prefrontal cortex. *Nature Neuroscience, 4,* 15–16.

Kernberg, O. F. (1975). *Borderline conditions and pathological narcissism.* Northvale, NJ: Aronson.

Kernberg, O. F. (1976). *Object relations and clinical psychoanalysis.* Northvale, NJ: Aronson.

Kernberg, O. F. (1979). Regression in organizational leadership. *Psychiatry, 42,* 24–39.

Kernberg, O. F. (1980). *Internal world and external reality: Object relations theory applied.* Northvale, NJ: Aronson.

Kernberg, O.F. (1984). *Severe personality disorders: Psychotherapeutic strategies.* New Haven, CT: Yale University Press.

Keysers, C., Xiao, D.K., Földiák, P., & Perret, D.I. (2001). The speed of sight. *Journal of Cognitive Neuroscience, 13,* 90–101.

King, R. (1985). Motivational diversity and mesolimbic dopamine: An hypothesis concerning temperament. In R. Plutchik & H. Kellerman (Eds.), Emotion (Vol. 3). *Theory, research, and experience* (pp. 363–380). New York, NY: Academic Press.

Kinney, D. K., Stengard, R. J., Renshaw, P. F., & Yurgelun-Todd, D. A. (2000). Perinatal complications and abnormal proton metabolite concentration in frontal cortex of adolescents seen on magnetic resonance spectroscopy. *Neuropsychiatric Neuropsychological Behavioral Neurology, 13*(1), 8–12.

Klauber, J. (1987). *Illusion and spontaneity.* London: Free Association Books.

Klein, M. (1946). Notes on some schizoid mechanisms. *International Journal of Psychoanalysis, 27,* 99–100.

Klein, M. (1975). Notes on some schizoid mechanisms. In *Melanie Klein: Envy and gratitude and other works 1946–1963* (pp. 1–24). New York, NY: Dell Books.

Knapp, P. H. (1992). Emotion and the psychoanalytic encounter. In T. Shapiro & R. N. Emde (Eds.), *Affect psychoanalytic perspectives* (pp. 239–264). Madiso n, CT: International Universities Press.

Knapska, E., Nikolaev, E., Boguszewski, P., Walasek, G., Blaszczyk, J., Kaczmarek, L., et al. (2006). Between-subject transfer of emotional information evokes specific pattern of amygdala activation. *Neuroscience, 103*(10), 3858–3862.

Kohut, H. (1971). *The analysis of the self.* New York, NY: International Universities Press.

Kohut, H. (1977). *The restoration of the self.* New York, NY: International Universities Press.

Kohut, H. (1984). *How does analysis cure?* Chicago: University of Chicago Press.

Kottler, J.A. (1993). *On being a therapist*. San Francisco: Jossey-Bass.

Kottler, J.A., & Blau, D.S. (1989). *The imperfect therapist: Learning from failure in therapeutic practice*. San Francisco: Jossey-Bass.

Kramer, S., & Akhtar, S. (Eds.). (1994). *Mahler and Kohut: Perspectives on development, psychopathology, and techniques*. Northvale, NJ: Aronson.

Lachmann, F. M., & Beebe, B. (1997). The contribution of self- and mutual regulation to therapeutic action: A case illustration. In M. Moskowitz, C. Monk, C. Kaye, & S. Ellman (Eds.), *The neurobiological and developmental basis for psychotherapeutic intervention* (pp. 91–121). Northvale, NJ: Aronson.

Lazarus, R. S. (1991). Progress on a cognitive–motivational–relational theory of emotion. *American Psychologist, 46*, 819–834.

LeDoux, J. (1996). *The emotional brain: The mysterious underpinnings of emotional life*. New York, NY: Simon & Schuster.

LeDoux, J. E., Romanski, L.M., & Xagoraris, A.E. (1989). Indelibility of subcortical emotional memories, *Journal of Cognitive Neuroscience, 1*, 238–243.

Lehky, A. R. (2000). Fine discrimination of faces can be performed rapidly. *Journal of Cognitive Neuroscience, 12*, 848–855.

Lemche, E., Giampietro, V. P., Surguladze, S. A., Amaro, E. J., Andrew, C. M., Williams, S. C. R., et al. (2006). Human attachment security is mediated by the amygdala: Evidence from combined fMRI and psychophysiological measures. *Human Brain Mapping, 27*, 623–635.

Lester, B., M., Hoffman, J., & Brazelton, T. B. (1985). The rhythmic structure of mother–infant interaction in term and preterm infants. *Child Development, 56*, 15–27.

Leucken, L. J., & Lemery, K. S. (2004). Early caregiving and physiological stress responses. *Clinical Psychology, 24*(2), 171–191.

Levin, F. M. (1997). Integrating some mind and brain views of transference: The phenomena. *Journal of the American Psychoanalytic Association, 45*(4), 1121–1151.

Lewis, M., & Miller, S. M. (1990). *Handbook of developmental psychopathology*. New York, NY: Plenum Press.

Lichtenberg, J. (1989). *Psychoanalysis and motivation*. Hillsdale, NJ: Analytic Press.

Linehan, M. M. (1993). *Cognitive–behavioral treatment of borderline personality disorder*. New York, NY: Guilford Press.

Lloyd, R. L., & Kling, A. S. (1991). Delta activity from amygdala in squirrel monkeys (Saimire sciureus): Influence of social and environmental context. *Behavioral Neuroscience, 105*(2), 223–229.

Loewald, H. W. (1973). On internalization. *International Journal of Psychoanalytic Association, 54*, 9–17.

Luborsky, L., & Crits-Christoph, C. (1990). *UnderstandingtTransference: The CCRT method*. New York, NY: Basic Books.

Luborsky, L., & Crits-Christophe, P. (1998). *Understanding transference: The core conflictual relationship theme method* (2nd ed.). Washington, DC: American Psychological Association.

Luna, B. (2009). The maturation of cognitive control and the adolescent brain. In F. Abitiz & D. Cosmeli (Eds.), *From attention to goal-directed behavior*. Berlin–Heidelberg: Springer-Verlag.

Luna, B., & Sweeney, J. A. (2001). Studies of brain and cognitive maturation through childhood and adolescence: A strategy for testing neurodevelpmental hypotheses. *Schizophrenia Bulletin*, *27*(3), 443–455.

Lyddon, W. J., & Sherry, A. (2001). Developmental personality styles: An attachment theory conceptualization of personality disorders. *Journal of Counseling & Development*, *79*, 405–414.

Mackey, S. K. (1996). Nurturance: A neglected dimension in family therapy with adolescents, *Journal of Marital and Family Therapy*, *22*(4), 489–508.

Mackenzie, K. R. (1997). *Time-managed group psychotherapy: Effective clinical applications*. Washington, DC: American Psychiatric Association.

MacNeilage, P. F. (1990). The "postural origins" theory of neurobiological asymmetries in primates. In N. Krasnegor, D. Rumbaugh, M. Studdert-Kennedy, & B. Lindblom (Eds.), *Biobehavioral foundations of language development* (pp. 165–188). Hillsdale, NJ: Erlbaum.

MacNeilage, P. F., Rogers, L. J., & Vallortigara, G. (2009). Origins of the left and right brain. *Scientific American*, *301*, 60–67.

Magnavita, J. J. (Ed.). (2004). *Handbook of personality disorders: Theory and practice*. Hoboken, NJ: Wiley.

Mahler, M. S. (1966). Notes on the development of basic moods: The depressive affect. In R. M. Lowenstein, L. M. Newman, M. Schre, & A. J. Solnit (Eds.), *Psychoanalysis—A General Psychology: Essays in Honor of Heinz Hartmann* (pp. 152–168). New York, NY: International Universities Press.

Mahler, M. S., Pine, F., & Bergman, A. (1975). *The psychological birth of the human infant*. New York, NY: Basic Books.

Main, M., & Solomon, J. (1990). Procedures for identifying infants as disorganized/disoriented during the strange situation. In M.T. Greenberg, D. Cicchetti, & E. M. Cummings (Eds.), *Attachment in the preschool years: Theory, research, and intervention* (pp. 121–160). Chicago: University of Chicago Press.

Masterson, J. F., & Lieberman, A. R. (Eds.). (2004). *A therapist's guide to the personality disorders: The Masterson approach*. Phoenix, AZ: Zeig, Tucker & Theisen.

McCabe, P. M., & Schneiderman, N. (1985). Psychophysiologic reactions to stress. In N. Schneiderman & J. T. Tapp (Eds.), *Behavioral medicine: The biophysical approach* (pp. 99–131). Hillsdale, NJ: Erlbaum.

McGaugh, J. L. (2004). The amygdala modulates the consolidation of memories of emotionally arousing experiences. *Annual Review of Neuroscience, 27*, 1–28.

McGilcrest, I. (2009). *The master and his emissary: The divided brain and the making of the Western world*. New Haven, CT: Yale University Press.

McKenna, C. (1994). Malignant transference: A neurobiologic model. *Journal of the American Academy of Psychoanalysis, 22*, 111–127.

McWilliams, N. (1994). *Psychoanalytic diagnosis: Understanding personality structure in the clinical process*. New York, NY: Guilford Press.

McWilliams, N. (1999). *Psychoanalytic case formulation*. New York, NY: Guilford.

McWilliams, N. (2004). *Psychoanalytic psychotherapy: A practitioner's guide*. New York, NY: Guilford Press.

Meichenbaum, D., & Gilmore, J. B. (1984). The nature of unconscious processes: A cognitive–behavioral perspective. In K. S. Bowers & D. Meichenbaum (Eds.), *The unconscious reconsidered* (pp. 273–294). New York, NY: Wiley.

Meloy, J. R. (1988). *The psychopathic mind: Origins, dynamics, and treatment*. Northvale, NJ: Aronson.

Merriam-Webster's dictionary. (1989). E. W. Gilman (Ed.). Springfield, MA: Author.

Middelberg, C. V. (2001). Projective identification in common couples dances. *Journal of Marital and Family Therapy, 27*(3), 341–352.

Miehls, D. (1997). Projective identification in sexual abuse survivors and their partners: Couple treatment implications. *Journal of Analytic Social Work, 4*(2), 5–22.

Millon, T. (1981). *Disorders of personality: DSM-III, Axis II*. New York, NY: Wiley-Interscience.

Mishna, F. (2007). Meeting them "where they are at": Intensive school-based psychotherapy for children who have been maltreated. *Psychoanalytic Social Work, 14*(2), 15–42.

Mitchell, S.A., & Aron, L. (1999). *Relational psychoanalysis: The emergence of a tradition*. Hillsdale, NJ: Analytic Press.

Mlot, C. (1998). Probing the biology of emotion. *Science, 280*, 1005–1007.

Monk, C. S., Klein, R. G., Telzer, E. H., Schroth, E. A., Mannuzza, S., Moulton, J. L., III, et al. (2008). Amygdala and nucleus accumbens activation to emotional facial expressions in children and adolescents at risk for major depression. *American Journal of Psychiatry, 165*, 90–98.

Morgan, M. A., & LeDoux, J. E. (1995). Differential contribution of dorsal and ventral medial prefrontal cortex to the acquisition and extinction of conditioned fear in rats. *Behavioral Neuroscience, 109,* 681–688.

Morris, J. S., Ohman, A., & Dolan, R. J. (1998). Conscious and unconscious emotional learning in the human amygdala. *Nature, 393,* 467–470.

Moskowitz, M., Monk, C., Kaye, C., & Ellman, S. (Eds.). (1997). *The neurological and developmental basis for psychotherapeutic intervention.* Northvale, NJ: Aronson.

Muran, J. C., & Barber, J. P. (Eds.) (2010). *The therapeutic alliance: An evidence-based guide to practice.* New York, NY: Guilford Press.

Murray, L. (1991). Intersubjectivity, object relations theory, and empirical evidence from mother–infant interactions. *Infant Mental Health Journal, 12,* 219–232.

Neafsey, E. J. (1990). Prefrontal cortical control of the autonomic nervous system: Anatomical and physiological observations. *Progress in Brain Research, 85,* 147–166.

Nebes, R. D. (1971). Superiority of the minor hemisphere in a commissurotomized man for the perception of part-whole relationships. *Cortex, 7,* 333–349.

Nesse, R. M., & Lloyd, A. T. (1992). The evolution of psychodynamic mechanisms. In J. H. Barkow, L. Cosmides, & J. Tooby (Eds.), *The adapted mind: Evolutionary psychology and the generation of culture* (pp. 601–626). New York, NY: Oxford University Press.

Nijenhuis, E. R. S., van der Linden, J., & Spinhoven, P. (1998). Animal defensive reactions as a model for trauma-induced dissociative reactions. *Journal of Traumatic Stress, 11,* 242–260.

Nobre, A. C., Coull, J. T., Frith, C D., & Mesulam, M. M. (1999). Orbitofrontal cortex is activated during breaches of expectation in tasks of visual attention. *Nature Neuroscience, 2,* 11–12.

Norden, J. (2007). *Understanding the brain: Parts 1–3.* The Great Courses. Chantilly, VA: The Teaching Company.

Northoff, G. (2010). Region-based approach versus mechanism-based approach to the brain. *Neuropsychoanalysis, 12*(2). Retrieved January 11, 2012, from http://www.neurospa.org.

Northoff, G., Bermpohl, F., Schoeneich, F., & Boeker, H. (2007). How does our brain constitute defense mechanisms?: First-person neuroscience and psychoanalysis. *Psychotherapy and Psychosomatics, 76,* 141–153.

Novey, S. (1959). The technique of supportive therapy in psychiatry and psychoanalysis. *Psychiatry, 22,* 179–187.

O'Neill, J. (2002). Therapy technique may not matter much. *NASW News, 47*(5), 3.

Ogden, P., Minton, K., & Pain, C. (2006). *Trauma and the body: A senso-rimotor approach to psychotherapy*. New York, NY: Norton.

Ogden, T. H. (1982). *Projective identification and psychotherapeutic technique*. New York, NY: Academic Press.

Oosterman, M., & Schuengel, C. (2007). Physiological effects of separation and reunion in relation to attachment and temperament in young children. *Developmental Psychobiology, 49,* 119–128.

Panksepp, J. (1999). Emotions viewed by psychoanalysis and neuroscience: An exercise in consilience. *NeuroPsychoanalysis, 1,* 15–28.

Panksepp, J. (2000). Affective consciousness and the instinctual motor system: The neural sources of saddness and joy. In R. D. Ellis & N. Newton (Eds.), *The caldron of consciousness: Motivation, affect and self-organization—an anthology*. Amsterdam, Netherlands: John Benjamin.

Panksepp, J. (2009). Brain emotional systems and qualities of mental life: From animal models of affect to implications for psychotherapeutics. In D. Fosha, D. J. Siegel, & M. Solomon (Eds.), *The healing power of emotion: Affective Neuroscience, development, and clinical practice* (pp. 1 –16). New York, NY: Norton.

Parad, H. J. (Ed.). (1958). *Ego psychology and dynamic casework*. New York, NY: Family Service Association of America.

Parad, H. J., & Miller, R. R. (Eds.). (1963). *Ego-oriented casework*. New York, NY: Family Service Association of America.

Passorotti, A. M., Sweeney, J. A., & Pavuluri, M. N. (2009). Neural correlates of incidental and directed facial emotion processing in adolescents and adults. *Social Cognitive Affective Neuroscience, 4*(4), 387–398.

Pearson, L. L., Cohn, D. A., Cowan, P. A., & Cowan, C. P. (1994). Earned- and continuous-security in adult attachment: Relation to depressive symptomatology and parenting style. *Development & Psychopathology, 6,* 359–373.

Peper, M., & Karcher, S. (2001). Differential conditioning to facial emotional expressions: Effects of hemispheric asymmetries and CS identification. *Psychophysiology, 38,* 936–950.

Perry, B. D., Pollard, R. A., Blakely, T. L., Baker, W. L., & Vigilante, D. (1995). Childhood trauma, the neurobiology of adaptation, and "use-dependent" development of the brain: How "states" become "traits." *Infant Mental Health Journal, 16,* 271–291.

Perry, R. J., Rosen, H. R., Kramer, J. H., Beer, J. S., Levenson, R. L., & Miller, B. L. (2001). Hemispheric dominance for emotions, empathy, and social behavior: Evidence from right and left handers for frontotemporal dementia. *Neurocase, 7,* 145–160.

Petrovic, P., Petersson, K. M., Ghatan, P. H., Sone-Elander, S., & Ingvar, M. (2000). Pain-related cerebral activation is altered by a distracting cognitive task. *Pain, 85,* 19–30.

Phillips, H. (2004). Teenagers fail to see the consequences. *New Scientists.* Available online at http://www.newscientist.com/article/dn6738-teenagers-fail-to-see-the-consequences.

Piaget, J. (1963). *The origins of intelligence in children.* New York, NY: Norton.

Pilkonis, P. (1988). Personality prototypes among depressives: Themes of dependency and autonomy. *Journal of Personality Disorders, 2,* 144–152.

Pipher, M. (1994). *Reviving Ophelia: Saving the selves of adolescent girls.* New York, NY: Brosset/Putnam.

Pipp, S., & Harmon, R. J. (1987). Attachment as regulation: A commentary. *Child Development, 56,* 648–652.

Pizzagalli, D. A., Regard, M., & Lehmann, D. (1999). Rapid emotional face processing in the human right and left brain hemispheres: An ERP study. *NeuroReport, 10,* 2691–2698.

Pollak, S. D., Cicchetti, D., Hornung, K., & Reed, A. (2000). Recognizing emotion in faces: Developmental effects of child abuse and neglect. *Developmental Psychology, 36*(5), 697–688.

Pollak, S. D., & Sinha, P. (2002). Effects of early experience on children's recognition of facial displays of emotion. *Developmental Psychology, 38*(5), 784–791.

Porges S. W. (1997). Emotion: An evolutionary by-product of the neural regulation of the autonomic nervous system. *Annals of the New York Academy Science, 807,* 62–77.

Porges, S. W. (2001). The polyvagal theory: Phylogenetic substrates of a social nervous system. *International Journal of Psychophysiology, 42,* 123–146.

Porges, S. W. (2003). Social engagement and attachment: A phylogenetic perspective. *Annals of the New York Academy of Science, 1008,* 31–47.

Porges, S. W. (2004). Neuroception: A subconscious system for detecting threats and safety. *Zero to Three, 32,* 19–24.

Porges, S. W. (2007). The polyvagal perspective. *Biological Psychology, 74,* 116–143.

Porges, S. W. (2011). Music therapy, trauma, and the polyvagal theory. In S. W. Porges (Ed.), *The polyvagal theory: Neurophysiological foundations of emotions, attachment, communication and self-regulation* (pp. 246–254). New York, NY: Norton.

Porges, S. W. (2011, March). *Safety as a transformative state: Mindfulness from a poly vagal perspective*. Lecture presented at the conference of the UCLA–Lifespan Learning Institute, Los Angeles, CA.

Racker, H. (1968). *Transference and countertransference*. New York, NY: International Universities Press.

Raine, A., Ishikawa, S. S., Arce, E., Lencz, T., Knuth, K. H., Bihrle, L. L., et al. (2004). Hippocampal structural asymmetry in unsuccessful psychopaths. *Biological Psychiatry, 55*(2), 185–191.

Raine, A., Meloy, J. R., Bihrle, S., Stoddard, J., Lacasse, L., & Buchsbaum, M.S. (1998). Reduced preforontal and increased subcortical brain functioning assess using postitron emission tomography in predatory and affective murderers. *Behavioral Sciences and the Law, 16*, 319–332.

Raine, A., Park, S., Lencz, T., Bihrle, S., Lacasse, L., Widon, C. S., et al. (2001). Reduced right hemisphere activation in severely abused violent offenders during a working memory task: An fMRI study. *Aggressive Behavior, 27*, 111–129.

Raine, A., Reynolds, C., Venables, P. H., Mednick, S. A., & Farrington, D.P. (1998). Fearlessness, stimulation-seeking, and large body size at 3 years as early predispositions to childhood aggression at age 11 years. *Archives of General Psychiatry, 55*, 745–751.

Rapaport, D. (1953). On the psychoanalytic theory of affects. *International Journal of Psycho-Analysis, 34*, 177–198.

Ratey, J. J. (2001). *A user's guide to the brain: Perception, attention, and the four theaters of the brain*. New York: Random House.

Rauch, S. L., van der Kolk, B. A., Fisler, R. E., Alpert, N. M., Orr, S. P., Savage, C. R., et al. (1996). A symptom provocation study of posttraumtic stress disorder using positron emission tomography and script-driven imagery. *Archives of Psychiatry, 53*, 380–387.

Redl, F. (1963). Psychoanalysis and group therapy: A developmental point of view. *American Journal of Orthopsychiatry, 33*, 135–147.

Redl, F., & Wineman, D. (1951). *Children who hate: The disorganization and breakdown of behavioral controls*. Glencoe, IL: Free Press.

Redl, F., & Wineman, D. (1952). *Controls from within: Techniques for the treatment of the aggressive child*. Glencoe, IL: Free Press.

Rosen, A. (1996). Anxiety disorders as they impact on couples and families. In F. W. Kaslow (Ed.), *Handbook of relational diagnoses and dysfunctional family patterns* (pp. 139–150). New York, NY: Wiley.

Rosenzweig, M. R. (1996). Aspects of the search for neural mechanisms of memory. *Annual Review of Psychology, 47*, 1–32.

Ross, N. (1975). Affect as cognition: With observations on the meanings of mystical states. *Review of Psycho-Analysis, 2,* 79–93.

Rothschild, B. (2000). *The body remembers: The psychophysiology of trauma and trauma treatment.* New York, NY: Norton.

Rothschild, B., & Rand, M. (2006). *Help for the helper: Self-care strategies for managing burnout and stress.* New York, NY: Norton.

Rowe, C. E., & MacIsaac, D. S. (1988). *Empathic attunement: The "technique" of psychoanalytic self psychology.* Northvale, NJ: Aronson.

Ruder, D. B. (2011). The teen brain. *Harvard Magazine.* Retrieved May 14, 2011, from http://harvardmagazine.com/2008/09/the-teen-brain.html.

Rutan, J. S., Stone, W. N., & Shay, J. J. (2007). *Psychodynamic group psychotherapy* (4th ed.). New York, NY: Guilford Press.

Sander, D., Grafman, J., & Zalla, T. (2003). The human amygdala: An evolved system for relevance detection. *Review of Neuroscience, 14*(4), 303–316.

Sandler, J. (1976). Counter-transference and role-responsiveness. *International Review of Psychoanalysis, 3,* 43–47.

Sapolsky, R. M. (1994). *Why zebras don't get ulcers: A guide to stress, stress-related diseases, and coping.* Boston: Freemen.

Sapolsky, R. (2005). *Biology and human behavior: The neurological origins of individuality.* The Great Courses (2nd ed., Parts 1 & 2). Chantilly, VA: The Teaching Company.

Schamess, G. (1984). Boundary issues in countertransference: A developmental perspective. *Clinical Social Work Journal, 9*(4), 244–257.

Schamess, G. (1996). Structural theory and ego psychology. In J. Berzoff, L. M. Flanagan, & P. Hertz (Eds.), *Inside out and outside in: Psychodynamic clinical theory and practice in contemporary multicultural contexts* (pp. 50–101). Northvale, NJ: Aronson.

Schamess, G. (2006). Therapeutic processes in clinical supervision: Part II. *Clinical Social Work Journal, 14*(4), 427–445.

Schlegel, A., & Barry, H. (1991). *Adolescence: An anthropological inquiry.* New York, NY: Free Press.

Schmale, A. (1964). A genetic view of affects: With special reference to the genesis of helplessness and hopelessness. *Psychoanalytic Study of the Child, 10,* 287–310.

Schore, A. N. (1994). *Affect regulation and the origin of the self: The neurobiology of emotional development.* Hillside, NJ: Erlbaum.

Schore, A. N. (1998, February). *Early trauma and the development of the right brain.* Paper presented at the conference of the UCLA–Lifespan Learning Institute, Los Angeles, CA.

Schore, A. N. (1997c). Interdisciplinary developmental research as a source of clinical models. In M. Moskowitz, C. Monk, C. Kaye, & S. Ellman (Eds.), *The neurobiological and developmental basis for psychotherapeutic intervention* (pp. 1–71). Northvale NJ: Aronson.

Schore, A. N. (2003a). *Affect dysregulation and disorders of the self.* New York, NY: Norton.

Schore, A. N. (2003b). *Affect regulation and the repair of the self.* New York, NY: Norton.

Schore, A. N. (2012). *The science of the art of psychotherapy.* New York, NY: Norton.

Schure, M. (1965). Affects and cognition. *International Journal of Psychoanalysis, 50,* 647–653.

Schwartz, J. M., Stoessel, P. W., Baxter, L. R., Martin, K. M., & Phelps, M. E. (1996). Systematic changes in cerebral glucose metabolic rate after successful behavior modification treatment of obsessive–compulsive disorder. *Archives of General Psychiatry, 53*(2), 109–153.

Schweinsburg, A. D., Nagel, B. J., & Tapert, S. G., (2005). fMRI reveals alteration of spatial working memory networks across adolescence. *Journal of the International Neuropsychological Society, 11,* 631–644.

Semrud-Clikeman, M., Fine, J. G., & Zhu, D. C. (2011). The role of the right hemisphere for processing of social interactions in normal adults using functional magnetic resonance imaging. *Neuropsychobiology, 64,* 47–51.

Shaw, S. K., & Dallos, R. (2005). Attachment and adolescent depression. *Attachment & Human Development, 7*(4), 409–424.

Sheafor, B. W., & Horejsi, C. R. (2008). *Techniques and guidelines for social work practice.* Boston: Allyn & Bacon.

Sheline, Y. I., Wang, P. W., Gado, M. H., Csernansky, J .G., &Vannier, M. W. (1996). Hippocampal atrophy in recurrent major depression. *Proceedings of the National Academy of Science, USA, 93,* 3908–3913.

Sherry, D. F., & Schacter, D. L. (1987). The evolution of multiple memory systems. *Psychological Review, 94,* 439–454.

Siegel, D. J. (1999). *The developing mind: Toward a neurobiology of interpersonal experience.* New York, NY: Guilford Press.

Siegel, D. J. (2003). Toward an interpersonal neurobiology of the developing mind: Attachment, "mindsight," and neural integration. *Infant Mental Health Journal, 22,* 67–94.

Siegel, D. J. (2007). *The mindful brain: Reflection and attunement in the cultivation of well-being.* New York, NY: Norton.

Siegel, D. J. (2012). *Pocket guide to interpersonal neurobiology: An integrative handbook of the mind.* New York, NY: Norton.

Silverman, R. C., & Lieberman, A. F. (1999). Negative maternal attributions, projective identification, and the intergenerational transmission of violent relational patterns. *Psychoanalytic Diaglogues*, *9*(2), 161–186.

Silverstein, O., & Rashbaum, B. (1994). *The courage to raise good men*. New York, NY: Viking.

Smith, B. L. (1990). The origins of interpretation in the counter-transference. *Psychoanalytic Psychology*, *7*(Suppl.), 89–104.

Solms, M., & Turnbull, O. (2002). *The brain and the inner world: An introduction to the neuroscience of subjective experience*. New York, NY: Other Press.

Sowell, E. R., Thompson, P. M., Tessner, K. D., & Toga, A. W. (2001). Mapping continued brain growth and gray matter density reduction in dorsal frontal cortex: Inverse relationships during postadolescent brain maturation, *Journal of Neuroscience 21*(22), 8819–8829.

Spear, L.P. (2000). The adolescent brain and age-related behavioral manifestations. *Neuroscience and Biobehavioral Review*, *24*, 417–463.

Spence, S., Shapiro, D., & Zaidel, E. (1996). The role of the right hemisphere in the physiological and cognitive components of emotional processing. *Psychophysiology*, *33*, 112–122.

Spezzano, C. (1993). *Affect in psychoanalysis: A clinical synthesis*. Hillsdale, NJ: Analytic Press.

Sroufe, J. (1991). Assessment of parent–adolescent relationships: Implications for adolescent development. *Journal of Family Psychology*, *5*, 21–45.

Sroufe, L. A. (1989). Relationships, self, and individual adaptation. In A.J. Sameroff & R.N. Emde (Eds.), *Relationship disturbances in early childhood* (pp. 70–94). New York, NY: Basic Books.

Sroufe, L .A. (1996). *Emotional development: The organization of emotional life in the early years*. New York, NY: Cambridge University Press.

Stauffer, K. A. (2010). *Anatomy & physiology for psychotherapists: Connecting body and soul*. New York, NY: Norton.

Sroufe, L. A., Egeland, B., Carlson, E. A., & Collins, W. A. (2005). *The development of the person*. New York, NY: Guilford Press.

Steinberg, L. (2004). Risk taking in adolescence: What changes and why? *Annals of the New York Academy of Sciences*, *1021*, 51–58.

Steinberg, L. (2005). *Adolescence* (8th ed.). New York, NY: McGraw-Hill.

Steinberg, L. (2007). Risk taking in adolescence: New perspectives from brain and behavioral science. *Current Directions in Psychological Science*, *16*(2), 55–59.

Steinberg, L., & Lerner, R. M. (2005). *Handbook of adolescent psychology*. New York, NY: Wiley.

Steiner, J. (1979). *Psychic retreats: Pathological organizations in psychotic, neurotic, and borderline patients*. London: Routledge.

Stenberg, G., Wiking, S., & Dahl, M. (1998). Judging words at face value: Interference in a word processing task reveals automatic processing of affective facial stimuli. *Cognition and Emotion, 12*, 755–782.

Stern, D. N. (1977). *The first relationship*. Cambridge, MA: Harvard University Press.

Stern, D. N. (1985). *The interpersonal world of the infant*. New York, NY: Basic Books.

Stern, D. N. (2004). *The present moment in psychotherapy and everyday life*. New York, NY: Norton

Stern, D. N., Hofer, L., Haft, W., & Dore, J. (1985). Affect attunement: The sharing of feeling state between mother and infant by means of modal influency. In T. M. Field & N. A. Fox (Eds.), *Social perception in infants* (pp. 249–268). Norwood, NJ: Ablex.

Steuerwald, B. L., & Kosson, D. S. (2000). Emotional experiences of the psychopath. In C. B. Gacano (Ed.), *The clinical and forensic assessment of psychopathy: A practitioner's guide* (pp. 111–135). Mahwah, NJ: Erlbaum.

Stewart, K .L. (Ed.). (1990). *Symposium on music therapy and trauma: Bridging theory and clinical practice*. New York, NY: Satchnote Press.

Stolorow, R. D., Brandchaft, B., & Atwood, G. (1987). *Psychoanalytic treatment: An intersubjective approach*. Hillsdale, NJ: Analytic Press.

Stolorow R. D., & Lachmann, F. (1975). Early object loss and denial: Development considerations. *Psychoanalytic Quarterly, 44*, 596–611.

Strean, H. S. (1996). Applying psychoanalytic principles to social work practice: An historical review. In J. Edward & J. Sanville (Eds.), *Fostering healing and growth: A psychoanalytic social work approach* (pp. 1–22). Northvale, NJ: Aronson.

Strupp, H. H. (1989). Psychotherapy: Can the practitioner learn from the researcher? *American Psychologist, 44*, 717–724.

Sullivan, R. M., & Gratton, A. (2002). Prefrontal cortical regulation of hypothalamic–pituitary–adrenal function in the rat and implications for psychopathology: Size matters. *Pschoneuroendrocrinology, 227*, 99–114.

Suslow, T., Ohrmann, P., Bauer, J., Rauch, A. V., Schwindt, W., Arolt, V., et al. (2006). Amygdala activation during masked presentation of emotional faces predicts conscious detection of threat-related faces. *Brain and cognition, 61*(3), 243–248.

Sweeney, M. S. (2009). *Brain: The complete mind*. Washington, DC: National Geographic Society.

Tarullo, A. R., & Gunnar, M. R. (2006). *Child maltreatment and the developing HPA axis: Hormones and behavior*. Available online at www.sciencedirect.com.

Tatkin, S. (2007, March). *Couples therapy: Addiction to "alone time"—avoidant attachment, narcissism, and a one-person psychology within a two-person psychological system*. Paper presented at the 2007 Couple's Conference, Anaheim, CA.

Teasdale, J. D., Howard, R. J., Cox, S. G., Ha, Y., Brammer, M. J., Williams, S. C. R., et al. (1999). Functional MRI study of the cognitive generation of affect. *American Journal of Psychiatry, 156*, 209–215.

Teicher, M. H., Andersen, S. L., & Hostetter, J. C., Jr. (1995). Evidence for dopamine receptor pruning between adolescence and adulthood in striatum but not nucleus accumbens. *Developmental Brain Research, 89*, 167–172.

Tomkins, S. S. (1962). *Affect imagery consciousness. Vol. I. The positive affects*. New York, NY: Springer.

Tomkins, S. S. (1963). *Affect imagery consciousness. Vol. II. The negative affects*. New York, NY: Springer.

Tomkins, S. S. (1970). Affect as the primary motivational system. In M. Arnold (Ed.), *Feelings and emotions: The Loyola symposium* (pp. 101–110). New York, NY: Academic Press.

Toth, S. C., & Cicchetti, D. (1998). Remembering, forgetting, and the effects of trauma on memory: A developmental psychopathologic perspective. *Developmental Psychopathology, 10*, 580–605.

Trevarthen, C. (1993a). The function of emotions in early infant communications and development. In J. Nadel & L. Camaioni (Eds.), *New perspectives in early communicative development* (pp. 48–81). New York, NY: Cambridge.

Trevarthen, C. (1993b). The self born in intersubjectivity: The psychology of an infant communicating. In U. Neisser (Ed.), *The perceived self: Ecological and interpersonal sources of self-knowledge* (pp. 121–173). New York, NY: Cambridge.

Trieschmann, A., Whittaker, J. K., & Brendtro, L. K. (1969). *The other 23 hours*. Piscataway, NJ: Transaction.

Tronick, E. Z. (1989). Emotions and emotional communication in infants. *American Psychologist, 44*, 112–119.

Tronick, E. (2007). *The neurobehavioral and social–emotional development of infants and children*. New York, NY: Norton.

Tronick, E. Z., & Weinberg, M. K. (1997). Depressed mothers and infants: Failure to form dyadic states of consciousness. In L. Murray & P. J. Cooper (Eds.), *Postpartum depression and child development* (pp. 54–81). New York, NY: Guilford Press.

Tucker, D. M. (1992). Developing emotions and cortical networks. In M. R. Gunnar & C. A. Nelson (Eds.), Minnesota symposium on child psychology. Vol. 24. *Developmental behavioral neuroscience* (pp. 75–128). Hillsdale, NJ: Erlbaum.

Tull, M., Jakupcak, M., McFadden, M. E., & Roemer, L. (2007). The role of negative affect intensity and fear of emotions in posttraumatic stress symptom severity. *Journal of Nervous and Mental Disorders, 195*(7), 580–587.

Ugrumov, M. V. (1997). Hypothalamic monoaminergic systems in ontogenesis: Developmental and functional significance. *International Journal of Biological Development, 41*, 809–816.

Vaillant, G. E. (1971). Theoretical hierarchy of adaptive ego mechanisms. *Archives of General Psychiatry, 24*, 107–118.

Vaillant, G. E. (1977). *Adaptation to life*. Boston: Little, Brown.

Vaillant, G. E. (1992). *Ego mechanisms of defense: A guide for clinicians and researchers*. Washington, DC: American Psychiatric Association.

van der Hart, O., Nieuwenhuis, E. R., & Steele, K. (2006). *The haunted self: Structural dissociation and the treatment of chronic traumatization*. New York, NY: Norton.

van der Kolk, B. A. (1987). The psychological consequences of overwhelming life experiences. In B. A. van der Kolk (Ed.), *Psychological trauma* (pp. 1–30). Washington, DC: American Psychiatric Association.

van der Kolk, B. A., & Fishler, R. E. (1995). Dissociation and the fragmentary nature of traumatic memories: Overview and exploratory study. *Journal of Traumatic Stress, 8*(4), 505–525.

van der Kolk. B. A. (2006). Clinical implications of neuroscience research in PTSD. *Annals of the New York Academy of Sciences, 1071*, 277–293.

van der Kolk, B. A., & Greenberg, M. S. (1987). The psychobiology of the traumatic response: Hyperarousal, constriction, and addiction to traumatic reexposure. In B. A. van der Kolk (Ed.), *Psychological trauma* (pp. 63–87). Washington, DC: American Association.

van der Kolk, B. A., McFarlane, A. C., & Weisaeth, L. (Eds.). (1998). *Traumatic stress: The effects of overwhelming experience on mind, body, and society*. New York: Guilford Press.

van der Kolk, B. A., & van der Hart, O. (1987). The intrusive past: The flexibility of memory and the engraving of trauma. *American Imago, 48*(4), 425–454.

Voeller, K. K. S. (1986). Right-hemisphere deficit syndrome in children. *American Journal of Psychiatry, 143*, 1004–1009.

Vuilleumier, P., Richardson, M. P., Armony, J. L., Driver, J., & Dolan, R.J. (2004). Distant influences of amygdala lesion on visual cortical activation during emotional face processing. *Nature Neuroscience, 7,* 1271–1278.

Wallin, D. J. (2007). Attachment in psychotherapy. New York, NY: Guilford Press.

Wallis, C. (2005, August 8). Is middle school bad for kids? *Time Magazine,* 48–57.

Wallis, C., Dell, K., & Park, A. (2004, May 10). What makes teen brains tick: A flood of hormones, sure. *Time Magazine,* 56–65.

Waska, R. (2007). Projective identification as an inescapable aspect of the therapeutic relationship. *Psychonanalytic Social Work, 14*(2), 43–64.

Weiss, J., Sampson, H., & the Mount Zion Psychotherapy Research Group. (1986). *The psychoanalytic process.* New York, NY: Guilford Press.

Weissman, H., Epstein, I., & Savage, A. (1983). *Agency-based social work: Neglected aspects of clinical practice.* Philadelphia: Temple University Press.

West, M., & Sheldon, A. (1998). Classification of pathological attachment patterns in adults. *Journal of Personality Disorders, 2,* 153–159.

Wexler, B. E., Warrenburg, S., Schwartz, G. E., & Janer, L. D. (1992). EEG and EMG responses to emotion-evoking stimuli processed without conscious awareness. *Neuropsychologia, 30,* 1065–1079.

Whalen, P. J. (1998). Fear, vigilance, and ambiguity: Initial neuroimaging studies of the human amygdala. *Current Directions in Psychological Science, 7,* 177–188.

Whalen, P. J., & Phelps, E. A. (2009). *The human amygdala.* New York, NY: Guilford Press.

Wilkinson, R. B., & Walford, W. A. (2001). Attachment and personality in the psychological health of adolescents. *Personality and Individual Differences, 31,* 473–484.

Winnicott, D. (1958). The capacity to be alone. *International Journal of Psycho-Analysis, 39,* 416–420.

Winnicott, D. (1963). The development of the capacity for concern. In D. Winnicott, *The maturational processes and the facilitating environment* (pp. 73–82). New York, NY: International Universities Press.

Winnicott, D. (1975). *Through paediatrics to psychoanalysis.* New York, NY: Basic Books.

Wittling, W. (1997). The right hemisphere and the human stress response. *Acta Physiologica Scandinavica, 640*(Suppl.), 55–59.

Wittling, W., Block A., Schweiger, E., & Genzel, S. (1998). Hemisphere asymmetry in sympathetic control of the human myocardium. *Brain and Cognition, 38,* 17–35.

Wittling, W., & Pflluger, M. (1990). Neuroendocrine hemisphere asymmetries: Salivary cortisol secretion during lateralized viewing of emotion-related and neutral films. *Brain and Cognition, 14,* 234–265.

Wolfsdorf, B. A., & Zlotnick, C. (2001). Affect management in group therapy for women with posttraumatic stress disorder and histories of childhood sexual abuse. *Journal of Clinical Psychology, 57*(2), 169–181.

Wolfson, A. R., & Carskadon, M. A. (1998). Sleep schedules and daytime functioning in adolescents. *Child Development, 69*(4), 875–887.

Yalom, I. D. (1975). *The theory and practice of group psychotherapy* (2nd ed.). New York, NY: Basic Books.

Yehuda, R. (1999). Linking the neuroendocrinolgy of post-traumatic stress disorder with recent neuroanatomic findings. *Seminars in Clinical Neuropsychiatry, 4,* 256–265.

Yoon, B.-U., Morillo, C. A., Cechetto, D. F., & Hachinski, V. (1997). Cerebral hemispheric lateralization in cardiac autonomic control. *Archives of Neurology, 54,* 741–744.

Young, E. A., & Breslau, N. (2004). Cortisol and catecholamines in post-traumatic stress disorder. *Archives of General Psychiatry, 61,* 394–401.

Zagon, A. (2001). Does the vagus nerve mediate the sixth sense? *Trends in Neuroscience, 24*(11), 671–673.

Zetzel, E. R. (1949). Current concepts of transference. *International Journal of Psychoanalysis, 37,* 369–376.

Index

freeze behaviors, 95
freeze response, in clinical work, 113
Freud, A., 38
Freud, S., 12, 22, 30, 37, 38, 194
frontal cortex, amygdala and, 68*t*
frontal lobes
    adolescent *vs.* adult brains and, 199*t*
    memory storage and, 7

Gacano, C. B., 97
Gallese, V., 16
Gilmore, J. B., 37
goal setting, managed care and, 246
grandiosity, 15
gray matter, adolescence and pruning of, 202
Green, R. L., 30
Greenough, W. T., 202
grief, 23
group culture, 222
group development stages, 219–21
    formative stage, 220
    mature stage, 220–21
    reactive and termination stages, 220
group dynamics, 221–23
    group culture and norms, 222
    leadership, 221
    roles, 222–23
group norms, 222
group spokesman, projective identification and, 258
group therapy
    brain functions within treatment modality of, 217–43
    case example, 228–43
    growth opportunities through, 243
    ultimate goals of, 219, 243
group work, countertransference issues in, 258

Hartmann, H., 38
Hebbian principle, 41
hierarchical functions
    defined, 67
    levels of consciousness, 69–70
    memory systems, 71–73
    modes of engagement, 70
    somatic and emotional self states, 70–71
hindbrain, 6, 7*f*

hippocampal formation, anatomy of, 29*f*
hippocampus, 28*f*, 29, 29*f*
    amygdala and, 68*t*, 69
    memory systems and, 71, 72, 73
homeostatically balanced, 35
    autonomic nervous system, 11, 125, 140
    defenses, 41, 43*t*–44*t*
    meaning of, 251
Horejsi, C. R., 39
hormones
    adolescent *vs.* adult brains and, 201*t*
    regulation of, within bloodstream, 30
Hornung, K., 203
Horowitz, L., 138, 173, 258
Hugdahl, K., 120
Hurricanes Katrina and Rita, case of
    Cori's survival from, 4–5, 9, 10, 12, 15, 19, 24–27, 35, 215
hypothalamic-pituitary-adrenal (HPA) axis
    amygdala and, 68*t*
    stress management and, 70
hypothalamus, 7*f*, 28*f*, 29

identification, 225
imitation, 224–25
implicit cognitions, 77
implicit memory, 30, 31
    attachment styles and, 78
    insecure attachments and, 79
    self state and degrees of, 76–77
individualism, adolescence and American culture's emphasis on, 196
insecure attachments
    extreme projective identifications and, 253
    implicit memories and, 79
    internalized model, description of, 219
    styles of, 77
insecure-avoidant attachment, parasympathetic branch of ANS and, 13
insecure resistant/ambivalent attachment, sympathetic branch of ANS and, 13
insula
    amygdala and, 68*t*, 69
    neuroception and, 96
    right, "heightened therapeutic moment" and, 256
internalization, 225
internalized object relations, 13, 21

parasympathetic segment, of autonomic nervous system, 11

"parent blaming," steering away from, mental health treatment and, 189

parents, American culture and adolescents' connections to, 196

parietal lobe, 7

patterns, 114

peer influence, adolescence and, 197

periaqueductal gray (PAG), fight, flight or freeze behaviors and, 95–96

peripheral nervous system, 2f, 8

peripheral organs, primary parasympathetic influence on, 92

permeability of interpersonal emotional boundaries, Mary as adult client case illustration and, 277

Perry, B. D., 121

personality disorder, not otherwise specified, 187

personality disorders
criteria and diagnosis of, 114–15
developmental cause of, 116
models of self and other in, 116–17
suggested relationship between arousal branches of ANS and DSM diagnostic categories, 118t
traits of, 117

personality organizations, anger expressions and, 96

"personality systemic" model, 116

phobias, amygdala and, 72, 82t

Piaget, J., 194

pituitary gland, 28f

play situations, children and displacement of emotions into, 215

Plutchik, R., 39

PNS-dominated personality disorders, 118t

Pollak, S. D., 203

polysubstance issues, 188

polyvagal system
anxious-ambivalent attachment and, 128
function shutdown and, 121

polyvagal theory, 90–93, 113

pons, 7f

Porges, S. W., 32, 33, 90, 91, 92, 93, 94, 95, 96, 98, 103

posttraumatic stress disorder (PTSD), 13, 148, 149
compromised amgdala functioning and, 75
personality organizations and, 96, 97

poverty, adolescence and, 197

prefrontal cortex
adolescent *vs.* adult brains and, 199t, 200t
stress and altered development of, 204

prefrontal limbic areas, reorganization of adolescent brain and, 202

preoccupied attachment category, proposed DSM depressive personality disorder compared to, 160t

preoccupied attachment in adulthood, case example of, 154–59

primitive affects, group development and, 221

process of change
defined, 226
therapeutic, in group work, 226–28

progesterone, compromised amgdala functioning and, 75, 76

projective identification, 22, 244, 247, 248–55, 256, 258
adaptive, 245, 248, 249–51
maladaptive or defensive, 251–55
therapeutic encounter and, 261, 262
traumatized individuals and potential functions of, 258

pruning of disused neural connections, adolescent brain and, 198, 202

psychobiological dysfunction, autonomic nervous system and, 114

psychological work, in groups, 224

psychopathy
compromised amgdala functioning and, 75, 76
developmentally acquired, hypofunctioning ventro-medial cortex and, 204
personality organizations and, 96, 97, 98

psychotherapy, long-term goal of, 24

PTSD. *see* posttraumatic stress disorder (PTSD)

Racker, H., concordant-complementary identification of, 256–57

altered development of prefrontal cortex and, 204
amygdala and, 66, 67, 68
defense mechanisms and, 121
object constancy and, 253–54
stress hormones, amygdala functioning and, 78
stress response, neurohormones and, 20
styles, 114
substance abuse, 188
supervisee
going over almost verbatim material with, 247
selected supervision issues and, 245–48
supervisee-supervisor dynamics, mirroring of dynamics in clinician-client relationship and, 246
supervision
meeting with intern regarding Mary as adult client, 260–61
parallel process in, 270–75
selected issues in, 245–48
transference-countertransference and, 255, 256
supervisor
degree of self-disclosure between supervisee and, 245
selected supervision issues and, 245–48
supervisory process, integrating selected neurobiological concepts into, 245–77
sympathetically driven defenses, 41, 46t–48t
sympathetic nervous system (SNS), 3, 94
sympathetic segment, of autonomic nervous system, 11
synapses, adolescent brain and formation of, 202
"synaptic shadows," 279
synchrony, 23

Tatkin, S., 116
templates, 114
temporal lobe, 7
termination stage, of group development, 220
testosterone, compromised amgdala functioning and, 75, 76
thalamus, 7f, 28f, 29, 30

"theory of mind," amygdala and, 82t
therapeutic alliance
Mary as adult client case illustration and, 276, 277
neurobiological perspective on, 278–79
rupture of, 278
as strongest predictor of treatment success, 278
therapeutic encounter, projective identification during, 261, 262
therapeutic factors in group therapy, 223–24
learning and psychological work, 224
self-revelation, 223
supportive factors, 223
therapeutic processes of change in group, 226–28
clarification, 227
confrontation, 226–27
interpretation, 227–28
working through, 228
therapeutic withdrawal, Mary as adult client case illustration and, 269
threat management, amygdala and, 66, 67
threat response, ambiguity and, 74–75
threats, personality organization and, 97
toxic affects, in clinical situation, 258
traits, 114
transference, 32, 225–26, 244, 248, 255–56
clarification and, 227
group therapy and, 239–40
projective identification and, 258
reenactments, affect-laden, 20
schema approach to, 22
transfer of affect, 127
trauma, 91
amygdala and, 9, 66, 68, 69, 72
unresolved, ruptured therapeutic alliance and, 278, 279
traumatic memories
defensive projective identification and, 251
dissociation and "off-loading" fragments of, 252
transference and, 255–56
treatment alliance, as curative factor, 246
Tronick, E. Z., 21
trust, in group work, 222